AMERICA, GUNS, AND FREEDOM

A JOURNEY INTO POLITICS AND THE PUBLIC HEALTH
& GUN CONTROL MOVEMENTS

MIGUEL A. FARIA, JR., M.D.

MASCOT
BOOKS

AMERICA, GUNS, AND FREEDOM

A JOURNEY INTO POLITICS
AND THE PUBLIC HEALTH
& GUN CONTROL
MOVEMENTS

MIGUEL A. FARIA, JR., M.D.

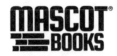

www.mascotbooks.com

AMERICA, GUNS, AND FREEDOM:

A Journey Into Politics and the Public Health & Gun Control Movements

For more information, please contact:
Mascot Books
620 Herndon Parkway #320
Herndon, VA 20170
info@mascotbooks.com

Library of Congress Control Number: 2018911270

CPSIA Code: PBANG0619A
ISBN-13: 978-1-64307-217-3

Printed in the United States

For Helen, Regina,
Elena, and Gabriela

CONTENTS

FOREWORD   1

INTRODUCTION: MY JOURNEY   5

PART 1: PUBLIC HEALTH AND GUN CONTROL—
"GUN VIOLENCE AS AN EPIDEMIC"   9

PRELUDE: Gun Violence as a Public Health Issue   11

CHAPTER 1: Gun Control and Expedient Medical Politics   15

CHAPTER 2: The Politics of Gun Control and the Subversion of Medical Science   22

CHAPTER 3: The Perversion of Soviet Science
in the Service of the State—Unlearned Lessons   29

CHAPTER 4: The AMA Enters the Fray for Gun Control   37

CHAPTER 5: Defanging the CDC's Gun Control Apparatus   52

PART 2: WITHIN THE BELLY OF THE BEAST   65

CHAPTER 6: Public Health, Social Science, and the Scientific Method (Part I)   67

CHAPTER 7: Public Health, Social Science, and the Scientific Method (Part II)   79

CHAPTER 8: A History of Public Health—From Science to Politics   90

PART 3: DEBUNKING BIASED INFORMATION DISSEMINATED IN MEDICAL JOURNALS AND THE LAY PRESS · 103

CHAPTER 9: Statistical Malpractice—"Firearm Availability and Violence" · 105

CHAPTER 10: Statistical Malpractice—Educational and Socioeconomic Factors · 113

CHAPTER 11: Debunking the Typical Ecologic Study Linking Gun Ownership with Violent Crime · 123

CHAPTER 12: Who Could Complain About Innocuous Public Databases? · 128

PART 4: THE AMA AND THE MEDICAL POLITICIANS ENTER PARTISAN POLITICS · 135

CHAPTER 13: Re-enters the AMA with Dwindling Membership but With Lots of Money · 137

CHAPTER 14: Outlandish and Biased Medical Journalism · 146

CHAPTER 15: AMA Exhorts Doctors to Spy on Patients' Gun Ownership · 164

PART 5: THE SECOND AMENDMENT IN MODERN SOCIETY · 175

CHAPTER 16: Women, Guns, and the Need for Self-Protection · 177

CHAPTER 17: Children, Shootings, and Juvenile Delinquency · 200

CHAPTER 18: Self-Defense: Lethal Threat May Require Protective Lethal Force · 210

PART 6: TYRANNY AND THE EUROPEAN SOCIAL DEMOCRACIES · 221

CHAPTER 19: The Naïveté of Americans and the Gun Control Fallacies of the European Social Democracies · 223

CHAPTER 20: Gun Control in Australia and Great Britain · 240

CHAPTER 21: Gun Control and the Hallmarks of Tyranny · 263

PART 7: MASS SHOOTINGS AND THE MEDIA 277

CHAPTER 22: Shooting Rampages, Mental Health,
and the Sensationalization of Violence 279

PART 8: AMERICA, GUNS, AND FREEDOM 313

CHAPTER 23: America, Guns, and Freedom—A Recapitulation of Liberty 315

CHAPTER 24: America, Guns, and Freedom—An International Perspective 331

CHAPTER 25: Offense is the Best Defense for Advocating Gun Rights 345

EPILOGUE 367

APPENDIX A: DRACONIAN GUN LAWS AND KNEE-JERK DEMOCRACY IN NEW ZEALAND 373

APPENDIX B: KNIFE CONTROL IN GREAT BRITAIN? 375

ACKNOWLEDGMENTS 379

REFERENCES/NOTES 381

ABOUT THE AUTHOR 435

BIBLIOGRAPHY 437

INDEX 441

FOREWORD

Few medical doctors in their careers attain a worldview that encompasses much more than their own special repertoire of medical knowledge and expertise. Medicine's demands on our time, mental reserves, and sheer physical presence leave little time for reflection on world history and politics. It is for that reason that Dr. Miguel A. Faria, Jr. is so remarkable because during his professional career, he practiced one of our profession's most demanding specialties—neurosurgery. It is remarkable that he found time and energy during his busy career as a brain surgeon to reflect on the state of medicine and freedom in America, to say nothing of writing and publishing his observations.

In an age ruled by superficiality and vulgarity, Dr. Faria stands out as a true 21st century Renaissance man. His scholarly grasp of history—particularly the ancient recurring theme of tyranny—sharpens his understanding, and also that of his readers, of today's efforts to quell freedom and advance the statist dreams of liberal progressives. His insider's view as a practicing surgeon, informed policy advocate, and even public servant likewise hone his understanding of the public health establishment's disgraceful role in dismantling our liberty.

Dr. Faria's latest book recounts the history of the public health establishment's calculated attack on the American civil right of gun ownership, relating it to the larger picture of liberal encroachment on American institutions—academia, the media, even the American family. He relates that history as one of its creators because Dr. Faria was and is at the heart of the resistance to this outrageous power play by the public health establishment and organized medicine.

At about the same time in the mid-1990s, Dr. Faria and I were both involved in our state medical associations as delegates to their policy-making bodies; he in Georgia and I in California. We both soon encountered the extreme bias and intolerance of organized medicine as our independent efforts to bring balance to the then-nascent firearm policy debate in medicine were met with hostility, duplicity, and finally, exclusion from the debate. Dr. Faria has recounted the details of his own battles in his 1997 book, *Medical Warrior: Fighting Corporate Socialized Medicine* (Hacienda Publishing).

Here Dr. Faria approaches his sweeping subject—America and its traditions of freedom and gun ownership—from a perspective that few of us can claim. He and his family lived under a Communist dictatorship before fleeing to America (see another selection from his prolific authorship, *Cuba in Revolution: Escape From a Lost Paradise* [Hacienda Publishing, 2002]). The turmoil and deprivation of the Castro regime, which persists today, gave him a deep and indelible reverence for the notion of liberty and the promise of America to honor it. As with other immigrants I have known, Miguel is a truer American than many of us who were born here.

His introduction to firearm policy began during his stint as editor of the *Journal of the Medical Association of Georgia*. Asked by noted author and legal scholar David Kopel to consider some articles written by Edgar Suter, M.D. for publication, Dr. Faria and his editorial colleagues at *JMAG* were intrigued by the serious criticisms Dr. Suter presented of the state of public health firearm research. Dr. Suter showed convincing evidence that the flood of firearm research papers starting to appear in medical journals was part of a coordinated effort by the public health community to discredit firearm ownership in America.

These were serious charges, but Dr. Faria, always seeking truth and not afraid to challenge orthodoxy, published Dr. Suter's articles as well as similar articles from other noted authors. These mold-breaking and—at the time—daring articles in a previously obscure state medical association journal were the shots heard 'round the medical world and beyond. They launched the movement that eventually discredited the public health community's dishonorable descent into junk science in the service of gun control.

Dr. Faria paid the price for his honesty and courage, being considered too controversial for the staid and timorous titans of the medical society. He lost his position as editor of *JMAG*, but their loss became our gain as he went on to other editorial posts. The whole episode made Dr. Faria a celebrity in the powerful community of Second Amendment advocacy. Indeed, it was after Dr. Faria's victory at *JMAG* that I met him in Washington, D.C. in 1996, both of us sitting at the witness table in front of the House Appropriations Subcommittee. We were giving testimony about the latest public health scandal—a program of gun control advocacy at the federal government's Centers for Disease Control and Prevention. Rather than give away my friend Miguel's story here, I shall let him tell it as only he can. He will tell you facts that have been deliberately distorted and concealed from public view for years by the mainstream media, an eager collaborator in the public health establishment's war on liberty. I will leave the reader with this final thought: You are privileged to learn the true story of public health's war on gun owners from a learned insider, a sharp observer of human nature, and a true patriot. We are blessed indeed to be Dr. Faria's students.

— Timothy W. Wheeler, M.D.

Timothy Wheeler, M.D. is a retired southern California head and neck surgeon, founder of Doctors for Responsible Gun Ownership (DRGO) in 1994, serving as its director until 2016. He is coauthor of two books: one with Dr. David C. Stolinsky, *Firearms: A Handbook for Health Professionals* (Claremont, CA: The Claremont Institute, 1999); and the second with Dr. E. John Wipfler, III, *Keeping Your Family Safe: The Responsibilities of Firearm Ownership* (Bellevue, WA: Merrill Press, 2009).

INTRODUCTION:
MY JOURNEY

*The condition upon which God hath given liberty to man is
eternal vigilance; which condition if he break, servitude is at once
the consequence of his crime and the punishment of his guilt.*

—John Philpot Curran (1750—1817),
Ireland, 1790

In this book I recount a personal journey as contemporaneously as possible
with the hope that I succeed in creating an interesting chronological narrative
that the reader will enjoy as both history and contemporary politics.

I have also attempted to use, sparingly, the communication concept of
the SOCO—"the single over-riding objective"—in the form of repetition of
some important points in different chapters so that the reader can take not just
a single objective, but multiple salient messages that can be recalled for future
use in conversation, debate, or writing letters to the editor. For the benefit of
the reader, I have sometimes italicized these useful and memorable objectives.

Interestingly enough, the SOCO communicating tool was developed
by the Centers for Disease Control and Prevention (CDC) media relation
officials to communicate essential points (usually facts but sometimes, as in
the case of gun control, propaganda) to the media, repeating "over-riding
objectives" for the media to emphasize and get across to the public.

As for our use, as Johann Wolfgang von Goethe (1749—1832), the
great literary polymath, once declared, "Truth has to be repeated constantly,
because Error also is being preached all the time, and not just by a few, but by
the multitude. In the Press and Encyclopaedias, in Schools and Universities,
everywhere Error holds sway, feeling happy and comfortable in the knowledge

of having Majority on its side." I don't know about the majority, but for the rest of the observation, Goethe is quite correct, and we must do what we can to contravene propagandistic errors attempting to pass as scientific facts.

This book is not a treatise on criminal justice or a medical textbook on public health, but a detailed narrative relating my personal experience of nearly three decades in the trenches fighting for a more balanced treatment of the issue of "guns and violence" against the opposition of the medical establishment—headed by the American Medical Association (AMA) and "organized medicine," including the major medical journals controlled by these organizations—and the public health establishment (PHE).

Public health researchers have their studies published in their own journals and in AMA publications, where the information is further disseminated to the medical community. It is a mutually beneficial political relationship, but not necessarily in the best interest of patients, society, science, or medicine. Propagandizing views—on utilitarian, population-based, redistributive ethics; gender and transgender politics; gun control; and environmental issues—are repeated so often in so many medical journals and publications that PHE opinions become "fact" in the minds of physicians and other medical personnel. Those views, as well as the alleged social responsibility of the individual to society and the collective, rather than to the individual and his family, are progressive (socialistic) views they want to impose on society, using public health and medicine as vehicles. This book will deal mostly with the gun control issue, but I will also touch on other points in the narrative and demonstrate their interconnection to the issue of public health and gun control.

Thus, when the medical and public health establishments adamantly refused to present a more balanced view of the role of guns in society and to publish both sides of the gun control debate, I joined others in exposing the bias and misinformation printed in the medical journals and attempted to correct the public record.

The fact that I served as a delegate from Bibb County to the House of Delegates of the Medical Association of Georgia for several years and subsequently, in 1993, as editor of the *Journal of the Medical Association of Georgia* provided me with a unique opportunity to fight from within the belly of "organized medicine."

I did not know at the time that wouldn't be the only occasion I would be afforded such an opportunity. The next time, as the reader shall see, would be from within the belly of an even more strident entity.

As editor of a state medical publication sponsored by the so-called "organized medicine," I was disturbed to find a massive barrage of gun control propaganda being published by the AMA and public health officials. I was expected to go with the flow, but I refused. Instead, I attempted to balance this barrage of propaganda by presenting the other side of the issue. For my attempt at journalistic independence and fairness, I was to pay dearly.

Yet, ultimately, I was profusely rewarded, as the reader will learn from the pages that follow. Moreover, I was to learn that I was not alone. There were other physicians out there, scattered throughout the land, willing to speak out. Thus, I came to be aided in my labors by a precious few, a small band of medical warriors, willing to fight. Initially, they had worked in the effort independently and we were unknown to each other. Among them were Dr. William C. Waters IV, who had been active in Georgia; and Dr. Edgar A. Suter and Dr. Timothy W. Wheeler in California.

I learned from the noted civil rights lawyer, criminologist, and scholar David Kopel that Dr. Edgar Suter—at the time chairman of Doctors for Integrity in Policy Research (DIPR)—had been unsuccessful having his work published in the medical literature, even though he had done a superb job analyzing the works of Florida State University professor of criminology Gary Kleck, public health researcher Dr. Arthur Kellermann (both of whom we will hear a lot more about in subsequent chapters), and other noted criminologists and public health researchers. Suffice to say, Dr. Suter had been unable to breach what he called "the monolithic wall of censorship of the established medical journals." Kopel asked me, as newly appointed editor of the *Journal of the Medical Association of Georgia*, if I would be willing to take a look at Dr. Suter's work. I replied that if he submitted his work, it could possibly fit under the AMA's campaign against domestic violence, which by that time had evolved into "gun violence"—but only if the manuscript passed the *Journal's* peer review process. Dr. Suter's work was scrutinized by two reviewers, including one member of the editorial board of the *Journal*.

The medical reviewers and I found the work of Dr. Suter scholarly, yet fascinating and provocative. The fact that his work had not been previously published, but instead had been censored, was shocking to me as well as to the peer reviewers. This was at the time when *The New England Journal of*

Medicine (*NEJM*), the *Journal of the American Medical Association* (*JAMA*), and most state medical journals were busy publishing material on this very topic of "guns and violence."

What happened following the publication of Dr. Suter's work, the events that unfolded, and the political ramifications that ensued are recounted in this book, which is both a personal saga as well as the story of public health and gun control and its interrelation with politics.

PART I

PUBLIC HEALTH AND GUN CONTROL—
"GUN VIOLENCE AS AN EPIDEMIC"

PRELUDE

GUN VIOLENCE AS A PUBLIC HEALTH ISSUE

In the aftermath of the Sandy Hook tragedy on December 14, 2012, when 22 children and six adults were shot to death, the liberal media and gun control activists, just as they had done in the wake of the Columbine School shooting of April 20, 1999, saw and used the tragedy as an opportunity to clamor for more stringent gun control—gun control that punishes the law-abiding gun owners, but does not stop criminals and madmen who obtain their guns illegally and do not obey the laws.

The heinous Las Vegas shooting on October 1, 2017 further changed the dynamics of the gun control debate 180 degrees, from a favorable pro-gun atmosphere before the shooting, when the Republican Congress was ready to take up several pro-gun measures including Concealed Carry Reciprocity and easing restrictions on gun suppressors, to postponing consideration of those measures "indefinitely." Some Republicans—e.g., Newt Gingrich, Paul Ryan (R-WI), and other GOP congressmen, even President Donald Trump—suggested that some gun control measures may be considered, caving in to the knee jerk calls from the press and the vociferous Democrats, including Hillary Clinton, Nancy Pelosi (D-CA), and John Lewis (D-GA), that drastic gun control measures needed to be taken.

In 2012, though, the gun control activists and their allies in the media used a different approach. It had been exactly 15 years since Congress passed a law curtailing the excesses the public health establishment (PHE) had repeatedly exercised in promoting gun control via political lobbying and biased gun research. So seizing the tragic occasion of the Sandy Hook shooting, the activists clamored for ending the congressional "ban" on gun research. Following the Las Vegas shooting in 2017, they would do the same, joined by the medical journals.

Supposedly, an intolerant Congress had thwarted science. Public health researchers complained that gun and violence research had "slowed to a trickle in the past 15 years." In January 2013, barely one month after the Sandy Hook tragedy, President Barack Obama issued an executive order ordering the CDC to "conduct or sponsor research into the causes of gun violence and the ways to prevent it." Obama also requested $10 million in funding for the CDC's gun violence research programs. Congress stood its ground and denied the funding.[1] Reading media accounts and the editorials in the medical journals such as *Lancet* and *Journal of the American Medical Association* (*JAMA*), one was led to believe that Congress opposed scientific investigation and that supporters of the so-called "ban" were a bunch of intolerant gun nuts from the NRA who were against science and progress.[2]

The fact is that the story has not been fully told because the media has spun and distorted the facts to feed their preconceived anti-gun notions. The whole truth was, and remains, that public health officials had been ordered by Congress not to use taxpayer money to conduct politicized, biased, and result-oriented gun research, which always reached the preordained conclusion of promoting gun control. The so-called ban is not a complete prohibition written in stone, but, as the reader shall see, a reasonable restriction preventing the use of junk science to effect public policy. Also, unbeknownst to most of the public, public health officials had been prohibited from unlawfully using public funds, intended for teaching conferences and research, for illegal lobbying activities and attempting to influence public policy towards the implementation of gun control. That systematic illegality, which has not been given the attention it deserves, was prohibited at the same time as restrictions were placed on conducting politicized gun research.

And so, since 2012, the clamor has remained and still is directed at criticizing Congress for going purportedly "against science" and scientific gun research. The effort now is to "lift the ban" on research (and lobbying). Dr. David Satcher, who was in charge of the CDC in the 1990s at the time the restrictions were passed by Congress, lamented in a recent interview that "Any time we restrict research, it is dangerous for public health and democracy. It is sad when you really think about it. We are in an environment when children are dying and we are playing political games."[3] There you have it: The very senior public health official, who had been at the center of the problem, is two decades later still propagandizing with emotional sound bites. Which side was really misusing science? This book will provide the answer.

Regarding the congressional prohibition, as we will demonstrate in this book, it was the public health officials who brought this upon themselves. They were not using science or medicine in their research. They were the ones using politics and subverting science in pursuit of their ideology and to satisfy their voracious greed for public money. What follows in the chapters of this book is the history of public health and the public health establishment's drive to use biased, politicized, result-oriented research to promote stringent gun control—using public funds that were intended for educational and research purposes. What was their goal? Ultimately, to assist the government in imposing civilian disarmament upon American citizens, perverting the purpose of science and medicine in the process. The medical politicians have joined in force with the PHE in calling for the resumption of the CDC gun violence research.[4] Their disingenuous mantra is that "gun violence is a public health issue," and that it has become "an epidemic that needs eradicating."

CHAPTER I

GUN CONTROL AND EXPEDIENT MEDICAL POLITICS

The greatest evil is not now done in those sordid 'dens of crime'
that Dickens loved to paint. It is not done even in concentra-
tion camps and labor camps. In those we see its final result.
But it is conceived and ordered (moved, seconded, carried,
and minuted) in clean, carpeted, warmed and well-lighted
offices, by quiet men with white collars and cut fingernails and
smooth shaven cheeks who do not need to raise their voice.

—C.S. Lewis (1898—1963),
British novelist, essayist, and lay Christian theologian

In 1991, the American Medical Association (AMA) became involved in a widely publicized campaign against domestic violence. Launched for public relations and media consumption, the AMA's campaign went hand in hand with a previously articulated (1979) U.S. Public Health Service objective of complete eradication of handguns in America, beginning with a 25 percent reduction in the national inventory by the year 2000.[1]

Despite the purported safeguards of peer review and the imprimatur of the prestigious medical journals, and the alleged claims to objectivity and impartiality by government-funded researchers in public health, particularly at the Centers for Disease Control and Prevention (CDC), I became completely convinced that gun research and the portrayal of firearms in the medical literature was biased and unreliable because sound scholarship had been abandoned for the allure of government money in the form of grants, the political expediency of the times, and the progressive, liberal ideology evinced by public health officials and researchers.[2-4]

Science or Ideology in Public Health

It's difficult to comprehend the travesty of supposedly honest researchers allowing ideology and personal self-interest to influence the outcome of their scientific and medical research, but this was exactly what was happening in the area of injury prevention in public health. In unguarded moments, they even admitted their bias influenced their work, and in some cases their entire careers. For instance, CDC official Dr. Patrick O'Carroll was quoted in the *Journal of the American Medical Association (JAMA)* propounding:

> 'Bringing about gun control, which itself covers a variety of activities from registration to confiscation was not the specific reason for the section's creation,' O'Carroll says. 'However, the facts themselves tend to make some form of regulation seem desirable,' he says. 'The way we're going to do this is to systematically build a case that owning firearms causes death.'[5]

Although, in a letter to the editor, O'Carroll later claimed he was misquoted, Dr. William C. Waters IV, then Eastern Director of Doctors for Integrity in Policy Research (DIPR), pointed out that Dr. O'Carroll did not claim to be misquoted when in the same article, he blurted, "We are doing the most we can do, given the political realities."[6]

Prejudice against gun ownership by ordinary citizens is pervasive in the PHE, even when professing objectivity and integrity in scientific research. Deborah Prothrow-Stith, then dean of the Harvard School of Public Health, in a moment of lucidity encapsulated the typical attitude of her professional colleagues, many of them working in "injury prevention" and purportedly tackling the problem of "guns and violence" from a scientific perspective: "My own view on gun control is simple. I hate guns—and cannot imagine why anybody would want to own one. If I had my way, guns for sport would be registered, and all other guns would be banned."[7]

Dr. Mark Rosenberg, former director of the CDC's National Center for Injury Prevention and Control (NCIPC), told *The Washington Post* in 1994, "We need to revolutionize the way we look at guns, like what we did with cigarettes. Now it [sic] is dirty, deadly, and banned."[7]

A few public health officials like Dr. C. J. Peters, at one time the head of the CDC's Special Pathogens Branch, expressed concerns about the direction public health had taken and reported to the *Pittsburgh Post-Gazette*, in the midst of the controversy over taxpayer-funded gun (control) research, "The CDC has got to be careful that we don't get into social issues." He added, "If we're going to do that, we ought to start a center for social change. We should stay with medical issues."[7]

Public health officials and CDC researchers should have listened to Dr. Peters' advice. Instead they continued to insist, "gun violence is an epidemic that must be eradicated." PHE officials conveniently neglected the fact that guns and bullets were inanimate objects that do not follow Koch's Postulates of Pathogenicity, the time-proven, logical series of scientific steps that should be carried out by medical investigators to definitively prove a microorganism is pathogenic and directly responsible for causing a particular disease. Koch's Postulates state: "First, the germ must be found growing abundantly in every patient and every diseased tissue. Second, the germ must be isolated and grown in the laboratory. Third, the purified germ must cause the disease again in another host." In injury prevention and the study of "guns and violence," the public health establishment threw science into the wastebasket, confusing microbiology and pathology with sociology and politics.

Yet, these public health researchers don't understand sociology or criminology. They delve into areas in which they have not been trained and, consequently, know little about. In short, they are out of their depths and simply fail to recognize the importance of individual responsibility and moral conduct—namely, that behind every shooting there is a person pulling the trigger who should be held accountable for his actions. The portrayal of guns in the medical literature by the AMA, the various schools of public health, and until 1996, the CDC and NCIPC, paralleled the sensationalized violence in the mainstream media, exploiting understandable concerns about domestic violence and rampant street crime, but failing to produce unbiased, accurate and objective information expected of scientific research.

While the CDC has tempered its stand on guns and violence research in the last two decades following the restrictions of 1996 (events that will be described in other chapters), the rest of the PHE—supported financially by wealthy gun control proponents such as Michael Bloomberg and George Soros, as well as progressive, gun prohibitionist organizations such as the Joyce Foundation—continue to promote gun control masquerading as social or public health scientific research.[8]

Why would the AMA suddenly jump in and become involved in this politically expedient but potentially explosive issue of gun control as a public health issue? The 1991 effort by the AMA to increase membership, although expensive, was highly unproductive. The AMA attempted to reverse the decades-long trend of dwindling membership to achieve at least a majority membership of American physicians, but it was utterly unsuccessful, unable to keep pace with its attrition rate and holding then to a 38 percent membership of American physicians. Doctors did not like the politicization of the AMA and were jumping ship. Three decades earlier, the AMA had commanded a 75 percent supermajority. By 2011, AMA membership had dropped to a barebones 15 percent, and of those remaining, many of them were employed in public health, not in private practice as in former times.[9]

This tactic of launching a highly visible campaign against domestic violence entwined with a major gun control effort was (and remains) essentially a public relations ploy judged to be one sure way to get endless, politically correct, and praiseworthy publicity; attract membership; and score public relations points while ingratiating itself with the liberal media.

The truth was that when it came to the topic of guns and violence, sound scholarship was ignored or frankly discarded by the AMA and "organized medicine" leadership. When it came to the topic of guns and violence, free inquiry and the free flow and exchange of information were banned from AMA publications. Following the lead of the AMA/CDC/NCIPC, many doctors, particularly pediatricians, jumped on the gun control bandwagon, giving the pseudo-scientific research and gun control policy pronouncements an aura of respectability. Along the way, as the AMA-public health bandwagon traveled down the slippery slope of promoting only politically correct views while censoring dissenting views, the AMA and "organized medicine" damaged its credibility and lost the respect of the vast majority of physicians.

A Sinister Objective—The Use of Public Health as a Tool for Gun Control

As early as 1985, the CDC had conducted and published in the mainstream medical journals, including *The New England Journal of Medicine* (*NEJM*) and the AMA subsidiary journals, dozens of articles all supporting stricter gun control policies. This biased and faulty research, funded at taxpayer expense, accelerated after the inception of the NCIPC. Why this faulty research and dissemination of biased, unscientific information? In a comprehensive and widely discussed *Tennessee Law Review* article, "Guns and Public Health," criminologist and civil rights attorney, Don B. Kates and associates wrote, "Based on studies, and propelled by leadership from the Centers for Disease Control and Prevention (CDC), the objective has broadened so that it now includes banning and confiscation of all handguns, restrictive licensing of owners of other firearms and eventual elimination of all firearms from American life, excepting (perhaps) only a small elite of extremely wealthy collectors, hunters or target shooters. This is the case in many European countries."[10]

In the chapter "Bad Medicine: Doctors and Guns," Kates and associates described a particularly egregious example of editorial bias and censorship by *The New England Journal of Medicine.*[7] In 1989, two studies were independently submitted for publication to *NEJM*. Both authors were affiliated with the University of Washington School of Public Health. One study by Dr. John H. Sloan and associates was a *selective* two-city comparison of homicide rates in Vancouver, British Columbia and Seattle, Washington.[11] The other paper was a *comprehensive* comparison study between the U.S. and Canada by Dr. Brandon Centerwall.

Predictably, the editors of the *NEJM* chose to publish the Sloan article with inferior but orthodox data that claimed erroneously that severe gun control policies had reduced Canadian homicides, and rejected Centerwall's superior study showing that such policies had not affected the rate of homicides in Canada. In fact, the homicide rates had been lower in Vancouver before the restrictive gun control laws were passed, and rose after the laws were passed. The Vancouver homicide rate increased 25 percent after the institution of the 1977 Canadian law. Sloan and associates also glossed over the disparate ethnic compositions of Seattle and Vancouver. When the rates of homicides for whites were compared in both of the cities, it turned out that the rate of homicide in Seattle was actually lower than in Vancouver, while the fact that blacks and Hispanics had higher rates of homicides in Seattle was not mentioned by the investigators. In searching for societal solutions to the problem of crime and violence not only socioeconomic but also cultural factors such as race and ethnicity must be considered, as different approaches may be required.

Centerwall's paper on the comparative rates of homicides in the U.S. and Canada was eventually published in the *American Journal of Epidemiology*, but his valuable research was not made widely available to the public.[12] In contradistinction to his valuable gun research data, Centerwall's other research pointing to the effects of TV violence affecting homicide rates has been made widely available, but his data exculpating gun availability and homicide rates have not.[13-15]

It had become clear that the AMA and the PHE had set themselves the dishonest task of circumventing the constitutional right of Americans to keep and bear arms, as enshrined in the Second Amendment to the U.S. Constitution, by using biased and flawed "guns and violence" research, misusing and subverting the time-honored medical profession in the process. Kates and associates wrote, "In this connection, the term 'gun control' needs some clarification. That term could mean no more than noncontroversial measures to prohibit gun misuse or gun possession by high-risk groups. In the literature we are analyzing, however, 'guns are not...inanimate objects, but in fact are a social ill,' and controlling them implies wholesale confiscation from the general public so as to radically reduce gun availability to ordinary people."[20]

As a neurosurgeon who spent incalculable hours in the middle of the night treating neurological victims of gunshot wounds, I too deplored the high level of violence, particularly the rampant crime in American inner cities. Yet, as physicians and public health workers, we should have the moral courage to pursue the truth and find viable solutions through the use of unbiased, sound, scholarly research. Public health researchers have an obligation to write their conclusions based on objective data and scientific information, rather than on ideology, emotionalism, political expediency, and budgetary considerations that include financial self-interest. These interrelated issues of ideology and budgetary considerations are reflected in the insatiable lust for ever-increasing public funds extracted from overtaxed Americans, and then allocated in good faith to public health officials, who frequently turned out to be biased researchers bent on establishing that guns are a social evil that should be eradicated from the general population.

CHAPTER 2

THE POLITICS OF GUN CONTROL AND THE SUBVERSION OF MEDICAL SCIENCE

No matter if the science is all phony, there are collateral environmental benefits...Climate change [provides] the greatest chance for bringing about justice and equality in the world.

—Christine Stewart,
Canada, Minister of the Environment. Speaking about Global Warming to the editors of the *Calgary Herald* as reported by Dr. Fred Singer in *Access to Energy*, December 1998

Science is concerned with the acquisition of knowledge and the pursuit of certainty, elusive as these noble goals may be; in contradistinction to bolstering ignorance, propaganda, or willful misunderstanding. After all, science is charged with the attainment of general and specific truths and the solving of the riddle of the mechanics and operations of the general laws of the universe.

None of this should be surprising for the etymology of science derives from the Latin *scientia*, "having knowledge." The "how-to" or operation of the natural laws are examined and tested through the scientific method which calls for the identification of a problem, the gathering of facts through observations and experimentation, and the testing and re-testing of ideas (that we call hypotheses) that need to be proven right or wrong within a reasonable degree of scientific certainty.

Recognizing True Science, Separating the Wheat from the Chaff

When in the 18th century, Edward Jenner inoculated and developed a protocol for immunizing his patients with a vaccine against smallpox; and in the 19th century, Louis Pasteur identified and characterized the gram positive bacillus that causes Anthrax and developed an immunization method against rabies; Robert Koch developed his famous postulates to prove or disprove that a particular microorganism causes a specific disease; and Joseph Lister developed sterilization techniques to fight nearly invisible, microscopic, and seemingly invincible (*animalcules*) pathogenic invaders—these scientists all laid precious building blocks of medical knowledge that led to the construction of the edifice of the germ theory of disease, and wholly or in part, used the scientific method to advance both science and medicine. These medical advances, directed toward the comfort and benefit of humanity, were not only rooted in science but also in moral principles, derived from our dual Graeco-Roman legacy of medical humanitarianism and philanthropy and Judeo-Christian morality of charity and hope.[1]

How does science work? One way is by formulating a methodology whereby a researcher defines and tests a hypothesis by devising an experiment, collects data, and then reaches a conclusion as to the validity—that is, the truthfulness or wrongness—of the tested hypothesis. Yet, before this conclusion is formed, the data must be collected and verified, and accurate observations must be made. The scientific method also requires diligence in avoiding selection bias and in ascertaining that the samples to be analyzed are adequate in size and that the control groups are properly matched. The researcher must be assured that the experiment is properly carried out and the data properly obtained, and that he or she is unbiased and an honest observer, not deceived by preconceived notions about the subject under study. Failing this, the conclusions drawn from the observations or experiments are null and void.

An example of what can happen when scientific research is riddled with illogical reasoning and errors in methodology and design, or tainted by dishonesty or biased information, was given sometime back by Dr. Jane Orient in a series of articles, "Practice Guidelines and Outcomes Research," published in the *Medical Sentinel*.[2,3] Dr. Orient demonstrated with pinpoint accuracy how managed care's outcome research was riddled with procedural errors and, in fact, was unscientific because it dealt not with objective patient treatment results and evaluations of specific scientific medical advances, but with subjective evaluations and health systems measurements leading to the preconceived goals of cost containment and rationing of medical care. Plainly speaking, the pseudo-research Dr. Orient criticized was not searching for the elusive alleviation of suffering, but instead to satisfy the fashionable cliché of "the proper allocation of scarce resources" and the realization of the bottom line for the managed care networks working under monopolistic government protection.

Another example of faulty research was displayed by the AMA's Council of Scientific Affairs when it endorsed—on the basis of pseudo "scientific research"—the ban on assault weapons.[4] Obviously, the Council had a public relations ax to grind rather than expert knowledge of the sciences of criminology and ballistics. Instead of doing its own scholarly work or at least relying on the expert work of Dr. Martin Fackler, the foremost wound ballistics expert in the United States, the Council unfortunately relied, for political purposes, on unscientific data and even sensationalized newspaper articles, one of which claimed that watermelons fired upon with "assault weapons" are appropriate human tissue simulants to demonstrate wound ballistics! It has been pointed out correctly, I might add, that if that were the case, an 18-inch drop of a watermelon would also be appropriate for the study of head injuries.[5]

Before proceeding further, allow me to clarify some general terms. A *theory* is a *general principle* that is proposed to explain observed facts. A *hypothesis*, on the other hand, is an *assumption* that must be defined in advance and then tested before it can subsequently be used as a theory to explain observed facts or natural phenomena. If after a hypothesis is properly tested, it's not supported by objective, scientific observations, it must be rejected. That is why Albert Einstein announced, "No amount of experimentation can ever prove me right; a single experiment can prove me wrong." On the other hand, if experimental data or observations support the hypothesis, the latter should be accepted, at least until the time when another given observation properly rejects it.

In science, *a posteriori* reasoning (whereby the attainment of knowledge occurs from observations and experience) is preferred over *a priori* reasoning, which relies on the deduction of knowledge from self-evident propositions, independent of observations or experience.

Above all, scrupulous researchers must avoid *post hoc, ergo propter hoc* reasoning, "after it, therefore because of it;" they must make sure their conclusions truly follow from their observations and experiments, rather than assume that a conclusion follows simply because a certain independent event preceded it. Take, for instance, the often-heard proposition, repeated time and again without dissent, in the medical literature on the subject of "guns and violence"—namely, that guns in the U.S. are responsible for high rates of suicide. When in reality, the overwhelming available evidence compiled from the discipline of clinical psychiatry is that untreated or poorly managed depression is the real culprit behind high rates of suicide.

Suicide and Crimes of Passion

Let me now say a word about suicide and gun availability. Both Drs. Arthur Kellermann and John H. Sloan have written about suicides and have attempted to link these fatalities to the availability of guns in articles published in *The New England Journal of Medicine*.[6,7]

It may seem too obvious to restate but yes, the overwhelming available evidence compiled from the psychiatric literature is that untreated or poorly managed depression is the real culprit behind the high rates of suicide. The evidence is authoritative on this point as classified in the *Diagnostic and Statistical Manual of Mental Disorders* of the American Psychiatric Association and any standard psychiatric text.

From the social science of criminology, in fact, we solve the seeming paradox that countries such as Japan, Hungary, and the Scandinavian countries, which boast draconian gun control laws and low rates of firearm availability, have higher rates of suicide than the U.S. In these countries, where guns are not readily available, citizens simply *substitute* other cultural or universally available methods to kill themselves, such as Seppuku (Hara-kiri) in Japan; drowning in the Danube in Hungary; suffocation (with poisonous gases, such as carbon monoxide from automobile exhausts) or hanging in Denmark and Germany; or drinking agricultural pesticides, which is commonly done in Sri Lanka and many other third world nations. In these countries, citizens commit suicide quite effectively by those methods at comparable or even higher rates than in the U.S.[8,9,10]

Gun violence studies do not fall within the discipline of biology, but within the spheres of sociology and criminology; and since guns and bullets are not biological entities, biological tools are inadequate to study them. The health advocacy of the PHE, the AMA, and "organized medicine" must come to terms with the fact that guns and bullets are inanimate objects that do not abide by Koch's Postulates of Pathogenicity (which prove definitely and scientifically that a microorganism is responsible for a particular disease), and recognize the fact that behind every shooting there is a person pulling the trigger who should be held accountable. The problem is more complex than just "easy availability" of firearms or guns and bullets as animated, virulent pathogens needing to be stamped out by limiting gun availability and, ultimately, eradicating guns from law-abiding citizens.

Within the context of gun availability, much has been said about the "crimes of passion" that supposedly take place impulsively in the heat of the moment or in the furor of a domestic squabble. Criminologists have pointed out that homicides in this setting are the culmination of a long simmering cycle of violence. In one study of the police records in Detroit and Kansas City it was revealed, for example, that in "90 percent of domestic homicides, the police had responded at least once before during the prior two years to a disturbance," and "in over 50 percent of the cases, the police had been called five or more times to that dysfunctional domicile."[11] Surely, these are not crimes of passion consummated impulsively in the heat of the moment by ordinary citizens, but the result of violence in highly dysfunctional families in the setting of repeated alcohol or illicit drug use; it is also the setting of abusive husbands who after a long history of spousal abuse finally commit murder, and increasingly, wives defending themselves against those abusive husbands, representing acts of genuine self-defense.[11]

Avoiding Pitfalls such as Ideological Bias and Political Expediency

Today, sadly, many government researchers who depend on government funds (naturally, extracted from reluctant taxpayers) are frequently placed in a conflict-of-interest situation, or position themselves in the dubious circumstances in which their credibility (and professional reputations) can be called into question. (I would also say honor, but the term is considered anachronistic and antiquated in such quarters.) Given the nature of research impacting directly on public policy, many of these researchers are veritably pressed to reach preordained conclusions about scientific projects in which government officials and political leaders have a vested political interest or an ideological ax to grind.

In these circumstances, particularly when politics and ideology are at stake, we end up not with objective research and the attainment of scientific truth, but with what Dr. Edgar Suter of Doctors for Integrity in Policy Research (DIPR), Dr. Timothy Wheeler, myself, and others have called politicized, results-oriented research.[5,8,12-14] This kind of pseudo-science, masquerading as scientific research, has adverse and detrimental effects on public policy in general, and science and medicine in particular.

Politicized, results-oriented research reached a pinnacle of sophistication and preordination with the work that was carried out by the Centers for Disease Control and Prevention (CDC) up to 1996, which prior to the 1970s enjoyed a high degree of respect and credibility with both the scientific community and the public because of its historic record fighting truly epidemiologic and contagious diseases afflicting humanity.

The problem from the late 1980s to 1996 stemmed from the gun control propaganda generated by the National Center for Injury Prevention and Control (NCIPC) and published in the medical journals, particularly the *Journal of the American Medical Association* (*JAMA*) and *The New England Journal of Medicine* (*NEJM*).

Those of us who studied this problem found that systematically and methodically, the conclusions were preordained. This meant that selected data were collected and observations made to reach foregone, politicized, result-oriented conclusions—the ends desired by the researchers and their sponsors.

How this travesty of unscientific, preordained "research" was carried out, published, and disseminated in the mainstream medical journals, and how this preordained "research" and unscientific information could result in adverse and detrimental effects on public policy will be the subjects of subsequent chapters. But first, let's review a lesson from history.

CHAPTER 3

THE PERVERSION OF SOVIET SCIENCE IN THE SERVICE OF THE STATE–UNLEARNED LESSONS

To be corrupted by totalitarianism, one does not
have to live in a totalitarian country.

—George Orwell (1903—1950),
quoted by Cuban freedom fighter, Guillermo Cabrera Infante
(1929—2005), in his memoirs *Mea Cuba*, page 45

The lessons of history clearly demonstrate to those who care to learn that whenever science and medicine become subordinated to the State, the results have been as perverse as they have been disastrous. This was the case with science in the former Soviet Union and its satellites, particularly during the 1930s through the 1950s, and in the case of Soviet psychiatry, extending until the very end of the USSR in 1991. In communist Cuba, the abuse of psychiatry continued until the 21st century.[1]

In the last several decades, we have witnessed the astounding growth of government at the expense of the individual. The threat of tyrannical government with the subordination of science for political purposes, including disarming law-abiding citizens, is disturbing, particularly in a society that at the same time is permissive to criminal elements. Moreover, the threat of tyrannical government and the misuse of science are ever present and never fully eliminated. Each generation must wage its own battles, but to do so its members must remain informed and vigilant, as well as knowledgeable about what took place in preceding generations.

Soviet Science—Genetics and Agriculture

As I observed in *Vandals at the Gates of Medicine* (1994), published in
the midst of the Clinton Administration's attempted takeover of the American
health care system, subversion of the biological sciences by the Marxist-
Leninist Soviet state began soon after the triumph of the October Revolution
under Vladimir Ilyich Lenin (1870—1924) and intensified under the even
more brutal rule of the Red Czar, Joseph V. Stalin (1879—1953). Under Stalin's
dictatorship, the Russian scientists that did not believe in the new collectivist Soviet science of Marxist genetics or opposed the teachings of the "new
science," were purged—either expelled from their teaching posts and research
positions, or consigned to the depths of the gulags and eventually, unceremo-
niously, killed in the labor camps, exterminated as "enemies of the people"
and the Soviet Motherland.

At the helm of Soviet science from the 1930s through the 1950s was
Trofim Denisovich Lysenko (1898—1976), a Soviet agronomist who, as
president of the Lenin Academy of Agricultural Science from 1938 to 1956
and director of the Institute of Genetics of the Soviet Academy of Sciences,
became the supreme leader in Soviet science, genetics, and agriculture.[2]

Lysenko heralded a sorrowful chapter in the subversion and perversion
of science. He placed genetics and science and agriculture at the political
whims of the Soviet totalitarian state. Lysenko vehemently rejected what he
called capitalist "bourgeois" science and repudiated the fundamental laws of
genetics that had been proposed by the celebrated Austrian monk, Gregor
Mendel (1822—1884), genetic principles that had been accepted and used
in the West in theoretic and applied biologic sciences. Lysenko proscribed
"bourgeois genetics" and during the immediate post–World War II period,
assisted by plant breeder I.V. Michurin, began a series of preposterous plant
crossbreeding experiments based on the theory of the inheritance of acquired
characteristics, a theory first promulgated in 1801 by the French biologist
and naturalist, Jean Baptiste Lamarck (1744—1829).

The Lamarckian theory of inheritance of acquired characteristics,
although a forerunner of Charles Darwin's theory of evolution, held that
new acquired traits in organisms developed as an immediate *need* to adapt
to the environment and were inherited by the offspring. This hypothesis had
already been rejected in the West by systematic, scientific observations, and

the sound, rigorous experimentation normally expected and conducted by Western scientists.

One experiment debunking the Lamarckian theory consisted of simply studying consecutive generations of rats whose tails had been amputated and checking successive offspring for evidence of shortening in their tail. Systematic observations revealed no such evidence. This simple experiment, in a free society, would have been enough to reject the Lamarckian hypothesis. But, that did not happen behind the Iron Curtain where Soviet science was subjugated to State politics and totalitarian socialist ideology. After all, Soviet politics and science were committed to forging the *novus homo*, "the New Socialist Man." Spearheading this effort was trusted party comrade Lysenko, who earnestly committed himself to the new science and to harvesting a "new Soviet crop." Lysenko's experiments promised the Soviet *nomenklatura* to make Siberia a huge granary at the disposal of the Soviet Union, a vehicle to export Lenin's world revolution, but it was not to be.[2]

Although for this preordained purpose Lysenko did create a hybrid plant through his extensive crossbreeding experiment, his grand experiment turned into a monumental failure. He had envisioned creating a new plant with lush foliage, juicy stems, and palatable leaves resembling lettuce or cabbage and, perhaps, having fruit-like tomatoes. Comrade Lysenko further expected the new hybrid to have tuberous underground roots with plump, nutritious, potato-like vegetables. In short, the entire plant would be edible—and a monument to Soviet genetics and agriculture.

What he, in fact, created was a plant variety—certainly a new species—but instead of the perfect crop as envisioned, the new plants had inedible stems and leaves, no fruit above ground, and rudimentary and unsavory roots. Comrade Lysenko's hybrid plants that were to feed the masses of the Soviet people were troublesome weeds not fit for human consumption.

Vast fields planted with the hybrid variety as allocated by Lysenko and the central planners and cultivated by the unfortunate prisoners of the gulags were lost. The promising Soviet experiment controlled by the State and headed by the great Lysenko proved a disastrous debacle. Lysenko, Michurin, and his willing and collaborating colleagues were finally dethroned and consigned to the dustbin of bogus scientific socialist theories—but not before their collaboration and perversion of Marxist biology was shown to the world to be quackery employed as a tool of the Soviet State.

Lysenko's legacy should not be readily forgotten, for it denotes a particularly sad chapter in the history of science. It reveals science's dark descent into the chasm of ignorance, intolerance, and totalitarian control by the most powerful and barbaric of former "cradle-to-grave" socialist workers paradises. Lysenko's preordained cornucopia in Soviet agriculture did not materialize; instead, the Russian people experienced starvation on a grand scale and unimaginable human suffering. Soviet science, subjugated to the Soviet socialist policy, did not support Lamarckian theory any more than the possibility of creating the New Socialist Man; yet, the madness went on for decades with science perverted, lives wasted, generations lost—all thrashed into the infamous cesspool of collectivism.

Millions of Soviet citizens died during this period under Stalin as a result of bogus science, the failure of central planning and collectivization policies, and most savagely, by the deliberate creation of State-planned famines to break the spirit of the individualist Kulaks—whether Georgians, Ukrainians, and ordinary Russians—all of whom opposed collectivization. In good time, those who went along with the State and collaborated with evil were made the scapegoats for the Soviet failures.

I need not remind the reader that while Lysenko perverted science in the Soviet Union, a German physician, his counterpart in the Third Reich, climbed the ladder of academia and did whatever was necessary to reach the top and serve the *Wehrmacht*. His name was Dr. Joseph Mengele, but that story has been told before, so let's return to Soviet style collectivism closer to our time.

Soviet Psychiatry and Rehabilitation

Throughout 70 years of barbaric existence, up to November 1989 with the fall of the Berlin Wall, the communist Soviet empire also bore witness to the perversion of psychiatry—another sad chapter, which plainly supports our contention that science and medicine must remain divorced from (and above) politics, and never become pliable tools of government power.

In the former Soviet Union, psychiatry, like genetics and other medical sciences, was used as a tool of the State. The imputation of mental illness to political dissidents has been practiced in collectivist and authoritarian societies for decades, particularly Soviet medicine. As enunciated by Premier Nikita Khrushchev in 1959, Soviet psychiatry was to serve the State: "Can there be diseases, nervous diseases among certain people in the communist society? Evidently there can be. If that is so, then there also will be offenses that are characteristic of people with abnormal minds. To those who might start calling for opposition to communism on this 'basis,' we say that now, too, there are people who fight against communism but clearly the mental state of such people is not normal."[3]

In other words, it is impossible for "normal" people in a socialist society to oppose collectivism or question orthodoxy in politics or science.[4,5] Supposedly, dissent or criminality is impossible in a workers' paradise because everyone in a socialist utopia is by definition content—so it follows those opposed to the socialist order are not really criminals or political dissidents requiring punishment, but insane madmen who require treatment, institutionalization, and rehabilitation in psychiatric facilities.

We have numerous examples, most notably the case of dissident Vladimir Bukobsky, who spent 10 years in Soviet hospitals being "rehabilitated" on psychiatric wards. Obviously, he was mad for rejecting Soviet communism, but despite the indoctrination and brainwashing sessions during his intensive "rehabilitation," Bukobsky would not cave in to the system. Like Aleksandr Solzhenitsyn, who spent years in the Soviet gulags in the 1960s and 1970s, Bukobsky survived and lived to see the day in 1992 when he was able to return to Russia from his exile in England to testify against the Soviet system in Russia's Constitutional Court.

Bukobsky's testimony corroborated the fact that Soviet psychiatry had existed at the disposal of state security and had been used as a political tool by the Soviet Union until well into the late 1980s and the rule of Mikhail Gorbachev (1985—1991).

So in passing, and in the context of psychiatry and rehabilitation, it is worth pointing out and remembering that while in constitutional republics, citizens have civil liberties and constitutional protections, they also have a duty to obey the laws. Yet, they are free to choose either to obey and conform to the laws and be left undisturbed, or to break the laws and face punishment. Transgressors are punished, usually by imprisonment, as prescribed by the law, and effectively isolated to protect society. (Rarely are they executed.)

Authoritarian states, on the other hand, allow no such choice. There the prisoners are "rehabilitated" or eliminated. Social(ist) democracies today want to follow the authoritarian path to "rehabilitation" with a human face, deploring the building of more prisons and refusing to hold individuals accountable. Social democrats, modern liberals, social planners, and other "progressives" do not want transgressors punished and held responsible for their criminal conduct; they opt instead for therapeutics and "rehabilitation," absolving the individual and instead blaming society. All the while, the nanny state of the social democracies accumulates more and more power unto itself not only in the bureaucracies of the socialist penal system but also, and even more importantly, in society at large. During this time, law-abiding citizens are subjected to the passage of more laws with more restrictions placed on personal freedom and the general loss of liberty, while the real criminals, even those convicted, are coddled. No wonder this is so; they serve as an excuse for increasing the political power of the State in the name of law and order.

Politicized Research and Politicized Diseases

How does this historic information relate to the gun control research in the United States today, and to our legacy of freedom? Let us state that in the decades of the 1970s to the 1990s, government agencies, e.g., the NCIPC funded by American taxpayers, were systematically producing flawed gun control research using *a priori* logic and junk science to arrive at predetermined conclusions. Hypotheses were tested but not rejected; *selected* facts were collected; valid information was omitted; and statistics were concocted based on skewed *biased* population samples—all of this was done to reach the predetermined conclusions that guns and not criminals are responsible for violent crime in our society; that firearms, even for home and family protection, have no place in modern society; and that firearms for self-protection should be banned and unavailable to ordinary citizens. The propaganda continues today in a more diluted form coming from the politicized schools of public health sprouting up all over the country, supported by donations of poorly informed but well-intended benefactors, or the obsessed inclinations of authoritarian elites, such as George Soros and Michael Bloomberg, who seem hell-bent on disarming their fellow citizens.

The promotion of gun control by authoritarian governments using politicized science as a vehicle should not be surprising. Authoritarianism always seeks to have a monopoly of force against the very citizens the government purports to serve. The use of public health as a tool of gun control is only one (albeit a most dangerous one) of many other examples of present-day attempts at the subordination of science and medicine to the State for political ends.

Anyone vaguely familiar with the politically protected disease HIV/AIDS, can discern the politicization of that once dreaded sexually transmitted disease by the PHE and "organized medicine" in collusion with the State. In the case of AIDS, the government, via its public health agencies—particularly the CDC and other subsidiary public health departments throughout the nation—tortured statistics until they falsely confessed about the nature of the epidemic and the delayed application of legitimate public health measures that were needed to limit the spread of the disease.

Even more disturbing is the comparison of how the issues of gun violence and AIDS were mishandled by the public health authorities. They urged (and still profess) that gun violence is a public health issue: "Gun violence is an epidemic, like a virus, that must be eradicated with strict public health measures, stringent gun control." While they insist on applying the public health model to gun violence, where it does not apply; in the 1980s and 1990s they refused to institute public health measures to control HIV/AIDS, a sexually transmitted disease where strict public health measures were essential and urgently needed to save lives.

The collusion was protected and promoted by media hype, misinformation, and sensationalism—as to obfuscate the issue and force the viewpoint that heterosexuals were as much at risk of contracting the HIV virus as homosexuals and illicit drug users. Supposedly, "we were all at risk."[6] AIDS rapidly became a government protected disease and no public health measures were implemented such as widespread testing, contact tracing, and closing gay bathhouses until very late in the course of the disease after hundreds of thousands had died.[7] Most troubling in the case of HIV/AIDS was the fact that contrarian views on the nature of the virus were silenced, and the scientists promoting divergent views were ostracized. Why the mendacity, at the risk of more cases and more lives? First, because AIDS had become politicized, a disease subject to politics first and public health measures second. Government agencies wanted to be able to obtain more funding from frightened and empathetic taxpayers, "since we were all at risk," and replicate their bureaucracies faster, perhaps faster than the virus could replicate itself! There was also the secret desire for social engineering, to change the social and cultural perspective of this tragic disease in the constant reconstruction of American society towards a more progressive and socialistic image.

Public health officials blamed it all on needing more money and more research. All this, mind you, despite the fact that more money was being spent in AIDS research and drug development than in any other disease including breast cancer, which AIDS funding surpassed by a margin of nearly 3:1, even though, in the previous decade, breast cancer killed almost three times as many women.

Another issue subject to politics first and science second is global warming (or climate change) whereby the politicized research of social-ly-minded scientists, fueled by the radical environmentalists and bolstered by a sympathetic media, promotes an anti-technologic agenda, duplicitously leading to further government intervention, statism, and collectivism. At the same time, international taxation (beginning with a carbon dioxide emission tax) would be promoted as to accomplish a new redistribution of wealth on a global scale aimed at fostering world socialism on a docile, disarmed world population.

(CHAPTER 4
THE AMA ENTERS THE FRAY
FOR GUN CONTROL

Of all tyrannies, a tyranny sincerely exercised for the good
of its victims may be the most oppressive. It may be better
to live under robber barons than under omnipotent moral
busybodies. The robber baron's cruelty may sometimes sleep,
his cupidity may at some point be satiated; but those who
torment us for our own good will torment us without end,
for they do so with the approval of their own conscience.

—C.S. Lewis (1898—1963),
British novelist, essayist, and lay Christian theologian

Having already alluded to the PHE's gun control agenda and the motives
behind it, allow me to elaborate from personal experience and now recount
my saga in medical politics.

In 1991, when the AMA and its allies in "organized medicine" launched
a campaign against domestic violence, as a member of the House of Delegates
of the Medical Association of Georgia and later as editor of the *Journal of the*
Medical Association of Georgia (*JMAG*), I joined in what seemed a worthwhile
cause. Researching the topic of domestic violence, to which gun crimes were
quickly added, and attempting to find workable solutions, I came to the inescapable conclusion and appalling reality that the medical literature on the
subject of guns and violence was flawed and severely biased. In fact, it was
completely one-sided, a one-way street.

The medical journals had failed miserably to objectively discuss both sides of the issue of guns and violence. This had happened despite the purported safeguards of peer-review and the alleged claims to balance and objectivity expressed by government-funded researchers in public health—and the medical journal editors who published their studies.

What I found, over the subsequent five years, particularly as editor of the *Journal of the Medical Association of Georgia* (between 1993 to 1995) was, frankly, that when it came to the issue of guns and violence, medical journals were presenting only one side, and censoring the other. The side that was being censored, despite the accumulating amount of data supporting it, was the side dealing with the beneficial aspects of firearm ownership and the benefits of self, family, and home protection by law-abiding citizens. Instead of providing a balanced and fair approach based on truth and objectivity, the medical literature echoed the emotionalism and rhetoric of the mass media, and thwarted free inquiry in scientific research. In most cases, it provided politicized, result-oriented, or preordained research based on what could only be characterized as junk science so as to bolster the agenda of the gun control lobby and the gun prohibitionists.

Why? Partly because that was the side advocated and where money was being allocated by the Clinton administration. Ideology also played a part with officials of the public health establishment. Opportunism and political expediency, as with almost every policy taken by the AMA in recent years,[1] comprised, at least initially, the lion's share of the reason that "organized medicine" entered the fray of gun control politics.

How? By going along with the PHE and propounding the erroneous but politically correct notion that guns and violence were public health issues and that crime was a disease, an epidemic rather than a major facet of criminology. Public health officials, AMA leaders, and willing political accomplices joined hands and espoused the preposterous but politically-expedient concept of guns and bullets as animated, virulent pathogens needing to be stamped out by limiting gun availability, and ultimately, eradicating guns from law-abiding citizens.

The fact that guns and bullets are inanimate objects that do not follow Koch's Postulates of Pathogenicity, which prove definitively and scientifically that a microorganism is responsible for a particular disease, was ignored. Further, the public health establishment failed to recognize that behind every shooting there is a person pulling the trigger who should be held accountable.

The portrayal of guns in the medical literature by the PHE reflected the sensationalized violence portrayed in the mainstream media and exploited our understandable concern for violence and rampant street crime, but it did not reflect accurate, unbiased, scientific, and objective information needed for optimum public policy.

Faulty and Biased Research

As it regards public funding of the NCIPC's gun research, public funds were severely misused in the 1980s up to 1996. As an example, various critics including Dr. Edgar Suter, Don B. Kates, and myself cited the work of one prominent gun control researcher, Dr. Arthur Kellermann of Emory University School of Public Health.

Since the mid-1980s, Dr. Kellermann (and associates), whose work was heavily funded by the CDC, published a series of studies purporting to show that persons who keep guns in the home are more likely to be victims of homicide than those who don't. Despite the "peer reviewed" imprimatur of his published research, Kellermann's studies, fraught with errors of facts, logic, and methodology, were published in *The New England Journal of Medicine* (*NEJM*) and the *Journal of the American Medical Association* (*JAMA*). His articles were published with great élan and fanfare (i.e., advanced notices and press releases were followed by arranged interviews and press conferences, compliments of *JAMA*, and in tandem with the AMA campaign against domestic violence) and to the delight of the like-minded, cheerleading, mainstream (liberal) journalists.

In a 1986 *NEJM* paper, Dr. Kellermann and associates claimed their "scientific research" proved that defending oneself or one's family with a firearm in the home is dangerous and counter-productive, claiming "a gun owner is 43 times more likely to kill a family member than an intruder."[2] This erroneous assertion was accurately termed Kellermann's "43 times fallacy" by Dr. Edgar Suter, chairman of DIPR.

In a critical review article published in the March 1994 issue of the *Journal of the Medical Association of Georgia* (*JMAG*), Dr. Suter not only found evidence of "methodologic and conceptual errors," such as prejudicially-truncated data and non-sequitur logic used in their pro-gun control arguments, but also "overt mendacity," including the listing of "the correct methodology which was described but never used by the authors."[3] Moreover, the gun control researchers failed to consider and "deceptively understated" the protective benefits of guns in the hands of law-abiding citizens protecting themselves, their families, and their property.

Dr. Suter wrote:

> *The true measure of the protective benefits of guns are the lives saved, the injuries prevented, the medical costs saved, and the property protected—not the burglar or rapist body count. Since only 0.1 percent to 0.2 percent of defensive gun usage involves the death of the criminal, any study, such as this, that counts criminal deaths as the only measure of the protective benefits of guns will expectedly underestimate the benefits of firearms by a factor of 500 to 1,000.[3]*

In 1993, in another peer-reviewed *NEJM* article (and the research again heavily funded by the CDC), Dr. Kellermann again attempted to show that guns in the home are a greater risk to the victims than to the assailants.[4] Despite valid criticisms of his previous works (including the 1986 study) by reputable scholars, Dr. Kellermann ignored their criticisms and again used the same flawed methodology and non-sequitur logic. He also used study populations with disproportionately high rates of serious psychosocial dysfunctions from three selected state-counties, unrepresentative of the general U.S. population. For example, 53 percent of the case subjects had a history of a household member being arrested, 31 percent had a household history of illicit drug use, 32 percent had a household member hit or hurt in a family fight, and 17 percent had a family member hurt so seriously in a domestic altercation that prompt medical attention was required.

Moreover, as Dr. Suter found, both the case studies and control groups in this analysis had a very high incidence of financial instability. In fact, in this study, gun ownership, the supposedly high-risk factor for homicide, was not one of the most strongly associated factors for being murdered. Drinking, illicit drugs, living alone, history of family violence, and living in a rented home were *all* greater individual risk factors for being murdered than a gun in the home.³ One must conclude there was no basis to apply the conclusions of this study to the general population.

Needless to say, all of those were factors that, as Dr. Suter pointed out, "would expectedly be associated with higher rates of violence and homicide." The results of such a study on gun homicides selecting that sort of unrepresentative population sample nullified the authors' generalizations, and voided their preordained, unscientific conclusions that could not be extrapolated to the general population.³

Although the 1993 *NEJM* study purported to show that the homicide victims were killed with a gun ordinarily kept in the home, the fact was, as criminologist Don B. Kates and associates pointed out in another critical study, 71.1 percent of the victims were killed by assailants who did not live in the victims' household using guns presumably not kept in that home.⁵

While Kellermann and associates began with 444 cases of homicides in the home, cases were dropped from the study for a variety of reasons, and in the end, only 316 matched pairs were used in the final analysis, representing only 71.2 percent of the original 444 homicide cases.

This reduction increased tremendously the chance for sampling bias. Analysis of why 28.8 percent of the cases were dropped would have helped ascertain if the study was compromised by the existence of such biases, but Dr. Kellermann, in an unprecedented move, refused to release his data and make it available for other researchers to analyze.⁶

Likewise, Professor Gary Kleck of Florida State University wrote to me in a personal communication [9/21/99] that knowledge about what guns were kept in the home was essential, but Dr. Kellermann never released the data. Kleck wrote, "The most likely bit of data that he [Kellermann] would want to withhold is information as to whether the gun used in the gun homicides was kept in the home of the victim."⁷

Methodology Flaws

Professor Kleck's analysis further disclosed several flaws in the methodology. First, "violent households" would be expected "to be more likely to own guns than people in less violent households, even if guns themselves made no contribution at all to the violence." Second, Kleck asserted, "because their study did nothing to distinguish cause from effect...," we know nothing about "risk-increasing or risk-decreasing, of keeping guns for self-protection." In other words, we do not know what percentage of gun uses were for self-protection and which ones were criminal. For example, 63 percent of the "victims" were men; yet we do not know how many of these homicides represent genuine acts of self-defense by women against abusive husbands or lovers, and committed as justifiable homicides.[8]

In fact, according to Kellermann and associates, "a majority of the homicides (50.9 percent) occurred in the context of a quarrel or a romantic triangle."[4] In this regard, it should be pointed out that other investigators had concluded that, "about half of shootings by one spouse or the other are defensive killings of husbands by victimized wives. So it misleadingly characterizes many cases in which guns save innocent lives as gun murders."[8]

Furthermore, only gun uses that resulted in death were analyzed, thus the Kellermann study ended up excluding the vast majority of gun uses that do not result in death, and which are more likely to be defensive uses by victims of crime, to protect themselves. In fact, as Professor Kleck points out in his critique, "at least three-fourths of all uses of guns in crime-related incidents are defensive uses by the crime victims."[8]

Kates and associates also pointed out, "The validity of the *NEJM* 1993 study's conclusions depend on the control group matching the homicide cases in every way (except, of course, for the occurrence of the homicide)."[9] However, in this study, the controls collected did not match the cases in many ways (i.e., in the amount of substance abuse, single parent versus two parent homes) contributing to further untoward effects, and decreasing the inference that can legitimately be drawn from the data of this study.

Be that as it may, "the conclusion that gun ownership is a risk factor for homicide derives from the finding of a gun in 45.4 percent of the homicide case households, but in only 35.8 percent of the control household. Whether that finding is accurate, however, depends on the truthfulness of control group interviewees in admitting the presence of a gun or guns in the home."[8]

Most importantly, Kellermann and associates once again failed to consider the protective benefits of firearms, and this time, arrived at the "2.7 times" fallacy.[3] In other words, this time they falsely claimed that a family member is 2.7 times more likely to kill other family members than an intruder.[4] Yet, a fallacy is still a fallacy and as such, it deserves no place in scientific investigations and peer-reviewed, medical publications, claiming scientific objectivity. These premeditated errors invalidated the findings of Kellermann's 1993 study, just as they tainted those of 1986.

The truth of the matter is that Kellermann and associates had gone along with the faulty *post hoc ergo propter hoc* reasoning, "after it therefore because of it," blaming guns for the rise of crime and violence in America. As a neurosurgeon who has spent incalculable hours in the middle of the night treating victims of gunshot wounds, I also deplore the rising violence and crime in America, but we must have the moral courage to find the truth and recognize the fact that there is another side to the story that is seldom promulgated.

The floodgates of dissension were opened when the March 1994 issue of the *Journal of the Medical Association of Georgia* asserted that physicians had a professional obligation to base their opinions on objective data and scientific information rather than on emotionalism or political expediency. After devoting an entire issue to the topic of guns and violence, we concluded that the objective cumulative data indicated that indiscriminate gun control disarms the law-abiding citizen but does not prevent criminals and street thugs from perpetrating crimes on unwary victims. Moreover, guns in the hands of law-abiding citizens deter crime and clearly afford the benefit of self-protection.[3,8]

The Problem with Scientific Surveys

Professor Gary Kleck has written extensively that false denial of gun ownership is a major problem in survey studies, and yet Kellermann and associates do not admit or mention that fact.[10,11] That is critical. It would take only 35 of the 388 controls *falsely* denying gun ownership to make the control gun ownership percentage equal that of the homicide case households. As Kates and associates wrote, "If indeed, the controls actually had gun ownership equal to that of the homicide case households (45.4 percent), then a false denial rate of only 20.1 percent among the gun owning controls would produce the thirty-five false denials and thereby equalize ownership."[5]

Consider the fact that Kellermann and associates' pilot study had a higher percent false denial rate than the 20.1 percent required to invalidate the study, and yet, they concluded there was no "underreporting of gun ownership by their control respondents," and claimed their estimates were therefore considered not biased.[4]

In the *Medical Sentinel*, we considered this type of bias in response to a *JAMA* 1996 gun ownership survey. In fact, as medical editor I urged investigators—especially those funded by the public—to share scientific data with other researchers. We called this academic request of research data impacting on the formulation of public policy, the open data policy for public review.[6] Returning to the *JAMA* survey, we reported how on question number 20 of that survey: "If asked by a pollster whether I owned firearms, I would be truthful? 29.6 percent disagreed/strongly disagreed."[12] So according to that survey, 29.6 percent would falsely deny owning a firearm. We know that nearly one-third of respondents intentionally conceal their gun ownership because they fear future confiscation by the police, as has happened in cities such as Washington, D.C., Detroit, and New York.

Again one must conclude, and it's worth repeating, that on the basis of these errors Kellermann's findings in his 1993 study are as invalid as the ones in 1986.[2,4]

Nevertheless, those errors crept into and permeated the lay press, the electronic media, and particularly, the public health literature and the medical journals, where they remained uncorrected and were repeated time and again and perpetuated. Also, because the publication of the data (and their purported conclusions) supposedly came from prestigious medical journals and objective medical researchers, it was given a lot of weight and credibility by practicing physicians, social scientists and law enforcement Those errors needed to be corrected to regain the lost credibility of public health in the area of gun and violence research.

Ignored or Neglected Benefits of Firearms

Thanks to the meticulous and sound scholarship of Professor Gary Kleck of Florida State University; the American economist and gun scholar, John R. Lott, Jr.; noted legal scholars, Don B. Kates and David Kopel, among others; and the medical studies conducted initially by Doctors for Integrity in Policy Research (DIPR) and continued by Doctors for Responsible Gun Ownership (DRGO), we know the benefits of gun ownership by law-abiding citizens had been greatly underestimated and far outstrip the illegal misuses of firearms. [3,5,8-11,13-15] In his monumental work, *Point Blank: Guns and Violence in America* (1991) and subsequent publications, Professor Kleck found that *the defensive uses of firearms by citizens amount up to 2 million to 2.5 million uses per year and dwarf the offensive gun uses by criminals. Between 25 and 75 lives are saved by a gun for every life lost to a gun. Medical costs saved by guns in the hands of law-abiding citizens are 15 times greater than costs incurred by criminal uses of firearms. Guns also prevent injuries to good people and protect billions of dollars of property every year.*[3,10,11]

Those findings were substantiated at least in part by a 1993 U.S. Department of Justice study made public in 1997 that confirmed Kleck's findings. The Clinton Justice Department study found that up to 1.5 million citizens used firearms annually to protect themselves and their property, and of those surveyed, 67.7 percent had effectively used a weapon to defend themselves against violent crime.[16]

More recently, Kleck was challenged for his figure of "up to 2 million to 2.5 million defensive uses of firearms per year." The gun prohibition-ist Violence Policy Center (VPC) was quoted in the *Los Angeles Times* as claiming that in 2012 only 259 criminals were killed by law-abiding citizens protecting themselves and their families. VPC suggested that this was a very small number in comparison to the fact that in the same year there were 1.2 million violent crimes committed.[17] Violent crimes are defined as murder, forcible rape, robbery and aggravated assault. The number is not only surprisingly small but also incorrect. Armed citizens shoot and kill more criminals yearly than do police, at least twice if not three times as many. Kleck found that good citizens kill between 606 to 1527 attackers and violent criminals in self-defense (or in justifiable homicides) every year. Citizens in fact have a better track record than the police in shooting the bad guys. This should not be surprising.

Contrary to what one might have been led to believe, "only two percent of civilian shootings involved an innocent person mistakenly identified as a criminal. The 'error rate' for the police, however, was 11 percent, more than five times as high."[17] The reason citizens do a better job than the police is that they are already on the scene. They witnessed what happened or were the actual victims, so they know who the bad guys are, while the police enter a scene in progress and must make judgments that occasionally turn out to be wrong.

So how did the VPC arrive at the figure of only 259 criminals killed by armed citizens? By ignoring facts and cherry-picking figures without performing in-depth analysis. Because the assignation of "justifiable homicide" is made by the FBI Uniform Crime Report from the preliminary data of the reporting officer, and not from final determination, "justifiable homicides" are underreported. Eventually up to 20 percent of "homicides" are judged to be "justifiable homicides." So as we reported earlier, the correct figure is that between 606 to 1527 criminals are killed by good citizens in self-defense (or in justifiable homicides) every year, not the paltry 259 figure reported by the VPC.[17]

The *Los Angeles Times* writer and the VPC also tried to play down Kleck's previously cited figure of up to 2 million to 2.5 million beneficial uses of firearms per year, citing a Federal Bureau of Justice Statistics' National Crime Victimization Survey (NCVS) that, according to him, puts the number much lower—about 67,740 times a year. We disagree on many counts. First, the NCVS is the only study to make such a claim, and Kleck and Suter among others have pointed out its unreliability because it is a study about victimization and not about defensive gun use. Second, to make matters worse, respondents in the NCVS are denied anonymity. As such, it vastly underestimates defensive uses of firearms by at least an order of magnitude.[17]

The VPC and its anti-gun activists also ignore or deny that up to 2.5 million criminal cases are foiled yearly because lawful citizens used guns to protect themselves, their families and their property. Most of those cases go unreported, but we know about them from Kleck's work, which has been supported by the complimentary studies by James D. Wright, Peter Rossi, and John R. Lott, as well as the various studies carried out by the Department of Justice over the years. In fact Kleck recently responded by reaffirming that at least 760,000 times per year beneficial uses of firearms continue to take place and in 90 percent of cases, there is not even the need to fire the defensive weapon; just displaying the firearm to the potential criminal is enough of a deterrence to avoid the commission of a crime, saving lives and property.[18]

The good guys (the cops and lawful citizens) do not kill unnecessarily, as violent criminals are prone to do, but only when they absolutely have to.

Violent offenders, many of them repeat criminals, kill in the commission of crimes and to get away with whatever they intend to do with little regard for life or property. Some kill for the sake of killing, therefore the body count is unreliable. As we have said previously, when quoting Dr. Edgar Suter:

> *The true measure of the protective benefits of guns are the lives saved, the injuries prevented, the medical costs saved, and the property protected—not the burglar or rapist body count. Since only 0.1 percent to 0.2 percent of defensive gun usage involves the death of the criminal, any study, such as this, that counts criminal deaths as the only measure of the protective benefits of guns will expectedly underestimate the benefits of firearms by a factor of 500 to 1,000.*[3]

As I was putting the finishing touches in this book, Professor Gary Kleck has published a report uncovering several CDC surveys from the 1990s that had been kept under wraps and never published (or even publicly disclosed within the CDC) confirming that nearly 2.5 million defensive uses of guns take place every year, matching almost exactly Professor Kleck's own studies that had concluded that guns are used defensively and beneficially much more frequently than offensively and criminally.

The surveys about defensive gun uses were conducted by the Behavioral Risk Factor Surveillance System of the CDC in the 1996, 1997, and 1998, and according to Kleck were "high quality telephone surveys of enormous probability samples of U.S. adults," and yet they were deliberately not disclosed to the public. Thus, we have no reason to modify our original figures, and we simply restate that at the very least 760,000 to up to 2 million to 2.5 million defensive (beneficial) uses of firearms take place by law-abiding citizens against potential criminals, as well as dangerous animals, yearly.[3,10,11,16,18] As to the seemingly wide range in the estimates of beneficial uses of firearms per year, the reader should not be surprised. We have already discussed the problems and shortcomings of scientific surveys in the previous section citing Professor Kleck's observations in this regard.

Regarding the much ballyhooed effect of gun violence on medical care, the actual U.S. health care costs of treating gunshot wounds was calculated to be approximately $1.5 billion in the mid-1990s, which was less than 0.2 percent of the annual health care expenditures. The $20 to $40 billion figure so frequently cited in the medical literature of the 1990s was a deliberately exaggerated estimate of lifetime productivity lost, where criminal predators are given productivity estimates as if their careers were suddenly expected to blossom into that of pillars of the community with projected salaries equal to those of health executive CEOs.[3] Exaggeration of the monetary costs of gun violence continues to the present. In 2002, unfazed by the criticism, public health researchers claimed that U.S. health care costs this time amounted to $100 billion per year, again using lifetime productivity lost and criteria selected to deliberately inflate figures. In 2017, NBC News came up with the more reasonable figure of $2.8 billion but without estimating the savings from the beneficial uses of firearms. Gun rights proponents countered that using the state of Arizona's figure of human life worth at $6.5 million, multiplied by the midrange number of defensive gun uses per year resulted in a net savings of approximately $1 trillion per year.[13]

Yet, despite these effective rebuttals to exaggerated figures, the medical politicians and public health advocates of "organized medicine" cling to the erroneous figures and extrapolations of Drs. Arthur Kellermann, Philip J. Cook, Jens Ludwig, and other public health researchers, and use whatever convenient but erroneous figures they can dig up in propounding health and gun control policies, to the detriment of the unknowing—and in some cases deliberately deceived—public.[13]

To make up for the lost ground on gun and violence research accumulating in the criminological and sociological literature in the last two decades, we have to look not only to the data collected by Kleck and disseminated in medical circles by Dr. Edgar Suter[3,13], but also to the work of Drs. Timothy Wheeler and David C. Stolinsky. In fact, the latter two scholars summarized the literature on the benefits of firearms and arrived at 2,163,519 defensive uses with firearms of all types and 1,545,371 uses with handguns annually.[19]

In his momentous and seminal book, *More Guns, Less Crime— Understanding Crime and Gun Control Laws* (1998), Professor John R. Lott, Jr., formerly of the University of Chicago and Yale University, expounded on the benefits of firearms from a different perspective. He collected and analyzed massive amounts of data proving further beneficial effects of armed citizens in terms of crime control. Despite the efforts of anti-gun opponents,

Lott's findings could not be suppressed or contravened by the popular press or academia. Those negativistic efforts, permeated heavily with bias, have proved unsuccessful. Lott has been proven correct.

Lott studied the FBI's massive yearly crime statistics for all 3,054 U.S. counties over 18 years (1977-1994), the largest national survey on gun ownership and state police documentation in illegal gun use, and he came to some startling conclusions, which have been summarized as follows:

1. *While neither state waiting periods nor the federal Brady Law is associated with a reduction in crime rates, adopting concealed carry weapons (CCW) laws cut death rates from public, multiple shootings (e.g., as those which took place in Jonesboro, Arkansas, and Springfield, Oregon, in 1998; the Columbine High School shooting in Littleton, Colorado, in 1999; or the 1993 shooting on the Long Island subway)—by a whopping 69 percent.*

2. *Allowing people to carry concealed weapons deters violent crime—without any apparent increase in accidental death. If states without right to carry laws had adopted them in 1992, about 1,570 murders, 4,177 rapes, and 60,000 aggravated assaults would have been avoided annually.*

3. *Children 14 to 15 years of age are 14.5 times more likely to die from automobile injuries, five times more likely to die from drowning or fire and burns, and three times more likely to die from bicycle accidents than they are to die from gun accidents.*

4. *When concealed carry laws went into effect in a given county, murders fell by eight percent, rapes by five percent, and aggravated assaults by seven percent.*

5. *For each additional year concealed carry gun laws have been in effect, the murder rate declines by three percent, robberies by over two percent, and rape by one percent.*[14]

These conclusions have proved long-lasting and dramatic.

In his subsequent books, *The Bias Against Guns: Why Almost Everything You've Heard About Gun Control is Wrong* (2003) and *The War on Guns: Arming Yourself Against Gun Control Lies* (2016), Lott rebutted critics and expounded on his findings, at the same time showing how the media and academia have disseminated erroneous information due to their preconceived notions and outright bias against guns.[15,20]

Pretending to Build Castles in the Air

Because of the complex nature of violence in our society, violence and crime prevention efforts should be addressed by the education and criminal justice systems, assisted by social institutions and churches, synagogues, and other religious institutions. What continues to be clear is that violence is not a disease and therefore it's not amenable for study or treatable with the traditional public health model. Public health measures have proved inappropriate or deliberately deceitful.

Medical politicians and public health officials involved in the systematic perversion of science—and who masquerade as unbiased, objective researchers—are wrong and misguided, or they are deliberately deceitful. The goal of the gun control research promulgated by the AMA-PHE axis, which today includes an excessive number of schools of public health sprawling throughout the land, appears to be designed to promote total conformity with the nanny and omnipotent State. They are hoping to do this by propounding the idea that guns (even for self and family protection) are socially unacceptable. They want to enact citizen disarmament using public health as the vehicle.

The problem is that if this happened lawful citizens would be at the mercy of criminals, who do not obey the law and who will continue to possess guns illegally. What public health officials pushing for civilian disarmament should realize is that we live in a real world inhabited by individuals, not pliable automatons. Although admittedly, Americans are possessed of all the foibles and weaknesses of human nature and live in a stressful world of inescapable conflicts, they have a constitutional right to gun ownership and a natural right to protect life, liberty, and property.

Yet, elitist gun prohibitionists want to create a utopia that has never existed, divorced from reality. Assuming their best intentions, the PHE officials and medical politicians of the AMA and "organized medicine" want to help forge a world in their own image, where ordinary citizens are unarmed and live in blissful conformity under the supposedly protector, benevolent State, where violence has been eradicated, homicides have been extinguished, and (false) security has been attained—veritably constructing a utopia of castles in the air.

Unfortunately, at worst, they are striving for a Big Brother State to rule unopposed and omnipotent, able to conduct social engineering at will, capable of reconstructing and enforcing the socio-economic leveling of society—e.g., authoritarian collectivism by seduction of the people into acquiescence, or, if necessary, by force. Obviously, they hope to create the Total State in which, as expected members of the ruling elite in this Platonic idealist State, they would be playing leading roles. In their imaginary Total State, the government of philosopher-kings would reign supreme because the people have been disarmed and programmed to be docile automatons.

The reality is that if this utopian socialist vision became a reality, it would herald a brave new world of totalitarianism, where individual citizens would be totally at the mercy of the State and its social engineers and central planners. In this unhappy scenario, citizens and society would have no check upon the power of the State—an entity which history instructs us, has not always been benevolent.

CHAPTER 5
DEFANGING THE CDC'S GUN CONTROL APPARATUS

Quis custodiet ipsos? ("Who is going to look after the keepers?")

—From the Roman poet Juvenal,
Satires VI, lines 347–8

As a physician, I have always been a staunch supporter of public health in its traditional role of fighting pestilential diseases and promoting health by educating the public, as to hygiene, sanitation, and preventable diseases, as alluded to in my 1994 book, *Vandals at the Gates of Medicine*. Physicians, medical innovators, and public health doctors and nurses combating truly epidemic and contagious diseases played a heroic chapter in the history of medicine.

Yet, on the opposite extreme, I deeply resent the workings of that unrecognizable part of the public health establishment (PHE), which has become politicized and biased, bent on moving society in the name of social justice toward an authoritarian, collectivist, and gun control direction. To accomplish this it has used preordained, tainted, result-oriented research based on what can only be characterized as junk science.

In the early 1990s, it became clear that the CDC's National Center for Injury Prevention and Control (NCIPC) was the focal point of the AMA and the PHE for promulgating the concept of "gun violence as a public health issue" for which the facilitators proposed to ask the government for more and more funds from the taxpayers to combat the "gun violence epidemic," espousing scientific gun research and providing workable solutions to the problem of violence.

The truth is that by this time not only the CDC's NCIPC, but also the whole PHE, buttressed by the sprouting schools of public health, supported by the AMA, "organized medicine," and their publishing empire, had become engrossed in a deeply politicized agenda—abjectly losing sight of their mission and becoming arms of the gun control lobby—to the detriment of traditional medicine and public health. This contention was well expressed in the words of Dr. William C. Waters, IV, Eastern Director of DIPR, who in a letter to Senator Arlen Specter, Chairman of the Subcommittee on Labor, Health, and Human Services and Education of the Senate Appropriations Committee complained:

> We believe that the NCIPC fails to do its job because of unscientific bias... First is the overt political activism of the NCIPC staff and their federally funded researchers. Second... is that there seems to be a tacit assumption—perhaps even foundational concept—among many public health researchers that firearm prohibition/control provides a ready solution to many of society's ills. We believe that this view is expressed in the NCIPC's approach to the problem of violence, since the research performed is fantastically narrow in scope, excludes most of what is known about violence in human societies... and is often performed using abysmally poor methodology... There seems to be a tendency on the part of those defending the NCIPC to simply reiterate figures depicting the problem of firearms violence/injury as justification for the agency's existence.

Smoking Guns at the CDC?

Concerned about this issue and possible violations of the public trust, several DIPR members communicated with key members of Congress, including eight Senators at the U.S. Capitol, thoroughly briefing their staff as to this serious issue. Other concerned DIPR members and physicians, in an effort to inform the public, appeared on local and syndicated radio and independent television shows, including the Washington, D.C.-based, National Empowerment Television (NET).

Despite considerable barriers, the monolithic wall of censorship of the mainstream media was pierced successfully not only by DIPR but also by the California-based Doctors for Responsible Gun Ownership (DRGO). In a memorable encounter in September 1995, Dr. Timothy Wheeler, director of DRGO, was invited and appeared on CBS's *This Morning* vis-à-vis Dr. Jerome Kassirer, a fierce gun control advocate and editor-in-chief of *The New England Journal of Medicine* (*NEJM*). Dr. Kassirer had defended the CDC/NCIPC gun control propaganda in a previous, one-sided *NEJM* editorial. Furthermore, Dr. Kassirer, who had already admitted he deplored "assault weapons" and even though possessing little understanding of the mechanics of these firearms, had gone on to state that when it came to "assault weapons," he supported the "no-data-are-needed policy" of the *NEJM*, asserting that if a little gun control does not work, then, certainly, more gun control is needed: "If we still found them wanting [draconian gun control laws] we would be justified in supporting even more stringent restrictions."[1] It was a brief exchange, but it was devastating for Dr. Kassirer, who this time in the one-on-one debate was debating publicly a well-informed opponent who wielded the weapons of facts and figures. It was a decisive victory for truth and honesty in science. Dr. Wheeler also showed on camera a major piece of evidence, the Injury Prevention Network Newsletter titled "Women, Guns, and Domestic Violence," supported in part by a grant from the CDC, and featuring an offensive cover of a menacing handgun firing a bullet that blasts away at the defenseless female symbol.

Within this newsletter, a section titled "What Advocates Can Do," among other things, exhorted purported researchers and CDC public health staffers to:

> *Put gun control on the agenda of your civic or professional organization. Release a statement to the media or explain in your organization's newsletter why gun control is a woman's (or nurses' or pediatricians'...) issue.*
>
> *Ask TV and print media to name the gun manufacturer in every story it runs involving gun violence.*
>
> *Make your support for federal, state, and local gun laws known to your representative. This may include: opposing repeal of the*

assault weapons ban; maintaining support for the Brady Law;
restricting ammunition availability by caliber and quantity;
increasing enforcement of federal firearm laws; maintaining
restrictions on issuance of concealed weapons permits... [Also]

Organize a picket at gun manufacturing sites, perhaps with
posters showing pictures of victims of gun violence. (Modeled
after the Madres de los Desaparecidos in Argentina and
Chile; this can evoke a very powerful moral image.)

Work for campaign finance reform to weaken the gun lobby's
political clout.

Boycott publications that accept advertising from the gun
lobby or manufacturers... Launch a program aimed at getting
pediatricians [involved]... Get media attention for your events.
Encourage your local police department to adopt a policy
prohibiting officers from recommending that citizens buy guns
for protection, etc., etc.

Remember, these were not just private citizens using their own money and exercising their constitutional right to free speech, but supposedly objective, unbiased researchers using taxpayer money (grants) for social, ideological, and political purposes—in this case, to influence Congress and help the Clinton administration implement draconian gun control measures, aimed at disarming law-abiding citizens, using the cover of public health and junk science as the vehicles.

Faced with this ominous threat—namely, the subversion of science by a government agency run amok—DIPR and DRGO worked harder than ever to expose the public health deception but had been unable to find a medical outlet for their critiques. That is, until the advent of my editorship of the *Journal of the Medical Association of Georgia* (1993–95) and subsequently the *Medical Sentinel* (1996–2002), a medical journal I founded for the Association of American Physicians and Surgeons (AAPS), an independent national medical organization.

But that was not all; in the Mercer University School of Medicine medical library I found even more smoking guns—e.g., other public health newsletters involved in deeply partisan and political activities. One titled *Nation's Health*, a newsletter by the American Public Health Association (March 1995), defended the partisan activities of the CDC/NCIPC and even listed a "1-800 number" with a special Western Union Hotline that automatically send messages to Congress in support of "threatened public health programs."

Concerned dissenting public health workers dissatisfied with the politicization of public health also provided additional smoking guns of published information circulated within the PHE and the schools of public health to us for review. In particular, I received public bulletins and articles from Russ Fine, PhD, MSPH, professor of medicine and director of the Injury Control Research Center at the University of Alabama at Birmingham. This was valuable additional material corroborating our initial discoveries. A few years later (1999) I was happy to receive the following correspondence from Dr. Fine:

> ... *My most sincere congratulations to you and the Medical Sentinel for the promulgation of a courageous, open, intellectually honest and 'disarming' policy. I challenge any and all other medical and scientific journals to adopt this cutting edge policy [open data policy] ... one that can only foster intellectual integrity and blaze the trail for the eventual elimination of the junk science that litters the scientific landscape and pollutes the well of honest, scientific discourse.*

And so it was that at the time we found the tentacles of politicized public health misusing taxpayer money, not only for political advocacy but also flagrantly violating the public trust as supposedly objective researchers, to legitimize fraudulent research conducted for political reasons. Moreover, it must be reiterated that at the same time these officials were pursuing their financial self-interest, protecting and promoting yet more public health programs as well as research grants for which they were the primary beneficiaries.

One of the most helpful lawmakers who assisted in the quest for the truth was the freshman Congressman Bob Barr (R-GA). Expressing his concern for public-funded research, he wrote to fellow Congressman Christopher Shays, chairman of the Subcommittee on Human Resources of the House Committee on Government Reform and Oversight:

> *I write to bring to your attention a matter that goes beyond impropriety, and in my judgment crosses the line to potential illegality. I have written David Satcher, the Director of the Centers for Disease Control (CDC) in Atlanta asking him to investigate whether certain taxpayer funded grant money is being used to advocate opposition or endorsement of federal legislation, and, among other things urges picketing activities.*
>
> *I consider these activities, involving federal taxpayer dollars, to be not only questionable but very likely illegal. I find it highly offensive that federally appropriated monies are being used for lobbying and urging civil disobedience and possible illegal activity... I would officially request that your committee investigate this matter.*

Congressman Barr also gave an impassioned and intellectually charged speech against the politicized, result-oriented research conducted by the CDC/NCIPC and in support of the Dickey Amendment on the floor of the House of Representatives.

Testifying in a Congressional Subcommittee—
Where There is Smoke...

Our efforts finally bore fruition. On March 6, 1996, three physicians— Drs. William C. Waters IV, Timothy Wheeler, and myself—representing two physician organizations, DIPR and DRGO (clearly indicating that the AMA/CDC/NCIPC axis did not represent the views of all physicians), along with noted civil rights attorney and criminologist Don B. Kates, were given the opportunity to testify before the House Appropriations Subcommittee on Labor, Health and Human Services, and Education. Congressman Jim

Istook Jr. (R-OK), who served in the Subcommittee and who had assumed leadership in this reform effort along with Congressman Bob Barr, was the co-author of the Simpson-Istook Amendment designed to curtail the amount of tax dollars going to publicly funded, lobbying organizations.

I will not recapitulate our entire testimony, which is in the Congressional Record.[2] Suffice to say, we testified about the misrepresentation of data, skewed study populations (selection and extrapolations), inappropriate research models for the subject under study, and arrival to preordained conclusions (result-oriented research)—all these biases evident in the immensely shoddy "gun control" research conducted by the CDC/NCIPC. The panel was also informed about how the NCIPC researchers breached accepted scientific practice by refusing to release and make available to other researchers their publicly funded, original data for further critical analysis. This was taking place despite their repeated denials that they were doing just that.

We pointed out and brought into evidence the inappropriate (and probably illegal) diversion of taxpayer money allocated to research being used for dissemination of partisan newsletters. We also disclosed the occurrence of politicized meetings and organizations in which NCIPC staff and funded researchers were active participants. For example, at the Handgun Epidemic Lowering Plan (HELP) held in Chicago, Illinois in 1993 (and again in 1995), NCIPC researchers and staff were faculty for this "strategy conference" in which "like-minded individuals who represent organizations...[the goal of which is to] *use a public health model to work toward changing society's attitude so that it becomes socially unacceptable for private citizens to have guns.*" Dr. Katherine Christoffel, one of the founders of this conference is well known for her anti-firearms activism and her profoundly revealing statements. For example, she has reached prominence with statements such as:

> *...Guns are a virus that must be eradicated. We need to immunize ourselves against them. [And] ...Get rid of the cigarettes, get rid of the secondhand smoke, and you get rid of lung disease. It's the same with guns. Get rid of the guns, get rid of the bullets, and you get rid of deaths.*[3]

In the case of Dr. Arthur Kellermann, it was reported that during his formal presentation at the (October 17, 1993) HELP conference, in an emotional moment admitted his personal anti-gun bias (a bias that, as we have seen, is evident in the pattern of his research). Although in a letter to the *Journal of the Medical Association of Georgia*, Kellermann denied making such a statement at that specific meeting, he did not actually repudiate his general anti-gun bias.[4] Dr. Kellermann's elitism (and true appreciation of the value of a gun for self-protection), nevertheless, is well encapsulated in the following retort directed at a question from a reporter and quoted in the *San Francisco Examiner*: "If that were my wife [being attacked], would I want her to have a .38 Special in her hand? 'Yeah,' says Dr. Kellermann."[5]

When the University of Iowa sponsored a conference in 1992 on firearms violence, that confab was funded in part with CDC/NCIPC funds. Those funds had previously been allocated not for gun control propaganda but for the study of rural injuries and farm occupational hazards. Interestingly, the only non-academic faculty member invited was Sarah Brady of Handgun Control, Inc. (HCI). The conference, subsequently titled "National Violence Prevention Conference—Bridging Science and Program," reconvened in 1995, using again, the same type of funding and hosted by the CDC/NCIPC and the University of Iowa Injury Prevention Research Center. In his invocation to the conference, Dr. Mark L. Rosenberg, Director of the NCIPC, who served as Chairman of the Executive Planning Committee vaunted:

> *Violence in America has reached epidemic proportions and presents our nation with a public health challenge as great as we have faced in the past... We believe that violence in our homes and communities is a great public health challenge that our nation can face and overcome as we enter the next millennium.*

From the foregoing, it becomes plainly evident how—oblivious to the lessons of history, the unchanging nature and intractability of man, his fallibility and imperfectability, not to mention the accumulating body of legitimate scientific evidence in the sociological, legal, and criminological literature—public health officials, had acted with incredible hubris. They seemed to truly, but erroneously, believe in the socialist notion of the perfectibility of man (*novus homo*), conceived and generated by the brute force of the omnipotent State (*der staat über alles*). One of their mantras is the call for social justice to assist in the social and political reconstruction of a new and more egalitarian society, ignoring the previous disastrous efforts that caused the death of 100 million lives in the 20th century by communism, once again demonstrating the pervasive arrogance of the ivory towers of medical academia.

Finally, in our testimony we shed light on the fact that much of the injury prevention research performed by the CDC/NCIPC was superfluous, already being performed by a myriad of other agencies within the maze of U.S. government bureaucracy; this included the *Departments of Transportation* (which studies automobile-related injuries), *Labor* (where Occupational Safety and Health Administration [OSHA] carries out studies on workplace injuries), *Justice* (which studies domestic violence), *Education* (that supervises violence prevention within school systems), *Health and Human Services* (that oversees the National Institutes of Health which conducts research on violence prevention, mental health, drug and alcohol abuse)—not to mention additional divisions, too many to list here within or outside the purview of these labyrinthine, alphabet soup departments.

We concluded our testimony with the consensual opinion that given the complex nature of violence in our society, violence and crime prevention efforts should be addressed by a fortified educational and criminal justice system—not to mention our social institutions, churches, temples, and synagogues. Violence is not a disease and not treatable or amenable to study with the traditional public health model. Moreover, based on the serious violations in the production of [un]scientific research, the numerous transgressions in the pursuit of social and political agendas (that seek ultimately citizen disarmament despite constitutional protections), and the overly redundant functions of the NCIPC—we recommended that the committee eliminate all funding for the NCIPC, starting with the fiscal year of 1997, and thereby realize a savings to taxpayers of nearly $50 million annually—and most importantly, effecting a major step forward, towards liberating science from the claws of partisan politics.

A Wise Prohibition Against the Misuse of Public Funds

In short, concerned citizens waged a protracted battle over the subversion and perversion of science in gun (control) research supported and conducted by the AMA/CDC/NCIPC establishment and promulgated by the medical journals. That battle reached high intensity through the spring and summer of 1996. Although we were not able to close the doors of the NCIPC, and that remained our goal for the next two years, our fight culminated in a significant defeat for the gun-prohibitionists. In July 1996, the House of Representatives voted to shift $2.6 million away from the NCIPC and earmarked those funds for other health research projects in the Omnibus Appropriations Bill. The redirected funding was the amount formerly allocated by the NCIPC to the discredited "gun (control) research." For the first time in a decade, Dr. Arthur Kellermann, the primary gun control investigator for the NCIPC, was not funded for his research by that agency. The amendment also stipulated that of the remaining allocations: "None of the funds made available for injury prevention and control at the Centers for Disease Control and Prevention may be used to advocate or promote gun control."[6]

In a "Dear Colleague" letter sent to all members of the House, Congressman Jay Dickey (R-AR), who sponsored the amendment, revealed what the NCIPC director said about their political agenda: "What we have to do is find a socially acceptable form of gun control." Also, in a letter to Senator Arlen Specter (R-PA), several senators who supported the effort to curtail the NCIPC's anti-gun activities noted that NCIPC Director Dr. Mark Rosenberg stated that he "envisions a long-term campaign, similar to tobacco use and auto safety, to convince Americans that guns are, first and foremost, a public health menace."[7]

Although, the re-direction of $2.6 million away from the NCIPC's gun control research was a modest and overdue effort to deprive the anti-gun lobby of a taxpayer-subsidized propaganda organ and a first step towards attempting to restore the integrity of public health research, it also sent the greater symbolic message: that citizens, including many scientists and physicians, are not going to sit idly by and allow the subversion and misuse of science and medical research for political ends. For the reasons enumerated and discussed, we thought the appropriate and obvious long-term course of action should have been to eliminate all funding for the NCIPC, prohibit the CDC from conducting "gun research," saving the taxpayers nearly $50 million annually—and most importantly, effecting a major step towards restoring credibility and integrity to public health, returning it to its former traditional role of stamping out infectious diseases and true epidemics, and depoliticizing medical research. We did not know then whether this victory would be fleeting and evanescent, or definitive and long lasting. That same year, the AMA directed its lobbyists to "strongly advocate" that funding for gun (control) research be fully restored to the CDC/NCIPC.[8]

An Uncertain Aftermath or a Lasting Victory?

As it turned out, it was to be a long-lasting victory, at least as it concerns the CDC/NCIPC, up to the time of the writing and publication of this book two decades later. As mentioned in the prelude of this book, in the aftermath of the Sandy Hook tragedy of December 14, 2012, gun control activists saw and used the tragedy as an opportunity to renew their efforts for gun control. Forgetting the long history of shoddy research and misuse of funding by the NCIPC of the CDC—the story that I've recounted in the foregoing chapters—the activists seized the occasion to clamor for ending the congressional "ban" on gun research. Congress was obstructing the pursuit of science in the form of gun and violence research, and it was high time the "ban" was lifted, they argued.

Included among the lamenters were not only former CDC Director David Satcher but also the defunded gun researcher Arthur Kellermann, who admitted that private foundations and the U.S. Department of Justice funded gun violence studies but at "a fraction" of what existed before the mid-1990s. He neglected to mention that the research done by the Department of Justice was more in line with scientific studies and providing real useful data, not the politicized junk science generated by the public health establishment. Kellermann, who later went to work for the RAND Corporation, went on to say, "I have to acknowledge that the (NRA) strategy of shutting down the pipeline of science was effective. It is almost impossible today to get federal funding for firearm injury prevention research."[9] He has no one to blame but himself and his fellow public health researchers, for generating such mountains of faulty and politically prejudiced research.

The whole truth was, and remains, that public health officials had been ordered by Congress not to use taxpayer money to conduct politicized, biased, and preordained gun research that regardless of data, methodology, and common sense, always concluded in advocating and promoting gun control. That is not science, but political advocacy of the worse type because it's both fraudulent and a betrayal of the public trust. Moreover, the so-called "ban" is not a research prohibition, but, as we have shown, a reasonable restriction, preventing the misuse of public funds to advocate or promote gun control— the use of junk science to effect misguided public policy. With good reason, public health officials at the CDC have also been prohibited from unlawfully using public funds, intended for teaching conferences and research, for illegal lobbying activities. Needless to say, these lobbying activities are based on political or ideological grounds, as well as self-servingly affecting their own financial self-interest in the form of grants or in asking for money to fund more studies that they themselves conduct.

Thus, those systematic violations of the public trust in advocacy, lobbying, and political activities were wisely prohibited and should remain so. But as we have seen, the story did not end there. In January 2013, barely one month after the Sandy Hook tragedy, President Barack Obama issued his executive order that the director of the CDC "shall conduct or sponsor research into the causes of gun violence and the ways to prevent it." Side stepping Congress, Obama also requested $10 million for resumption of the CDC's gun violence research program, which was wisely opposed by Congress. Reading the media accounts and the medical journal editorials, one is led to believe that Congress opposes scientific investigations. However, the story, as we have seen, is more complicated than what the liberal media spins and promulgates.[10]

The Democrats continue their efforts towards gun control using public health as a vehicle.[11] They have continued to use the same approach as they have used since the Sandy Hook tragedy of 2012, assisted with the compliant mainstream media. CBS and other media, in fact, admitted, "The restriction hasn't explicitly banned the CDC from conducting research on gun violence." But still they lamented, "It has been barred from using federal funding to 'advocate or promote gun control.' " Since when is science supposed to be misused to advocate or promote a public policy, especially the violation of a constitutional right? The mainstream liberal media very rarely bothers to consult anyone critical of the gun research that was propounded by the CDC and the public health establishment, or those of us who testified in favor of the restrictions even in an attempt to provide a sense of balance or an explanation for contrary views. Instead, gun prohibitionists, such as Daniel Webster, director of the Johns Hopkins Center for Gun Policy and Research, one of the most strident public health centers clamoring for gun control, is asked for his opinion. As is the usual case with these researchers, Dr. Webster gives tortuous explanations why more gun and violence research is needed, but does not mention the reasons why Congress imposed the restrictions in the first place.[11]

We scored a great victory in curtailing pseudoscience as a means of promoting gun control, but conservatives and gun rights advocates must remain vigilant in the political debate and watchful of the PHE's mantra of "gun violence as a public health issue." The ploy of calling for lifting the "ban" on science and gun research used by public health officials and the gun prohibitionists has had some effect. During his 2016 presidential campaign, Dr. Ben Carson, Secretary of Housing and Urban Development, was swayed to join the chorus of those calling for lifting the restriction.[12] And the late Congressman Jay Dickey (D-AR), the very proponent and author of the Dickey Amendment, in the wake of the mass shooting in Aurora Colorado of July 20, 2012, reversed his position on gun research and also called for lifting the "ban."[13]

We must also recall that the individual right "to keep and bear arms" was only upheld by the U.S. Supreme Court in two razor-thin majority decisions of five to four, and "reasonable" restrictions are drummed up almost daily by various states and municipalities, not to mention lower federal courts, to erode the individual right to gun ownership in the home. The right to keep and bear arms outside the home is still to be decided by the Supreme Court. In the next chapters, we will discuss constitutional and criminological issues affecting the Second Amendment.

PART 2

WITHIN THE BELLY
OF THE BEAST

CHAPTER 6

PUBLIC HEALTH, SOCIAL SCIENCE, AND THE SCIENTIFIC METHOD (PART I)

I am only one; but still I am one. I cannot do everything;
but still I can do something; and because I cannot do every-
thing, I will not refuse to do the something that I can do.

—Edward Everett Hale (1822—1909),
author of the classic, *The Man Without a Country* (1863)

The consequences of my actions prior to my testimony to the House Appropriations Subcommittee on Labor, Health, Education, and Human Services in 1996, particularly as it relates to my editorship of the *Journal of the Medical Association of Georgia* between 1993 and 1995, are described in my book, *Medical Warrior: Fighting Corporate Socialized Medicine* (1997). In that book I published the so-called "offensive" material I had written as editor of the *Journal* and in the chapter titled, "Editorial Lynching in the Deep South," I recounted my travails with the Medical Association of Georgia and "organized medicine" for daring to bring both sides of the issue of guns and violence to medical journalism.

After testifying before the House Appropriations Subcommittee on Labor, Health, Education, and Human Services in 1996, time elapsed. President Bill Clinton was elected to a second term in office. While the NCIPC had been restrained from producing tainted gun research by the congressional "ban," the various schools of public health, led by the Johns Hopkins Bloomberg School of Public Health (that bears the name of its benefactor, the anti-gun billionaire Michael Bloomberg), continued to propound gun control propaganda. The various schools were also encouraged and prompted by the AMA and "organized medicine" to crank up "gun and violence" research to take up the slack left by the NCIPC. Specific examples of those biased studies will be discussed later in Part III.

In November 2000, George W. Bush was elected President of the United States and was sworn into office in January 2001. Things were beginning to look up again. Then suddenly out of the blue, I received a telephone call from Dr. Timothy Wheeler sounding me out about a possible appointment at the CDC. He informed me that I might receive a phone call from the office of Health and Human Services Secretary, Tommy Thompson. Instead, I received a call from a White House staffer for President George W. Bush, asking and exhorting me to accept an appointment to serve on an oversight committee at the CDC. The reader could well imagine my surprise at the sudden role reversal and the responsibility I was being asked to shoulder. But how could I refuse?

I agreed to serve on the CDC Grant Review Committee at the National Center for Injury Prevention and Control, of all places! What a quirk of ironic fate. I felt I would be working from within the belly of the beast, at least as far as gun and violence research was concerned. In this and the next chapter I discuss my tenure there.

And so it was that during the years 2002—2004, I served on the Injury Research Grant Review Committee (IRGRC; later referred to as the "Initial Review Group") of the CDC. I participated not only in the major meetings in Atlanta but also in on-site reviews and inspections of Injury Research Centers (IRGs), including the Johns Hopkins Bloomberg School of Public Health. I was reviewing thousands of pages of grant applications requesting funding for medical and public health scientific research proposals. I deliberately let some time elapse before I sat down and wrote an analysis of my stint at the CDC, with the purpose of being able to take a step back and write from a distance, objectively.

I should also inform the reader that as far as specific grant proposals, I must write in generalities, for according to CDC rules, I cannot disclose specific details of any grant proposal requesting funding, or discuss the content of the review of any specific grant application in which I participated or that came to my knowledge while working in the capacity of grant reviewer. Judging by the results, secrecy at the CDC seems to be more strictly held than at Los Alamos during the Manhattan Project. So, my discussion necessarily will be lacking specific examples to illustrate the thread of my arguments. Nevertheless, I ask you to bear with me for there are enough general topics of scientific interest that will, I think, make it worth your while—that is, if you have an interest in the present interrelationship between public health, social science, and the purported relationship these disciplines bear today with medicine, including neuroscience, and the scientific method.

Before proceeding, and as a further introduction to this topic, I would like to quote several excerpts from a magnificent and now classic article on medicine and statistics titled "Statistical Malpractice" by Bruce G. Charlton, M.D., of the University of Newcastle upon Tyne, England. It is perhaps no coincidence that Dr. Charlton is associated with the same great university that gave us the Father of Modern Epidemiology, Dr. John Snow, the illustrious physician who in 1849 successfully applied the scientific method to epidemiology. In the process, Dr. Snow proved that cholera is a water-borne disease and reemphasized the need for hygiene, sanitation, and clean water for preserving public health. His discovery led to the conquest of epidemic diseases, such as dysentery and typhoid fever. Later in Chapter 8, I describe the golden age of public health and its regrettable turn for the worse in the misuse of science and epidemiology after the mid-20th century, which in turn resulted in Dr. Charlton's warning about the growing misuse of epidemiology and statistics. As my narrative unfolds, the relevance of these momentous passages will become obvious.

Science Versus Statistics:

> There is a worrying trend in academic medicine, which equates statistics with science, and sophistication in quantitative procedures with research excellence. The corollary of this trend is a tendency to look for answers to medical problems from people with expertise in mathematical manipulation and information technology, rather than from people with an understanding of disease and its causes.
>
> Epidemiology [is a] main culprit, because statistical malpractice typically occurs when complex analytical techniques are

*combined with large data sets. Indeed, the better the science,
the less the need for complex analysis, and big databases are
a sign not of rigor but of poor control. Basic scientists often
quip that if statistics are needed, you should go back and do a
better experiment. Science is concerned with causes but statistics is concerned with correlations.*

*Minimization of bias is a matter of controlling and exclud-
ing extraneous causes from observation and experiment
so that the cause of interest may be isolated and characterized. Maximization of precision, on the other hand, is the
attempt to reveal the true magnitude of a variable, which
is being obscured by the "noise" [from the] limitations of
measurement.*

Science by Sleight-of-Hand

*The root of most instances of statistical malpractice is the
breaking of mathematical neutrality and the introduction
of causal assumptions into the analysis without scientific
grounds.*

Practicing Science without a License

*Medicine has been deluged with more or less uninterpretable
"answers" generated by heavyweight statistics operating on big
databases of dubious validity. Such numerical manipulations
cannot, in principle, do the work of hypothesis testing.*

*Statistical analysis has expanded beyond its legitimate realm
of activity. From the standpoint of medicine, this is a mistake:
statistics must be subordinate to the requirements of science,
because human life and disease are consequences of a historical process of evolution, which is not accessible to abstract
mathematical analysis.*[1]

As the reader will remember, we discussed the scientific process in Chapter 2. I mentioned the importance in hypothesis testing and how this essential step can decide by observation and experimentation the validity of a hypothesis leading to a scientific theory. But how can you test a hypothesis if the testing is discarded and replaced by numerical manipulations? Gun studies in the hands of public health injury researchers fell into this trap, deliberately in many cases, just as Dr. Charlton warned. Their epidemiologic studies expanded beyond the legitimate realm of activity because medical science is about human behavior, life, and disease, not about numerical manipulations.

Keeping this in mind, the following narrative is intended to describe the workings and some of the problems I encountered in the honorific service as a grant reviewer at the CDC. Additionally, I hope these few critical observations will be of some help to honest researchers in the field and improve overall the quality of grants submitted and approved at the CDC/NCIPC.

Research appropriateness and cost-effectiveness of grant proposals is included and discussed because the allocation of public health research funding is of concern to the American public (taxpayers), who are already shouldering a significant burden of their own rising health care costs. Yearly, they are asked to increase that burden with more tax dollars for social and public health research programs that frequently provide little in terms of improving the lives of their families and even less in terms of contributing to social harmony.

Despite definite improvements in the last several years, it is my opinion, after working in the belly of the NCIPC beast, so to speak, that much work still needs to be done. Much public health research in the area of injury control and prevention is duplicative, redundant, expensive, and not cost-effective. Many of the grant proposals for the study of spousal abuse, domestic violence, inner city crime, and juvenile delinquency belong more properly in the sociological and criminological disciplines than in the realm of public health and medicine. When we discussed the lack of science in many of these proposals, several reviewers privately acknowledged and agreed that the scientific method, or for that matter the application of the public health model, was found wanting when applied to the study of violence and crime. We were in the minority and in any event, we had to work within the framework that was already in place. Funding continues to roll in to the CDC's NCIPC, and much of it continues to be squandered in useless grant proposals accepted to preserve and increase funding, and misapplied by public health researchers, who continue to introduce causal assumptions into their epidemiologic or ecologic analysis without the scientific basis for doing so. Numerical manipulations continue to be used to force the statistics to confess as to reach the desired conclusions.

Congressional Authorization

Perhaps the biggest problem of all has been created and promoted by Congress in the allocation of ever-increasing amounts of taxpayer dollars to public health "research" into so many areas of investigations, particularly injury control that, frankly, in many dismaying instances is of questionable scientific validity and even less cost effectiveness. Oversight, accountability, and clear demonstration of cost effectiveness had been clearly lacking. Yet, the Department of Health and Human Services (HHS) shares some of the blame, as the executive federal agency has considerable leeway in how these tax dollars are spent by the CDC and the rest of the publicly funded PHE.

Many of the grant proposals submitted in the name of "violence prevention" and other goals of the Healthy People 2010 agenda were generally geared toward promoting social engineering and enlarging the scope and collective role of government in the lives of citizens. For example, numerous times I opposed and voted against proposals that required intrusive home visits to families by social workers ("home observations"), raising serious concerns of privacy violation. Ditto for proposals establishing databases of dubious validity where hypotheses were not tested, but propounded as scientific facts. Behind many of the health proposals is a compulsive need to protect people from themselves, as if they were children requiring the helping hand of the health bureaucrats for their own survival. All of these collectivizing and patronizing social programs, unfolding year after year, are borne at the expense of personal freedom, not to mention taxpayers' pocketbooks.

Other proposals sponsored year after year also involved extending "social justice," expanding socialistic agendas, and perpetuating the welfare state rather than seeking genuine scientific advances and applying them to improve health. In some cases, these grant proposals (most of which are actually funded) use or misuse statistics, collect data of dubious validity, and even use "legal strategies" to reach social goals and formulate health care policies that the public health researchers believe may achieve "social justice" (e.g., wealth redistribution). Many of these studies aim at nothing less than the gradual radicalization of society, using "health" as a conduit.[2,3,4] "Scientific" peer review in many instances, frankly, was not working or was non-existent. The reader will be surprised to learn that I found probably as many lawyers and social workers as practicing physicians and nurses applying for public health "scientific" research grants!

Healthy People 2000, Healthy People 2010, and injury control programs (particularly "Grants for Violence") became vehicles for the creation of ever-increasing social programs and the remodeling of society in the image of the progressive public health officials, who wrote and implemented them.[5] "Health" and "science" are used as covers because, to a significant extent, many of these proposals had relatively little to do with improving the general health of the public and even less with science and had absolutely no scientific merit. Frequently, proposals under previous Grant Announcements (perhaps with some notable exceptions for Traumatic Brain Injury and Acute Care and Rehabilitation) were submitted to dovetail antecedent social "research" in which statistical significance was frequently not established in prior studies. But the money kept rolling in, and more shoddy research was funded, year after year.

There may be light on the horizon, though. I have looked at the planning of Healthy People 2020 in the early Trump administration period, and the language has been transformed for the better; we now read of salubrious health prevention measures rather than politics. Let's hope this change is real and not an ephemeral transformation. We must also keep in mind that while some changes for the better have occurred, the decentralized PHE still needs close watching.

Simple Statistical Tools Frequently Missing

From the scientific point of view, a trend most troubling is the misuse or nonuse of the very simple but very helpful traditional statistical tools in the statistician's armamentarium. I refer to the useful methodology of *relative risks* (RR), *confidence intervals* (CI), and the increasingly ignored *p-values*. These traditional statistical parameters are essential in determining the strength of statistical associations. These tools are actually tough tests that are applied to statistical studies to ascertain their validity. Although these tests don't establish cause and effect relationships, they are essential in the process of establishing statistical associations, particularly in these social "science" (sociological) investigations that are carried out now routinely under the aegis of public health research. Their time-proven places in statistics are being replaced by complex, inscrutable statistical methodologies, such as regression models, multivariate stratified computer analysis, and other complex statistical manipulations that, devoid of the required clinical experience, befuddles everyone including the statisticians themselves!

Fishing Expeditions in Search of Social Problems

Not infrequently I found it difficult to discern in any of the ever-proliferating health (social) proposals strong statistical associations leading to groundbreaking, scientific research. Fishing expeditions in hypothesis searching and solutions in search of social problems are frequent, while hypothesis testing is poorly formulated. One reason for this misuse of statistics universally ignored is that epidemiology should be applied to rare diseases that occur at high rates in a defined segment of the population preferably over a shortly defined period of time (e.g., lung cancer deaths in smokers or even better, an outbreak of salmonella or shigella poisoning at a convention hall on a specified date) and should not be applied to low rate of disease or injury extending over a long period of time over vast populations (e.g., ongoing studies of juvenile crime in the inner city or health consequences of environmental toxins over a large population). Moreover, investigation of these diseases or injuries should be carried out in conjunction with clinical investigation.

Koch's Postulates of Pathogenicity were completely forgotten or just plainly ignored by the public health establishment (PHE). Koch's Postulates, as the reader will recall, are the steps that a medical researcher follows in proving that a specific microorganism causes a specific disease: "First, the organism must be found in the diseased animal. Second, the organism is then grown and isolated in the laboratory in pure culture. Third, the organism from such culture should cause the disease in a susceptible host upon inoculation. Fourth, the pathogenic organism must be re-isolated from the diseased host and cultured again in the laboratory."[6]

Epidemiological studies, whether they are case control or ecologic studies, are unreliable population-based investigations that should not be routinely used for investigating the etiology and course of common diseases, not to mention preventing injuries and violence among the general population. And yet, despite these objections, epidemiologic studies are funded routinely to investigate the pathophysiology, course, and outcome of common diseases and injuries that occur slowly or repeatedly over extended populations.

Premature Disclosure of "Scientific Findings"

Moreover, the media picks up these reports prematurely and sensationalizes conclusions that often contradict one another as soon as they are published, sometimes in the same issue of the same journal! Disconcertingly, for example, we have learned from the PHE and the media that coffee can cause cancer as well as prevent cancer, and that silicone breast implants are harmless and that they are not! We continue to be bombarded with prematurely reported headline-grabbing studies to the detriment of the trust that the public has invested in science and medicine.

The public, befuddled and confused, loses faith in "science" and looks elsewhere for answers, conducting its own research on the internet, not always with salubrious results. Public health proposals commonly tout their complex statistical analyses (e.g., multivariate and regression analysis to eliminate confounding variables), yet basic and extremely important statistical tools, such as p-values, relative risks, and confidence intervals are frequently not even mentioned in the body of the research!

Relative Risk

Although *relative risk* (RR) does not establish cause and effect relationships, it is an invaluable tool in statistics. RR is used to determine if there is a difference in the rate of a disease process or injury between two given populations. A RR of 1.0 signifies no difference. A RR of 2.0 means that the exposed population has twice (100 percent) the rate of disease (a positive association) as compared to the other population. Statistics are not science, and a 100 percent increase in this context is a very small number that could be explained solely by the quality of the data, thus denoting a weak statistical association.

Likewise, a RR value of 0.5 carries a risk of half (50 percent) as compared to the other population (a negative association) and likewise conveys a weak statistical association. Thus, experienced statisticians ignore the statistical significance of a RR ranging between 0.5 and 2.0, which relates no significant risks between the rate of disease or injury in the two populations under study. These figures should always be noted, but can be safely ignored by the epidemiologist as establishing no cause and effect relationship. Remember: RR between 0.5 and 2.0 do not reach statistical significance. To find out if a RR value outside those limits truly carries any statistical significance, two other tools are used: the *p-value*, the killer test that determines whether the difference in the two study groups are due to chance, and the *confidence interval* (CI).[4]

A p-value of 0.05 corresponds to the *95 percent level of confidence* that traditionally has been set by scientists as the gold standard for epidemiological research. A 95 percent confidence interval represents a range of values within which we are certain the true value of the relative risk (RR) is found (with 95 percent confidence). One must be aware that many public health researchers want to lower this standard to 90 percent (increasing uncertainty) to increase the chance of reaching statistical significance and confirm the validity of their research findings.

Other researchers do not disclose p-values, neglecting the possibility that their findings are due to chance. Those researchers who report and pass the p-value (p<0.05) test usually disclose it in their studies; those who ignore it make their study suspect, and their conclusions may not have reached the touted statistical significance they profess to have obtained. As we shall see, the *95 percent confidence interval* (CI) corresponds to a p-value of 0.05, but low p-values, even as low as p=0.006 or p=0.009, do not establish causation; they only denote strong statistical associations not likely due to chance. As statistician, Steven Milloy, author of the epidemiologic primer, *Junk Science Judo,* has pointed out, "Statistics are not science and do not prove cause and effect relationships."[4]

The next step that should be performed to test RR for statistical significance is the 95 percent confidence interval (CI). Scientists know that the true RR value is found with a 95 percent level of confidence. When a relative risk is greater than 1.0, the range for both the lower and upper boundaries must be greater than 1.0 to satisfy the CI test. Conversely, when the RR is less than 1.0, to satisfy the CI test, the range of CI values must fall below 1.0 (again both lower and upper reported boundaries included). Neither statistical association must include 1.0 within the range. If 1.0 is included in either range, a statistical significance is not established.

Frequently, I found that one or more of these traditional tools (e.g., RR, p-value, CI) were not mentioned or were incompletely disclosed in public health research proposals, apparently to avoid disclosing the inconvenient fact that drawn conclusions do not reach the level of statistical significance. Why? Because weak statistical associations, if honestly reported, would have disqualified them from reaching their preordained conclusions. Therein lies

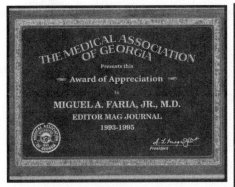

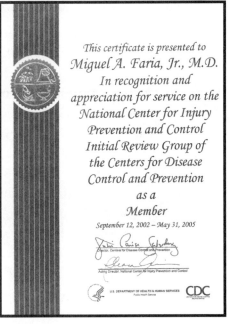

I received both an Award of Appreciation from the Medical Association of Georgia (1993-1995) despite my "controversial editorship" awakening the sleepy state medical journal that for the first time in years was read avidly by the membership, as well as a certificate of recognition and service from the National Center for Injury Prevention and Control of the CDC (2002-2005) for my service as a critical grant reviewer as discussed in the text.

the rub: Full reporting of values reaching no statistical significance may lead to no funding of further research grants! Thus, many shoddy grant research proposals in the violence prevention area of public health pad their numbers, increase uncertainty (90 percent CI), ignore p-values, and tout relative risks (RR) that have no statistical significance—to apply and re-apply for more funding for research grants. Remember, RR values between 0.5 and 2.0 denote no difference in rate of disease or injury between the two tested populations and carry no statistical significance. The difference may be due solely to the quality of the data.

Another situation arises when relative risks (Cohort Studies) or odds ratios (Case Control Studies) are mentioned, but then the discussion proceeds as if statistical significance had been reached (but it had not), and on the basis of statistically insignificant findings, *presto*, further social programs are proposed masquerading as ongoing public health studies. The money keeps rolling in. Broad hypotheses that should have been refined or discarded are kept and tested and re-tested. And, in subsequent studies, efforts at hypothesis searching are amplified to the point of becoming fishing expeditions, supported by poor data quality (e.g., data dredging) but are conducive to "positive" results. In the process, databases of dubious validity are compiled for further social research! Large data sets are hardly ever verified for accuracy and are used by some researchers in the hope of finding statistical association where none exist (e.g., data mining).[4]

In other words, much of this work entails reaching preordained solutions in search of problems, proposals in which narrow hypotheses are lost in nebulous seas of data. Immense sets of data are collected, tested, and re-tested, and statistics are tortured until finally they are made to confess to reach predetermined social objectives. These social goals are then put in place for dissemination to health policy makers, who believe that the conclusions have arisen via the arduous trials of the scientific method. More funding is allocated to implement public policy—and for more public health (social) research. And the beat goes on!

CHAPTER 7

PUBLIC HEALTH, SOCIAL SCIENCE, AND THE SCIENTIFIC METHOD (PART II)

No amount of experimentation can ever prove me
right; a single experiment can prove me wrong.

—Albert Einstein (1879—1955)

In the previous chapter we discussed in general terms some of the shortcomings I encountered in many of the grant proposals submitted during my stint as grant reviewer for the CDC's NCIPC in the years 2002—2004. There is no reason to believe that these epidemiologic and scientific shortcomings have been addressed and corrected in subsequent years. And from the outset, let me state the problems do not lie with the methodology requirements stated for the peer review process, but rather with the misuse of statistics and the lack of science in many, if not most, of the grant proposals for injury prevention. The methodology of grant review calls for the evaluation of research aims and long-term objectives, significance, and originality, as well as research design. These are appropriate criteria, but perhaps, for improvement, an additional criterion should be added: Show me the science—that is, the application of the scientific method!

Likewise, in the previous chapter, we also stressed Steven Milloy's axiom that statistics are not science, and cannot prove cause and effect relationships.[1] Yet statistics are a very useful tool of science that when properly applied establish correlations as to possible causes of disease processes. We were highly critical that such simple statistical tools as p-values were frequently missing in "scientific" grant proposals submitted for funding, although p-values are

important in establishing whether scientific findings reach statistical significance or are due to chance. We also discussed relative risks (RR) and the
confidence interval (CI) tests, as essential components of epidemiological
research. We also described shortcomings in strategic long-term proposals
in agenda-driven, public (social) health research.

Healthy People 2010

Healthy People 2010 is the United States' contribution to the World
Health Organization's (WHO) "Health for All" strategy. As such, many of
the proposals made in response to that contribution, sponsored by the PHE's
call for research papers, had frequently more to do with "social justice" in
the world, expanding socialism at home, and perpetuating the welfare state
than with making genuine advances in medicine and improving the health
of Americans. In some cases, these grant proposals use or misuse statistics,
collect data of dubious validity, and even use "legal strategies" to reach social
goals and formulate health care policies that the public health researchers
believe may achieve "social justice" in America or in the world at large. It is
worth restating that many of these studies are aimed at nothing less than the
gradual radicalization of society using "health" as a vehicle.[1-5] Healthy People
2010 in short was a veritable bureaucrat's dream, an overflowing cornucopia of
public (social) health goals geared toward social and economic reconstruction
of American society along socialistic lines—in the eyes of the PHE, a worthy
contribution to "Health for All" strategy.[6]

I also mentioned in the previous chapter the reader would be surprised
to learn that I found probably as many lawyers and social workers as practicing physicians applying for public health "scientific" research grants! No
wonder the science is lacking in many of the proposals, and frankly the peer
review process has been too lenient.

To further increase the chances of approval in the peer review process,
public health investigators now routinely ignore the basic traditional rules of
epidemiology such as RR, the p-value, and the CI test, which we previously
discussed. These are tough tests that would disqualify many low-caliber
research proposals. So the reader should not be surprised that in a competitive
world of funding grant proposals, many epidemiologists claim they are not

needed.[1] If high p-values (p>0.05), relative risk (RR) between 0.5 and 2.0, and confidence intervals too wide for comfort were disclosed, funding for health (social) programs may not be granted. Instead, epidemiologists and other public health researchers parade complex numerical computer manipulations such as regression models and stratified multivariate analysis that are designed to eliminate confounding variables. Nevertheless, confounding variables and other biases persist and junk science is the result. [1,2,5]

Here again is Dr. Charlton writing on this subject of statistical elimination for confounding variables:

> *[Science by sleight of hand] commonly happens when statistical adjustments are performed to remove the effects of confounding variables. These are manoeuvers by which data sets are recalculated (e.g., by stratified or multivariate analysis) in an attempt to eliminate the consequences of uncontrolled 'interfering' variables, which distort the causal relationship under study. There are, however, no statistical rules by which confounders can be identified, and the process of adjustment involves making quantitative causal assumptions based upon secondary analysis of the data base, but is illegitimate as part of a scientific enquiry because it amounts to a tacit attempt to test two hypotheses using only a simple set of observations.[7]*

The scientific process, like Koch's Postulates of Pathogenicity, indeed calls for much simpler methodology: [1] Observe a natural phenomenon. [2] Develop a hypothesis as a tentative explanation of what is occurring. [3] Test the validity of the hypothesis by performing a laboratory study and collecting pertinent data. Experimental trials (with randomization and control groups) are best. [4] Refine or reject the hypothesis based on the data collected in the experiment or trial. [5] Retest the refined hypothesis until it explains the phenomenon. A hypothesis that becomes generally accepted explaining the phenomenon becomes a theory.[4]

Let us return to the nuts and bolts of statistics and remember: For relative risks greater than 1.0 (no difference at all), the lower bound of the confidence interval test must be greater than 1.0. The inclusion of the value of 1.0 within the interval invalidates the 95 percent level of confidence.[1]

Likewise, for a relative risk less than 1.0 to satisfy the validity of the 95 percent level of confidence, the range of values must be less than 1.0. Again, the inclusion of the 1.0 value or higher invalidates the 95 percent statistical confidence in the study. (Next time you read a scientific study, check the statistics, make sure p-values, RR, and CI are disclosed in the scientific discussion.)[1]

Unfortunately, the public health establishment is going along in relaxing these inconvenient basic rules of statistics in order to continue to justify studies of little scientific validity but great social engineering potential. After all, the money keeps rolling in, year after year, for further research.

It is not surprising that even though the Injury Research Grant Review Committee (IRGRC; subsequently named the Initial Review Group [IRG]) members are asked to review the proposals for "scientific merit," the fact remains that—starting with the standard methodologies that rely largely on methods of population-based epidemiology, expansion of databases of dubious validity, complex statistical analysis subject to random errors and biases, complex numerical manipulations that are not mathematically neutral, and ending with "health" goals—little attention is paid in these proposals to the scientific method. More attention, in fact, is paid to social results and preordained, result-oriented or feel-good "research" than real, hard science. Science becomes a casualty in the politicized research battle.

Establishing Public Health Consensus

As of 2004, although the standing Initial Review Group (IRG) was composed of 21 members, there were so many grant proposals and so many members who apparently did not attend the meetings that the CDC con-tracted additional reviewers, "ad hoc" IRG consultant members to "assist" with the grant review process. Many of these consultants were former IRG members revolving back to the CDC and who tended to be sympathetic to the methodology, as well as to the social and political goals of the entrenched public health establishment. Thus, there was a current, an underlying conflict of interest intrinsic to this process. Moreover, many of the ad hoc members were statisticians, bureaucrats, epidemiologists or public health personnel, who had a direct or an indirect vested interest in approving the statistical studies of their colleagues rather than promoting medical science. Many of them were epidemiologists, who erroneously use statistics as if they were science proving cause and effect relationships without the corroborating findings of clinical medicine. In other words, Koch's Postulates of Pathogenicity, proving whether an organism causes a disease, were thrown out the window, and with it, of course, the required steps of the scientific method.

Statistics are a helpful tool of science that may disclose correlations, but they do not prove cause and effect relationships. Public health, as many workers have come to accept, has become a confusing mesh of socioeconomic programs injecting a heavy dose of politics into the undeserving body of science. It's no wonder then that these public health proposals are fraught with methodological errors and are subject to confounding variables that refuse elimination despite complex numerical computer manipulations. It is worth repeating that science establishes scientific facts; statistics establishes correlations.

Moreover, biases also enter the computations that cannot be corrected for because of poor data collection (data dredging) despite so-called mathematically neutral statistical "corrections." Someone had to step in front of the tanks in this milieu and proclaim that the emperor had no clothes, when it comes to the fact that science is lacking in many of these public (social) health proposals.

Many members and consultants of the Initial Review Group (IRG) have become entrenched bureaucrats in their ivory towers who want to go along to get along with their public health peers and push paperwork at their desks rather than serve as clinicians in the trenches, facing real sick patients to whom they must administer life-saving medical care.

The Department of Health and Human Services (HHS) should appoint to the IRG more clinicians, particularly practicing physicians and hard biological scientists, microbiologists, biochemists, physiologists, pathologists, anatomists, and fewer social "scientists," administrators, and bureaucrats. Although I met a few physicians, I did not meet a basic scientist in any of the above specialties—not one scientist involved in genuine research in the basic biological sciences! There must have been some, but if so, they were very few. This is a policy that must be established from above, from HHS, and implemented by the CDC as soon as possible.

Of course there are exceptions. I met several dedicated academicians and other fellow reviewers with whom I had the pleasure of working, both IRG members and consultants. Take for instance, Dr. Daniel O'Leary of the State University of New York, Dr. James F. Malec of the Mayo Clinic, and Dr. Patricia Findley of Rutgers University, who consistently placed science above other considerations in the panel's scientific discussions and conferences. There were others, but in the end, most reviewers readjust their views if they wish to be reappointed as consultants. They must ultimately conform to the basic work milieu of the NCIPC and work as to establish the much desired public health consensus in the approval process.

The CDC staff should have less influence in the review process by reducing or eliminating the need for ad hoc members, who are appointed at the discretion of its staff. These members are not only largely public health and social scientists rather than basic biological scientists or clinicians but also are contracted or appointed by the CDC and outnumber the standing IRG members at least three or four to one! My recommendation gives HHS the opportunity to bring in much-needed new blood and fresh ideas into the program.

Faulty Epidemiologic Methods Preferred Over More Scientific Studies

Furthermore, there is in the public health milieu a vested interest in promoting unreliable population-based statistical proposals because they lend themselves to the social study of spousal abuse, domestic violence, and adolescent crime that the NCIPC of the CDC is so fond of funding. And so, unfortunately, in the public health (social) research arena there is an overwhelming and disproportionate number of observational studies rather than experimental investigations. Clinical trials (e.g., controlled randomized, prospective trials), the most reliable of scientific research investigations, are few and far between. The vast majority of proposals are observational studies, which include in decreasing order of reliability, Cohort Studies (e.g., largely prospective but uncontrolled), Case Control Studies (retrospective and uncontrolled), and Ecologic Studies (e.g., population-based). Ecologic studies are so prone to error and so utterly unreliable as to give rise to the epidemiologic term of ecologic fallacy, a fallacy to which, in fact, all population-based studies are subject. [1,2]

There is also subliminal peer pressure to be lenient in the grant review process for accepting these proposals from other colleagues in the field because, although specific conflict of interest forms are signed and re-signed, many of the reviewers themselves receive federal money, and their own turn for review and approval will come sooner or later. To sum it up: CDC grant review committee members should be composed of more clinicians and more hard basic biological scientists, who are not receiving federal money, whether as ad hoc or standing members. New blood needs to be re-injected for new reviewers appointed by HHS and the CDC staff should not have the option of routinely re-appointing ad hoc members.

Another problem is the intrusive role played by a few CDC staffers and liaison officers working for the CDC in conjunction with the various injury control centers and schools of public health being supported by the CDC. One liaison officer I worked with exerted considerable pressure on committee members to approve a center with which he had a liaison. This happened specifically at a major center that I personally inspected with a team of reviewers. When the remote possibility of the center losing its funding came up, he stated this "is an excellent IRC (Injury Research Center)" and that "a score of 1.5 was necessary to assure funding of that center." That may be one of the reasons that center received one of the highest scores of all the centers reviewed, despite the fact the entire panel initially considered all of the large and small proposals (except for one) mediocre in methodology and lacking innovation and originality. The CDC staffer was supposed to be an observer and not discuss merit or budgeting (funding) with us. His job was only to make sure that we, the actual reviewers, consider and discuss the "scientific merits" of the program, for either referral or not, to the entire committee.

At the same time, I want to single out for praise among the CDC staff, Gwendolyn Haile Cattledge, PhD, deputy associate director for the science/scientific review administrator at the CDC in 2004, who was the embodiment of professionalism and competence during this time and all the time I worked with her. Likewise, I single for praise the then new director of the NCIPC, Ileana Arias, PhD, whom I only met briefly before her appointment. I thought she would have a bright future, and indeed she has moved to be the director of a division of Community Health Investigations.

Next, I would like to make the following observation: Congressional restriction of CDC use of funds for political lobbying and for shoddy gun (control) research efforts has been effective in reducing politicized, result-oriented gun research in the area of violence prevention. Yet, the temptation to resume this area of pseudo-scientific, result-oriented, political research is simmering just under the surface. Therefore, HHS should remain vigilant in this area—e.g., making sure this prohibition wisely ordained by Congress in 1996 is obeyed and followed as to preserve the integrity of true scientific research. This vigilance on the part of HHS is important. When I specifically asked a director of a prominent IRC if her center planned to do gun (control) research in the future, she stated that "no decision had been made but that they consider it a legitimate area of research and could very well resume doing so in the future." Indeed, they have; it is now an entire section at the Johns Hopkins Bloomberg School of Public Health. On the website, the Center for Gun Policy Research reads, "The Johns Hopkins Center for Gun Policy and Research is engaged in original scholarly research, policy analysis and agenda-setting public discourse. Our goal is to bring public health expertise and perspectives to the complex policy issues related to gun violence prevention."[8]

On the other hand, I have no direct criticisms of the largely good work the CDC has done in the proper application of epidemiology to medical and scientific research in the area of prevention and control of infectious and contagious diseases. That work should continue, particularly with the ever-increasing threat of virulent emerging infectious diseases caused by the Zika virus and other mosquito-borne virus encephalitides; ebola and other hemorrhagic fever viruses; as well as the looming threat of bioterrorism. I don't consider myself an enemy of public health. In fact, I admire the public health workers confronting major outbreaks and fighting serious epidemic diseases, but I do resent the politicization of public health and the misuse and fraudulent use of science for political purposes.

Too Much Money Available for Tempting Mischief

To this day Congress has expanded the budget of the NCIPC and continues to fund increasing amounts of taxpayer money for more injury and "violence" research, a large part of which is of dubious validity and duplication of work performed by other agencies that merely supports a burgeoning bureaucracy, expanding into other areas of research, health policy, and politics. With all this available funding, it stands to reason that more and more young people are going into the paperwork field of epidemiology and the social "sciences," rather than the experimental biologic sciences and clinical scientific research (e.g., microbiology, biochemistry, physiology, et cetera), or direct clinical patient care, where they will more certainly be needed for an increasingly growing and aging population.

If this trend towards the public (social) health field continues, we will have more young people attending law schools, the social sciences, and the schools of public health, and not enough in nursing, physician assistant programs (PAs), and medical schools. The resultant social scientists will not be doing basic science research (to provide us with new treatments for cancer and degenerative conditions of aging on the rise), or clinical medicine (to take care of our senior citizens surviving and living longer than ever) but working on purely computer epidemiological studies, carrying out armchair multivariate analyses with complex numerical manipulations and regression models. We need young people for the challenges of basic science (biological) research and attending medical, PA, and nursing schools. Yes, biological scientists, nurses, and physicians will drastically be needed for America's rapidly aging population of baby boomers, who have been retiring and soon will swell the ranks of septuagenarians and octogenarians. We need more nurses, clinicians, physicians at the bedside and public health workers out in the field as clinical epidemiologists in the arena of medical and mental health care delivery, rather than politicizing at the computer terminals!

Frankly, public health officials in politicized social research, directed at collectivist agendas and achieving "social justice," are still squandering taxpayer money. Not only is it a question of misallocation of health care resources and squandering money but also a question of the misallocation of medical personnel and the adoption of population-based ethics versus the reinstitution of the individual-based ethics of Hippocrates and direct patient care.[9,10,11]

Again, a major contributing factor to the growing problem of pseudo-scientific research is frankly too much available money, virtually allocated to a narrow area of research (injury prevention and the promotion of such "feel good" programs as were promoted in Healthy People 2010 agenda). I believe that cost ineffective research has been approved for the maintenance and expansion of budgets and in some cases the propagation of social welfare-type programs supported by junk science.

If I may be so bold, radical surgery is needed from the top to end politicized public health "injury research" and return to the field of science and genuine scientific investigations. Taxpayer money should be transferred from injury prevention and the social sciences (masquerading as public health) to the genuine good work that the CDC is doing in the field of infectious disease control, as originally intended.

Entering a School of Public Health?

In concluding this chapter, I would like to cite a book on medical history in which the author yearns for the day when the collectivist public health of a utopian future would supplant the individual-based practice of medicine. The tome is *The Story of Medicine* (1943) by Victor Robinson, M.D., an idealistic American socialist who was professor of the History of Medicine at Temple University in Philadelphia at the time of publication. He was very averse to what he termed "religious superstitions" in medicine, and expressed his yearnings for the expansion of secularist public health and the socialization of medical practice at the expense of traditional medical ethics and individual medical care.

As more schools of public health open—and no doubt there will be an excess of public health officials (bureaucrats) working and making work under that discipline—I hope medical and PA students (as well as nurses, the dedicated Florence Nightingales of the future) take notice of my own response to Dr. Robinson's yearnings. They should preserve their enthusiasm for their patient-oriented PA and medical schools and not switch by the present socialistic zeitgeist to the more fashionable and impersonal bureaucratic schools of public health. Most public health officials are desk workers, not epidemiologists in the field or in the trenches fighting outbreaks of deadly epidemics. But to those who do intend to do such fieldwork, as mentioned earlier, I tip my hat, for they also will be needed.

In the last two chapters of Dr. Robinson's *The Story of Medicine*, the acerbic medical historian sings the praises of public health, sociology and social work, while generally deploring the alleged shortcomings of American medicine—not always with justice to the participants or the times in which they lived. His secularist preaching denoted the fervor of a social moralist possessed with the zeal of righteous indignation. Towards the end of his book, Robinson calls for more social work and pleads for the socialized medicine of the future. He seems to forget or ignore the lessons of history revealing the more government intrusion in the social and economic life, the less the freedom available for the mental health of the people and the less humanitarianism and philanthropy that comes genuinely from the heart—and not from positive law, compulsion, and authoritarian socialism. Alas, the reader will remember the tragic story related in Chapter 3 of Comrade Lysenko that could have served as a splash of cold water on Robinson's dreaming face to awaken him to the realities of authoritarian socialism and collectivism.

Robinson ends his book with, "Preventive medicine, vastly extending the physician's horizon, is destined to change him from private practitioner to the nobler occupation of a worker for the public health and welfare."[12] And I say in response, that if and when that happens, and public health care workers dispense computerized health to the vast abstract humanity, who will be left then to console and minister care to the individual person, the real flesh and blood sick suffering patient at the bedside?

Now enter into the schools of public health those adventuresome souls responding to a professional calling to confront with courage infectious diseases and stem the tide of epidemics all over the globe; as for the rest, enter to the still noble professions of nursing, physician assistant, and medical schools, to confront the diseases, heal sickness, and ease the suffering of the individual patient.

CHAPTER 8

A HISTORY OF PUBLIC HEALTH– FROM SCIENCE TO POLITICS

Truth is the only merit that gives dignity and worth to history.

—Lord Acton (1834—1902),

classical liberal (today a conservative), historian, and British
Catholic MP in the Liberal Party of William Gladstone

Public health has had a magnificent and resplendent history. Sadly, some segments of the public health establishment (PHE) have strayed far from its glorious origin, initially modestly composed of independent physicians, nurses, dedicated epidemiologists and health care workers, to the present bloated, politicized and entrenched bureaucracy, which in certain areas seems to be more concerned with political agendas and their existence and budgets than the public health functions it has been charged by Congress to protect.

A Golden Age for Public Health

One could say the golden age of public health occurred in the late 19th and early 20th centuries, following the great discoveries of Edward Jenner (1749—1823), the English physician who developed a vaccine against small-pox (vaccination); Louis Pasteur (1822—1895), the French chemist who played a significant part both in the discovery of the germ theory of disease and in the development of immunizations; Joseph Lister (1827—1912), the British surgeon who developed antiseptic techniques in the treatment of wounds and in the implementation of surgical procedures; and Robert Koch (1843— 1910), the German physician, microbiologist and pathologist, who expounded on the concepts of microbes, the pathology of tuberculosis, and the development of microbiology. Following the lead of these physicians (except Pasteur, who was a chemist) and great public health workers, the men and women in the public health realm popularized the blessings of cleanliness, hygiene, and sanitation; carried out field work to determine sources of infectious diseases and outbreaks of epidemics; and even initiated the application of statistics for epidemiology as to aid private physicians in the life and death struggle against illness and disease, at home and in the work place. In that fashion, they all contributed greatly to the health of humanity.

The great discoveries of public health up to the early 20th century were independently conceived and largely decentralized events, the achievement of gifted individuals who followed in the tradition of independent physicians using their medical staff and frequently their own private fortunes. They were also in many occasions supported financially by charitable donations and the humanitarian goodwill of philanthropists and "captains of industry," wealth derived from the blessings of free market capitalism. The Industrial Revolution was winding down, the standard of living was improving dramatically, and medicine and public health were bestowing upon mankind the blessings of a better life and increasing longevity. Those were indeed the golden years of public health.

During the first half of the 20th century, the fountain of medical and public health discoveries gradually began to wane and the breakthroughs in medicine and science were made more and more by medical research corporations in the burgeoning, highly specialized fields of biochemistry, genetics, embryology, pharmacology, and other basic and clinical sciences.

Corporations and government bureaucracies entered the picture in great force in the wake of the New Deal of President Franklin D. Roosevelt. At that point in time, the leaders of the medical and public health establishments determined that rather than disband and pursue their work in specialized areas of study, they would continue to exist in the separate discipline of public health. But, to do so, they had to generate work to keep them busy, commence new projects, and seek new sources of funding. Those individuals drifted towards the government sector.

In the meantime, the private sector had also been squeezed by the unparalleled growth of government; it responded to the drying up of individual discoveries in medicine and the less available private funding from philanthropic individuals (who were also squeezed with increasing graduated taxation) with more efficient for-profit research and development (R&D) and technical specialization. With the concomitant growth of government, the public health segment became allied and more entwined with the State, and over time, became fully dependent on the federal government and enmeshed in its burgeoning, self-perpetuating bureaucracies.

Public Health Enters the Realm of Partisan Politics

Then, things began to change rapidly. With the release of the Kerner Report of 1968, the leaders of the public health establishment (PHE) crossed their Rubicon, many of them virtually leaving the realm of science to enter that of politics. They began to take political stands on issues only tangentially related to medicine or health, regardless of the wishes of the increasing membership. The PHE, boldly incarnated in the "American Public Health Association (APHA), embraced the federal government's Kerner Report on the 'root causes' of poverty and announced that social policy rather than public health, per se, would henceforth become its main focus."[1]

By the late 1960s and up to the early 1980s, the PHE began requesting and receiving more resources in the form of taxpayer money and used the resources, not always for the betterment of the health of the population, but frequently and increasingly for its own financial sustenance and political agendas. We must remember that by this time most infectious diseases in the industrialized world had been eradicated or nearly extinguished (e.g., poliomyelitis, smallpox, tetanus, and diphtheria) or fairly well controlled (e.g., most childhood diseases, as well as tuberculosis, leprosy, and syphilis). The wonders of medicine, the industrial revolution, free enterprise capitalism, and hygiene and sanitation, had done their job.

With more government money coming down the pipe and fewer infectious diseases to contend with, the PHE rapidly became a bloated bureaucracy, more concerned with increasingly radical political agendas and budgets than with the public health as charged by Congress. This is where James T. Bennett and Thomas DiLorenzo's book, *From Pathology to Politics: Public Health in America*, comes in. This eloquent and encyclopedic little book provides verifiable documentation of how the APHA has strayed far from its former beneficial path to that of a politicized, radical organization. *From Pathology to Politics* is an eye-opening indictment of the PHE and its perverse politicization of science and medicine. I am indebted to this tome for much of the information in this chapter.

The American taxpayer works the first four months of each year just to pay taxes to Uncle Sam. A significant portion of this amount went to fund unneeded public health projects and other boondoggles concocted by experts using nothing but junk science to promote their political agendas. Ever-increasing amounts of money in the billions of dollars per year went into projects aimed at establishing "social justice" and wealth redistribution schemes. Perhaps, this allocation could have been justified if the money had been used for the intended purposes it was allocated for by Congress and the American taxpayers. The reality was quite different.

Instead of being used to combat infectious disease and to fund needed research, Bennett and DiLorenzo charge much of the allocated money was used by the PHE for political purposes—e.g., promoting regulations in the workplace, calling for and establishing more bureaucracies, promoting greater government involvement in the lives of citizens, and lobbying to procure ever larger amounts of money for politically correct researchers. The claim of the PHE is they were protecting the public (from ourselves), while negating individual autonomy and resenting citizen empowerment.[1]

At one time, the PHE depended on campaigns of public education, but during this progressivist period, it did not. It preferred and depended on raw power and government coercion to enforce paternalistic policies on citizens, who apparently do not know any better. When education was called forth, it was immediately followed by calls for "reform," and the establishment of more agencies and bureaucracies, more regulation, more money extracted from the taxpayer, greater restrictions on civil liberties, more welfare programs, and a greater role of government in all aspects of our lives.

Public Health at the Far Left of Politics

The PHE incarnated in the American Public Health Association (APHA) cared more for the socialistic political agenda to which it subscribed than for the public health to which it is theoretically beholden. Politics always came first, and in politics, the PHE stood to the far left of even the most liberal legislators and the most strident political pressure groups.

Since many of their battle cries proclaimed they wanted reform "for the children," an illustrative example cited by Bennett and DiLorenzo is particularly revealing. In the name of protecting the Earth's ozone layer, the APHA joined the EPA and the FDA in proposing a ban on asthma inhalers because they purportedly contained chlorofluorocarbons, or CFS, that supposedly deplete the ozone layer. Even the AMA, which frequently sides with the PHE, for example in gun control, dissented. The AMA pointed out inhalers relieved the symptoms of children with asthma and in many cases were lifesaving. The plea to prevent the ban on lifesaving inhalers was even seconded by the leftist Congressional Black Caucus representing thousands of inner-city asthma sufferers, as well as a number of other liberal legislators. Nevertheless, the APHA, to the far-left of the political spectrum, and other public health-related agencies, such as the EPA and the FDA as well as the American Lung Association, continued to support the ban, showing more concern for environmental ideology and dubious science than for the health of asthmatic children, including those in the inner cities who they always claim to protect in their bureaucratic proposals.

As a result of this brouhaha raised by the PHE, the hardship on families of asthmatic children was extended for two decades and the cost of the new asthma inhalers when they arrived (without the chlorofluorocarbons) went up exponentially, adding financial hardship to medical woes.[2]

Another area where the APHA had shown duplicity was in welfare reform. After controlling for other variables, Bennett and DiLorenzo pointed out that studies had shown children on welfare had lower cognitive abilities, were more likely to drop out of or fail to graduate from school, had lower educational achievement, had high teenage crime rates, and were more likely to be illegitimate. Nevertheless, the APHA leadership, again to the far left of the political spectrum (many of them unreconstructed 1960s radicals rather than mainstream liberals, as Bennett and DiLorenzo correctly assert), strongly opposed the beneficial bipartisan bills of the 104th Congress to reform welfare.

Even though Congress and President Clinton went on to enact welfare reform in 1996, the APHA went on the record continuing to oppose the reforms, countering with all its heart and soul the phasing out of welfare spending by "working with coalition partners concerned about the children."[2]

The PHE and the APHA continued to support social policies that had already been discredited as failures. For example, the APHA leaders subscribed to the erroneous beliefs that "being on welfare is conducive to improving public health; government income redistribution programs can improve public health; individuals should not be held responsible for their health (government should be)," and so on.[3]

The APHA also strongly favored government control of medical care and, as Bennett and DiLorenzo described, has publicly stated it is opposed to the expansion of free market medical care. Totally out of step with the American people and other health care researchers and policy makers, the APHA "even criticized the failed Clinton health care plan in 1993—which would have abolished the private health insurance industry and placed the federal government in charge of most of the health care market—as being 'too market oriented.'"[4] In other words, the APHA favored fully nationalized, single payer, government controlled health care.

Bennett and DiLorenzo wrote: "It was apparent by the mid-1970s that the American Public Health Association was being directed not by main-stream liberals, but by radicals who place much greater reliance on political activism in the name of public health than had their predecessors."[5] As examples of good medical care, the APHA pointed to Nicaragua (in the 1980s under the communist Sandinista regime) and specifically singled out the Cuban health care system, as a "political and economic role model for the United States, especially with regard to health care."[6]

To pay for a nationalized, single payer health care system in the United States, the APHA rejected published scholarship and the economic facts revealing how exorbitant the cost of such a system would be for American tax-payers. Their answer for funding came straight out of Karl Marx's *Communist Manifesto*, "increasing progressive taxation."[7]

And again, while continuing to profess a concern for "the children," the

APHA rejected the solid scholarship behind the fact that day care centers were plagued by outbreaks of epidemics and other infections. Citing the work of Dr. Stanley Schuman, Bennett and DiLorenzo recounted how "day care centers are responsible for the recent outbreaks of diarrhea, dysentery, giardiasis, and epidemic jaundice—reminiscent of the pre-sanitation days of the seventeenth century. Other serious day care hazards include cytomegalovirus, shigellosis, hepatitis, Hib (Haemophilus influenzae), and ear infections."[8] For the APHA, it is frequently political ideology and socioeconomic theories that count, not the public health of the community.

The APHA response to these problems—namely, the same as what Hillary Rodham Clinton tried to label America's "silent crisis"—was to reject the idea of having a variety of day care centers based on the market place and parental choice, but to have a "single, government-controlled, monopoly system of 'quality' day care."[9] It should be noted that during the Obama administration, the APHA somewhat tempered its position and pragmatically supported ObamaCare.[10]

Regardless of the issue being discussed, the PHE always chooses the far left, socialistic side of the debate. Rather than acting as an organization of professionals advocating for the interest of the public health, they have become a political pressure group, always pushing for greater government control in all aspects of our lives. Despite contrary scholarship, the APHA, as pointed out by Bennett and DiLorenzo, believes that free market capitalism is generally hazardous to health and that socialism and nationalized health care provide all the answers to the world's woes.

The APHA remains committed to its own self-aggrandizement and within the larger context, increasing and magnifying the power of the State at the expense of the individual. To the extent that the State is acting to protect us from ourselves in the area of public health, injuries and disease prevention—coercion may be used and individual autonomy can be restricted for the common good.

Public Health Stands for Strict Gun Control

In the area of scientific research, the APHA has used *preordained, results-oriented, politicized research based on what can only be characterized as junk science and systematically ignores opposing scholarship.* The example provided by the authors on the issue of public health and gun control is instructive. Bennett and DiLorenzo wrote:

> *The CDC-funded gun control research simply ignores a large body of data that contradict its pro-gun control position. For example, 'in the 25 years from 1968 to 1992, American gun ownership increased almost 135 percent (from 97 million to 222 million), with handgun ownership rising more than 300 percent. These huge increases coincided with a two-thirds decline in accidental gun fatalities.'[11]*

Obviously, increased gun availability in ordinary, law-abiding citizens does not translate to more crime. Yet, the PHE was at the forefront of gun control stating that easy gun availability cause suicides and homicides.

Moreover, the PHE continues to ignore the fact that up to 2 million to 2.5 million defensive uses of firearms take place by ordinary citizens in the U.S. every year thwarting crime and protecting life and property, as has been demonstrated conclusively by the sound scholarship of Professor Gary Kleck of Florida State University. The PHE has also ignored the evidence gathered by criminologist John Lott demonstrating that *the expansion of concealed carry gun laws caused a decline in firearm violence, because law-abiding citizens with firearms are able to defend themselves and their families and deter crime in those states that have enacted those laws.* Inconvenient facts and statistics that do not support PHE views are thus rejected or ignored.

Yet, at the time of this writing in 2017, the APHA remains committed to applying the public health model (e.g., gun violence as an epidemic) to gun control. After every mass shooting they resume their call for Congress "to lift the ban on gun research," but nothing is said about preventive mental health measures. APHA members are urged to write to Congress using a prepared form letter and to "personalize their message." As of September 4,

2017, the APHA website, urged:

"As a constituent and American Public Health Association advocate, I write to urge you to take immediate action to address the epidemic of gun violence in the United States…We cannot allow senseless gun violence and mass killings to continue…

"We must take a comprehensive public health approach to address this ongoing crisis. For too long, we as a nation have failed to take on this devastating problem and we cannot afford to wait any longer…

"Providing adequate and unrestricted funding for the Centers for Disease Control and Prevention and other scientific agencies to research the causes of gun violence…

"Expanding the collection and analysis of data related to gun violence and other violent deaths by increasing the funding for CDC's National Violent Death Reporting System…

"Reinstating the federal ban on assault weapons and large-capacity ammunition magazines…"[12]

The sheer amount of money involved in public health research and the increasing number of bureaucracies and agencies in the PHE are of themselves corrupting influences. One can be sure much of the research that has been conducted by the PHE, particularly the APHA, whether for HIV/AIDS, carcinogens, or gun control, has had "an underlying ideological bias against capitalism." As shown by Bennett and DiLorenzo, the great cancer health threat of the 1970s was found to be "an anti-capitalist, ideological crusade funded with tax dollars and carried out by various segments of the public health profession."[13] Other public health-related agencies, and not just the APHA, supported this cancer scare. The EPA has supported a variety of cancer scare episodes with the cooperation of most of the PHE.

One particularly flagrant example was the Alar scare, a bogus episode that caused many mothers to be unnecessarily fearful of giving apples and apple juice to children because of flawed studies purporting to show a link to cancer. The alleged culprit was said to be the chemical Alar that was used to preserve apple freshness. The Alar scare was in fact what turned out to be hazardous to the public health because people, particularly children, were discouraged from eating fruit and drinking juice, which, of course, are beneficial and have been shown to reduce cancer and other diseases.[14]

Public Health Plays "Fast and Loose" with Science

As Bennett and DiLorenzo state, the PHE also played "fast and loose" with the scientific method. Public health researchers claimed, "that a statistical association connotes causation."[15] This kind of "cooking" of the data is done to obtain preordained results and assign false causation to [environmental] diseases to various chemicals and drugs, and to bypass the hurdle of relative risk. Sloppy techniques are used routinely in data collection to arrive at preordained conclusions (e.g., results-oriented research). We have already described in previous chapters how this was done by misapplying the public health model to the study of gun violence in order to arrive to the preordained conclusion that stricter gun control is needed.

Another meaningless source of public health anxiety is the supposed health threat caused by "disease clusters," ignoring more important risks, such as heredity and socioeconomic status. The PHE also has a predilection to ignore sound scientific principles, such as the principle in toxicology of hormesis, "the dose makes the poison." For example, medications are beneficial at lower doses intended to do what they are supposed to do, but at higher doses, they may result in fatal overdoses and lethal diseases. Ignoring this scientific fact, public health researchers, instead, conveniently uphold the "linear no-threshold model," asserting that miniscule exposure to chemicals or radiation (radon) is equivalent to massive exposure and is always related to dosage via extrapolation rather than by actual experimentation.[16]

A complete assault on the scientific method is the PHE's penchant to intentionally misuse relative risk (RR). In the case of secondhand smoke, Bennett and DiLorenzo point out that when the EPA wasn't able to obtain the statistically significant relationship it desired, the researchers took it upon themselves to increase the level of confidence from five to 10 percent. (By convention, epidemiologists have used the confidence level of 5 percent or less as being insignificant, p>.05.) This is referred to as the 95 percent level of confidence. But to obtain the desired results, the EPA, for example, used a 10 percent level of confidence as being significant (p>.10), in effect doubling the threshold, to obtain the desired result and statistical association.

And, when all else fails to reach the desired conclusion, public health researchers completely ignore the methodology of "relative risk" (RR) as we discussed in Chapters 6 and 7. Bennett and DiLorenzo relate that public health researchers have also used this methodology "to prove a preconceived notion rather than test a scientific hypothesis."[17]

Relative risk studies do not account for confounding variables, other factors that may cause disease. So it's not surprising that by deliberately misusing this methodology, "the politicization of science takes on bizarre proportions, such as the 'relative risk' bogus study that reported that women who wore brassieres all day are 12,500 times more likely to contract breast cancer than those who go braless."[18]

It is worth repeating that the APHA and the EPA also ignore contradictory studies that do not support or contravene their political agendas.

Moreover, Bennett and DiLorenzo agree with my assessment in the previous chapter asserting that "tax dollars for bureaucrats' budgets and research grants—is the driving force behind the corruption of public health science."[19] This assertion is entirely correct. "The whole purpose of the politicization of public health science is to expand the size and scope of the government agencies that sponsor this shoddy 'research,' to advance the careers of politicians and bureaucrats in the public health field, and to provide millions of dollars in research grants to government-funded researchers. It is all about money and power."[19]

When their studies are totally discredited, as in the case of the studies of particulate matter by the EPA, the public health agencies involved continue to push for their agendas apparently believing that science can be corrupted for a worthy cause.[20]

PHE's researchers, including those of the EPA, frequently refuse to make their data public, even though the data accumulated and obtained for their research was financed by grants funded by taxpayers.[20] We also raised this complaint in this book citing the examples of gun researchers. Another critic of the PHE, Michael Fumento, likewise deplored this refusal to release data in relation of public health workers at the EPA. Bennett and DiLorenzo did not forget our criticism of this issue and cited our denunciations in their book.[20]

In short, PHE expresses hypocrisy of the highest order when it criticizes industry-funded research as automatically flawed or labels it "biased" or "suspect" simply because the research was funded by the private sector. PHE researchers ignore the criticisms of their own research, even when it has been shown repeatedly to be flawed, biased and politicized, particularly in the areas pertaining to social and economic policy, yet relying on government funding. The PHE simply seeks to aggrandize the size and scope of government because it depends on public funding for its existence.[21]

In conclusion, the political partisanship and the far left politics of the PHE have led to a deteriorated state of affairs in some segments of public health. The medical politics of the AMA and "organized medicine" in collusion with the PHE have exerted and will continue to exert left-wing political pressure on society on many fronts. Public funding of these activities has continued to rise exponentially helping to remold society in their progressive collectivist image, and it's fair to say advancing socialism in the process.

The centralization and politicization of public health have helped to tilt the balance of power in society away from the individual and closer to the State. Fortunately, in one area, a most important one to be sure, the balance has returned towards individual freedom, and that has been in the restrictions placed by Congress on publicly funded, biased gun research—politicized research that attempted to circumvent the constitutional right of Americans by falsely portraying guns as a public health menace requiring eradication.

The state of affairs of the PHE needs serious revamping. Its functions should be surveyed and re-assigned, decentralized, and, as much as possible, returned to the private sector. The PHE structure, as it stands today, has outlived its usefulness in many areas of endeavor, and in some of these areas may actually be causing to the public more harm than good. Reforms could include funding through private philanthropies, reassignment to private research laboratories, and relocations to universities, all of which could be encouraged by tax credits for private entities, while gradually decreasing government funding for the public agencies. Most important, science must be divorced from politics, and the application of the scientific method insisted upon, as essential for the funding of grants and fundamental for a scientific pronouncement.

The worst thing Congress can do is to continue to support the PHE as a government-funded monopoly and indiscriminately continue to increase funding for all public health agencies, the EPA, and other bureaucracies that do not prove their science or that refuse to release their "scientific" data for public scrutiny. To not insist on these reforms will not only be counterproductive from a public-funding perspective but also very dangerous to our way of life and our health.

PART 3

DEBUNKING BIASED INFORMATION DISSEMINATED IN MEDICAL JOURNALS AND THE LAY PRESS

CHAPTER 9

STATISTICAL MALPRACTICE— "FIREARM AVAILABILITY AND VIOLENCE"

Truth has to be repeated constantly, because Error also is being preached all the time, and not just by a few, but by the multitude. In the Press and Encyclopaedias, in Schools and Universities, everywhere Error holds sway, feeling happy and comfortable in the knowledge of having Majority on its side.

—Johann Wolfgang von Goethe (1749—1832),
German poet, novelist, scientist, statesman

No matter what the tragedy might be, gun prohibitionists will find an angle to use it to push for gun control. In the aftermath of the September 11, 2001 catastrophe, among the organizations that did so were the Americans for Gun Safety (AGS) and the Violence Policy Center (VPC). At the time, like the VPC, AGS was a strident gun control organization that pushed the disingenuous cliché of "we need to close the gun show loophole."[1] This renewed effort continued, despite the fact that the government's National Institute of Justice 1997 study "Homicide in Eight U.S. Cities" had shown that less than two percent of criminals obtained their illegally-possessed firearms from gun shows.[2] AGS went further to erroneously claim it had found a link between terrorism and gun shows. The National Rifle Association (NRA) correctly tagged AGS "an anti-gun lobbying group with no members, no gun safety programs, and now, no credibility."[3] AGS has since folded into an organization titled Third Way, claims to be a nonpartisan think tank, and despite its name is a progressivist organization that under the subheading of social issues still opposes gun rights.[4]

As for the VPC, its head, Josh Sugarmann, was caught fabricating data to prove the absurd claim that concealed carry weapons (CCW) permits were responsible for home suicides. In fact, the report by the Michigan State Police only noted there were 56 suicides in 2010 committed by CCW holders, and it did not even list the method used by the licensees to commit suicide. Furthermore, the suicide rate for CCW holders was 13.3 per 100,000, which was lower than the rest of the population in Michigan at 16.3 per 100,000.[5]

Working Hand in Glove—Gun Activists and Public Health Researchers

Gun control organizations have worked hand in glove with the public health establishment disseminating their published propaganda. And here is a good example. Citing a Harvard School of Public Health study published in the February 2002 issue of the *Journal of Trauma*,[6] the VPC claimed, "The elevated rate of violent death among children in high gun ownership states cannot be explained by differences in state levels of poverty, education, or urbanization."[7] But the authors of the study, Miller and associates, did not put it quite so bluntly; they knew better, although they did their part to mislead. According to the abstract of the study, the authors asserted: "A statistically significant association exists between gun availability and the rates of unintentional firearm deaths, homicides, and suicides. The elevated rates of suicide and homicide among children living in states with more guns is not entirely explained by a state's poverty, education, or urbanization and is driven by lethal firearm violence, not by lethal non-firearm violence."[6]

President Bill Clinton once rhetorically explained that no one could prove that he had ever established administration policy based "solely" on the basis of campaign contributions, although in the case of China, the communist Chinese got their share of high-tech, strategic, missile-launching technology to pose a new threat to the U.S.

In the authors' abstract, the words "not entirely" become the key to understanding the preordained drift of their gun control agenda and the expected, result-oriented conclusions. The published study, indeed, is the typical, hackneyed public health result-oriented gun research repeatedly published in the medical literature claiming that "gun availability is responsible for firearm violence, 'intentional or unintentional.'"[6]

Thus, perhaps we should analyze further the meaning of the words "not entirely." What follows is a preliminary critique of the study, which we planned to finalize once we had received the primary, raw data requested from the authors for further analysis.

According to the study, the five states (all in the South) with the highest gun ownership—Louisiana, Alabama, Mississippi, Arkansas, and West Virginia—were more likely to have children dying from unintentional firearm injury (gun accidents), suicide (with or without firearms), and homicide than children in the five states with the lowest levels of gun ownership—Hawaii, Massachusetts, Rhode Island, New Jersey, and Delaware.

Why more mid-western and western states, such as North and South Dakota, Iowa, Wisconsin, Utah, Nebraska, and Alaska, that like southern states have relatively "easy gun availability" have low firearm death rates for children is left unexplained.

In fact, the whole study revolves around using the phraseology "not entirely" to exclude the much more important reasons for violence with or without firearms: the levels of poverty and education, not to mention the related cultural factors and the utter breakdown of the family in the pertinent states by welfare and other government policies.

Allow me to divert slightly at this juncture and expound on two related themes revolving around the subject of this study and establish a couple of observations, observations that were overlooked by the public health researchers and their consorts at the VPC.

Mass Shooting Incidents

Three major mass shootings occurred in the aforementioned "lowest gun ownership" states. Two of them, although they were adult, workplace shootings, occurred in Hawaii and Massachusetts—two of the states with draconian gun control laws and less "availability of firearms."

Likewise, several mass shootings, both adult workplace and children school incidents, have taken place in California, despite the stringent gun control laws and the supposedly less "availability of firearms" in that state.

The Xerox workplace incident in Honolulu, Hawaii (Nov. 2, 1999), the

San Diego, California, Santana School shooting (March 5, 2001), and the
Wakefield, Massachusetts, incident (December 26, 2000), all took place in
states with very restrictive gun control laws, where guns should not have been
easily "available" if the strict laws of these states were effective.

School shootings, of course, can also take place in states where firearms are available to law-abiding citizens. When they do, armed law-abiding
Americans at least have the capability to respond and stop the massacre before
more innocent victims are robbed of their lives. As we previously mentioned
(and will elaborate in later chapters), 600 to 1,500 criminals are killed yearly
by good citizens defending their lives, their families and neighbors, and their
property. Nevertheless, it is not the body count that makes the difference; it's
the defensive uses that count and make the difference, and admittedly, most
of the time the incidents do not result in the death of either the criminal or
the lawful citizen. As we learned in Chapter 4:

> The true measure of the protective benefits of guns are the lives
> saved, the injuries prevented, the medical costs saved, and
> the property protected—not the burglar or rapist body count.
> Since only 0.1 percent to 0.2 percent of defensive gun usage
> involves the death of the criminal, any study, such as this, that
> counts criminal deaths as the only measure of the protective
> benefits of guns will expectedly underestimate the benefits of
> firearms by a factor of 500 to 1,000.[8]

Law-abiding citizens can save lives. This was the case in 1998 in Pearl,
Mississippi, a state cited in the study where a schoolteacher used his firearm
to stop a school shooting by a student. Lives were thus saved. A few years later
in Virginia, two law school students overpowered and subdued a gunman
using their own weapons.

The point is that, as usual, the public health researchers ignored the
beneficial aspects of gun ownership and concentrated only in obtaining
supporting evidence for their long-known thesis that firearm availability is
responsible for violence in our society. Only data supporting their hypothesis are collected and analyzed. Contrarian data are ignored or discarded.

Law-abiding citizens obey the laws; criminals do not. When the government passes restrictive gun laws, those laws interfere in the lives of lawful citizens. Yet they do not stop criminals who are by definition bent on breaking them or the mentally deranged haunted by their own demons.

As stated previously, while neither state waiting periods nor the federal Brady Law has been associated with a reduction in crime rates, adopting concealed carry gun laws cut death rates from public, multiple shootings (e.g., those that took place in schools in San Diego, California; Pearl, Mississippi; and Littleton, Colorado) by an amazing 69 percent, according to criminologist John Lott, who now heads the Crime Prevention Research Center.[5] Not surprising, this type of data was not considered by public health researchers and did not enter into their analysis.

Television and Media Violence and Juvenile Delinquency

Another observation virtually ignored by the authors of the study, as well as their promoters at the VPC, is the effect of television and media violence on juvenile delinquency.

It should be of interest to the reader to learn that some of the most important breakthrough research papers on this topic first appeared in the 1970s and 1980s. The pioneering research was conducted and the paper written by Dr. Brandon Centerwall of the University of Washington School of Public Health.

Dr. Centerwall's studies found that homicide rates in Canada were not related to easy gun availability by ordinary citizens, as he had expected, but to criminal behavior associated with watching television.[9]

Centerwall found that homicide rates, not only in Canada but also in the U.S. and South Africa, soared 10 to 15 years after the introduction of television in those countries. In the U.S., there was an actual doubling of homicide rates after the introduction of television.

Moreover, Dr. Centerwall noted that up to half of all homicides, rapes, and violent assaults in the U.S. were directly attributed to violence on television. And that was when violence on TV was softer and much less graphic compared to the rampant and gory violence depicted today in the movies and on television.

Centerwall showed with elegant data that reducing gun availability did not reduce Canadian homicides. Homicide rates in Vancouver, for example, were lower before the gun control laws were passed in Canada, and in fact rose after the laws were passed. The Vancouver homicide rate increased 25 percent after the institution of the 1977 Canadian gun laws.

This valuable research, though, was not made widely available and was virtually consigned to the "memory hole" of the PHE. Fortunately, Dr. Centerwall's research pointing to the effects of television violence affecting homicide rates has been more widely publicized.[8]

In summer 2000, the media, including medical journalists, focused their attention on the associations of violence in television, music, video games, and movies to violent behavior in children and adolescents.

As a result, a consensus statement of experts released on July 26 and sponsored by the AMA and other medical groups proclaimed, "At this time, well over 1,000 studies—including reports from the surgeon general's office, the National Institute of Mental Health and numerous studies conducted by leading figures within our medical and public health organizations—point overwhelmingly to a causal connection between media violence and aggressive behavior in some children."[10]

The report continued, "Its effects are measurable and long-lasting... prolonged viewing of media violence can lead to emotional desensitization toward violence in real life."[10] Here is one good mark for the AMA and the National Institute of Mental Health. Additional studies have shown the deleterious effect of television and video game violence on children—namely a desensitizing effect and a potential to trigger aggressive behavior as the children go into adolescence.[11,12]

Why is all this background information being discussed about television violence and crime? Virtually, what we are seeing is life imitating art. Interestingly enough, the authors of the *Journal of Trauma* study discussed here, ignored relevant and important data impacting directly on their research.

Let us look at Table 1. Average Proficiency in Reading…

Table 1: Average proficiency in reading for 4th graders in public schools
(National Center for Education Statistics, 1994)

"High Juvenile Violence" State	Percentage of students reading for fun on their own time almost every day	Percentage of students watching television 6 or more hours per day
Alabama	41%	21%
Arkansas	41%	25%
Louisiana	38%	28%
Mississippi	39%	28%
West Virginia	39%	19%
Average	**39.6%**	**24.2%**

"Low Juvenile Violence" State	Percentage of students reading for fun on their own time almost every day	Percentage of students watching television 6 or more hours per day
Delaware	42%	26%
Hawaii	42%	20%
Massachusetts	46%	14%
New Jersey	43%	23%
Rhode Island	48%	16%
Average	**44.2%**	**19.8%**

As clearly shown in this table compiled from government statistics (1994), it turns out that, among other factors, students in the "high levels of juvenile violence" states, not only watch more television (24.2 percent) than those in the "low levels of juvenile violence" states (19.8 percent), but also do "less reading on their own time almost every day (39.6 percent versus 44.2 percent)."[13]

We will be looking at the factors that Miller et al. claimed were "not entirely" responsible for the high rates of unintentional firearm injury, homicide, suicide and overall violence in the mostly southern states. Incidentally, rather than using the biased, VPC shibboleths "highest" or "lowest gun ownership states," I have used the more objective terminology, "high" and "low levels of juvenile violence" states, for the purpose of this critique.[10]

On Feb. 28, 2002, I wrote Dr. Matthew Miller, the lead author of the study published in the *Journal of Trauma*, and requested that he kindly supply me with the primary, raw data that he and his associates used in reaching their conclusions.[14]

Like Kellermann and associates, as discussed in Chapter 4, the data was not made available. Unlike Kellermann, though, who at least responded with arguments, I did not even receive the courtesy of an answer to my request from the authors. In the next chapter I will analyze the authors' other published numbers, and see what they really reveal.

CHAPTER 10

STATISTICAL MALPRACTICE— EDUCATIONAL AND SOCIOECONOMIC FACTORS

The fundamental source of all your errors, sophisms and false reasoning is a total ignorance of the natural rights of mankind. Were you once to become acquainted with these, you could never entertain a thought, that all men are not, by nature, entitled to a parity of privileges. You would be convinced, that natural liberty is a gift of the beneficent Creator to the whole human race, and that civil liberty is founded in that; and cannot be wrested from any people, without the most manifest violation of justice.

—**Alexander Hamilton (1757—1804),**
The Farmer Refuted, 1775

In the previous chapter, we made some preliminary observations regarding the Harvard School of Public Health study published in the February 2002 issue of the *Journal of Trauma*.[1] At the time, the Violence Policy Center (VPC) lauded the study as "the most comprehensive study ever conducted on impact of gun availability." In its press release, the organization further stated, "The elevated rate of violent death among children in high gun ownership states cannot be explained by differences in state levels of poverty, education, or urbanization."[2]

For their part, the authors of the study asserted in their abstract, "A statistically significant association exists between gun availability and the rates of unintentional firearm deaths, homicides, and suicides. The elevated rates of suicide and homicide among children living in states with more guns is not entirely explained by a state's poverty, education, or urbanization and is driven by lethal firearm violence, not by lethal non-firearm violence."[1]

Now let's examine the factors that Miller and associates claim were "not entirely" responsible for the high rates of unintentional firearm injury, homicide, suicide and overall violence in the mostly southern states. As already noted, rather than using the biased VPC shibboleths "highest" or "lowest gun ownership states," I have used the more objective terminology "high" and "low levels of juvenile violence" states for the purpose of this critique.

Although it's not politically correct to bring race and ethnicity into the debate, let us state that illiteracy, broken homes, and violence, with or without firearms, have been shown to be more prevalent, whether linked to cultural, socioeconomic or other factors, to African-Americans and Hispanics (and less so to whites and Asians).[3]

A Table Worth a Thousand Words

The percentage of African American (and other significant minority) students enrolled in public schools in those states with high levels of juvenile violence were as follows:

Louisiana	47.6% (Hispanics, 1.3%)
Alabama	36.4% (Hispanics, 1.1%)
Mississippi	51%
Arkansas	23.5% (Hispanics, 3.0%)
West Virginia	4.2%

The percentage of other minorities in these states can be assumed to be insignificant because they were so small (e.g., less than one percent).

On the other hand, the percentage of African American (and other significant minority) students in states with low levels of juvenile violence were as follows:

Hawaii	2.4% (Hispanics, 4.6%; Asians, 72.2%)
Rhode Island	7.7% (Hispanics, 13.1%; Asians, 3.2%)
New Jersey	18.1% (Hispanics, 14.9%; Asians, 6.1%)
Delaware	30.6% (Hispanics, 5.4%; Asians, 2.2%)
Massachusetts	8.6% (Hispanics, 10.2%; Asians, 4.3%).[4]

As can be seen by these figures, New Jersey does have a relatively high percentage of Hispanics and a small Asian minority. Hawaii has only 2.4 percent blacks, while whites are 20.5 percent, and Asians, the least violent ethnic group, constitute 72.2 percent of the population.

Politically incorrect as it may be, blacks and Hispanics account for a much higher percentage of students in high levels of juvenile violence states, at 33.6 percent, whereas whites and Asians account for 66.4 percent.

Conversely, in the low levels of juvenile violence states, blacks and Hispanics account for only 23.1 percent, whereas whites and Asians account for a larger percentage of the enrolled students in public schools at 76.9 percent. These figures are important. Why is juvenile violence more prevalent with blacks and Hispanics than with whites and Asians?

In fact, previous studies have shown a significantly higher percentage of illiteracy and poverty in black and Hispanic populations. While the gap in the rates at which African-Americans and whites complete high school is narrowing, in the year 2000 there was still a seven percent gap between them. Unfortunately, government programs, such as No Child Left Behind, and welfare programs that increase government dependency have led to a widening in the gap in the first decade of 2000, instead of further narrowing of the gap, as I had hoped. The National Center for Education cites the following statistics from the U.S. Department of Education for 2013–2014: "black students graduated at a rate of 72.5 percent; Hispanics graduated at 76.3 percent; whites graduated at a rate of 87.2 percent; Asians/Pacific Islanders graduated at a rate of 89.4 percent."[5]

Yet, according to Cherrie Bucknor for the Center for Economic and Policy Research, the gap is narrower when using census statistics. Her study found that in 2013, "the black completion rate rose to its highest ever, 86.5 percent, and the black-white gap fell to 6.9 percentage points." Bucknor explained the reason for using census data was that all other statistics are calculated on a four-year period. The study conducted by the Center for

Economic and Policy Research used status completion rate, so that it included blacks who took longer than four years to complete schooling as well as those who received a GED.[6] Hopefully, the improvement in graduation rates will translate into less juvenile violence in those minorities striving to do better scholastically. Perhaps a much more important factor is family cohesiveness. African-Americans have suffered greatly from the breakdown of the family because of the many government dependency programs targeting them.

As far as the Scholastic Assessment Test (SAT) score averages, there are also significant differences between whites and other minorities. In the year 1999–2000, Asian Americans led the pack in mathematics with math, 565/verbal, 499; followed by whites, math, 530/verbal, 528; then Hispanics, math, 467/verbal, 461; and finally blacks, math, 426/verbal, 434.[7]

Since it has been said that a picture is worth a thousand words, let us look now at Table 2 (right) and compare such important factors as median household income and the level of poverty in the two sets of states.

Table 2: Median household income/poverty level for 1995
(National Center for Education Statistics, 1998)

"High Juvenile Violence" State	Median household income	Percentage of persons below the poverty level
Alabama	$25,991	20.1%
Arkansas	$25,814	14.9%
Louisiana	$27,949	19.7%
Mississippi	$26,538	23.5%
West Virginia	$24,880	16.7%
Average	**$26,234**	**18.9%**

"Low Juvenile Violence" State	Median household income	Percentage of persons below the poverty level
Delaware	$34,928	10.3%
Hawaii	$42,851	10.3%
Massachusetts	$38,574	11.0%
New Jersey	$43,924	7.8%
Rhode Island	$35,359	10.6%
Average	**$39,127**	**10.0%**

Suffice to say, when it comes to median household income, the "high level of juvenile violence" states ($26,234) average only two-thirds that of the "low levels of juvenile violence" states ($39,127).

As seen on the same table, the lower median household income corresponds with the lower socioeconomic status of the "high levels of juvenile violence" states (percent of persons below the poverty level, 18.9 percent versus 10 percent).[8]

While Criminological Evidence is Ignored, PHE Propaganda is Parroted

Yes, the death of any child by any cause is a tragedy. I, too, decry the high levels of violence in our society. As a neurosurgeon who has seen first-hand the effects of gunshot wounds on the central nervous system and actually having treated wounded victims of crimes, I too deplore the level of violence and crime in America, but physicians and public health officials should have the moral courage to recognize the fact there is another side to the story— namely, criminological and sociological data that is seldom promulgated by the media and needs dissemination in the medical literature. The medical politicians of the AMA and "organized medicine" must place objective science above partisan emotionalism.

We now know, for example, *that the defensive uses of firearms by lawful citizens, at up to 2 million to 2.5 million per year, dwarf the offensive gun uses by criminals. Between 25 and 75 lives are saved by a gun for every one life lost to a gun. Medical costs saved by guns in the hands of law-abiding citizens are 15 times greater than costs incurred by criminal uses of firearms. Gun safety programs for children, particularly the NRA's Eddie Eagle GunSafe® program, have resulted in a steady decline in unintentional injuries over the last several decades.*[9]

The number of guns in the civilian U.S. population has been increasing steadily for decades, and yet the number of fatal gun accidents has been falling for as long as statistics have been compiled (since 1903). In 1945, there were 350,000 firearms and eighteen fatal gun accidents per million Americans. By 1995, although the number of guns in the U.S. had more than doubled, incredibly there were only six fatalities per million Americans.

According to government figures, at least 45 to 50 percent of U.S. households have firearms in the home. And yet the latest U.S. statistics show that the rates of serious crimes, including homicides with firearms and aggravated assaults, have fallen to record 25-year lows—despite the fact that the number of guns in the hands of Americans have probably exceeded the 300 million mark, approximately one million firearms per million Americans.

Recently, the liberal media has been reporting that according to public polls, the number of households with firearms is falling, standing at about 33 percent. Obviously, they had not read what criminologists, like Professor Gary Kleck, found about gun polls and what we have reported in this book, namely that surveys about guns are unreliable because people fear telling the truth about their gun ownership. We found confirmation of this in a survey conducted by *JAMA*. For example on question number 20 of that survey: "If asked by a pollster whether I owned firearms, I would be truthful? 29.6 percent disagreed/strongly disagreed."[9] So according to this survey, 29.6 percent would falsely deny owning a firearm. We know from this survey and other data that nearly one-third of respondents intentionally conceal their gun ownership because they fear future confiscation by the police as has happened in cities such as Washington, D.C., Detroit, and New York.

Furthermore, we should ask ourselves why Switzerland, New Zealand, and Israel with modest gun control laws (as opposed to the draconian gun control laws in most of the rest of the world) and relatively easy availability of firearms, have low rates of homicide and violence, with or without firearms. It is because those countries in similarity with Japan that have stringent gun laws still have an intact family structure and cultural cohesion with civility and discipline traditionally passed from parents to children and preserved in the population.

Yes, we must lay the blame for the persistence of violence in America where it belongs, and it's not in "easy gun availability" but in many factors, as we have seen: broken families and the cycle of government dependency, the failure of progressive public education, and the general cultural disintegration that has been taking place for decades, particularly in the poorer southern states, and for which the federal government has been largely responsible.

Incidentally, if I have not been more pointed in addressing specific errors in my criticisms of this study by Miller and associates, it's because the raw, primary data that the authors supposedly used in formulating their conclusions were never made available for public review, despite my request to the authors.[10]

One expert who has already raised pointed objections to specific statistical errors in methodology in the study is Roger Schlafly, Ph.D., a mathematician. He wrote me about this study, as well as an article published in *The Economist*, "Bang, Bang, You're Dead" (March 2, 2002), vaunting the study of Miller and associates.

Schlafly states that in reality the highest childhood firearm death rates are in three rural states—Alaska, Montana, and Idaho—with much hunting but less accessible emergency care. He holds that the study actually used "adult fatality rates to estimate firearm ownership levels so that the only insight gained by the study is that child firearm fatalities are correlated with adult gun fatalities."

Schlafly also points out that although the authors mentioned gun survey data, Miller and associates instead used a modified "Cook's Index"—an index that they asserted excludes suicides and homicides among children 0–19 years of age from the calculations in the study and that they affirmed is highly correlated with gun availability measures.

The study thus ranked the states not only by "Cook's Index," the supposed proxy for firearm availability, but also to select the five "high-gun" and five "low-gun" states.

Roger Schlafly remarked, "I am a little baffled as to why this story would be news [in *The Economist*]. Wouldn't everyone expect that high-gun states would have more gun deaths than low-gun states? Isn't that obvious whether you are pro-gun or anti-gun? States with more cars probably have more car accidents also.

"The only thing I found surprising was that '16 times.' If one state had twice as many guns, then I'd expect about twice as many gun accidents. But why 16 times? I doubt that any state has 16 times as many guns (per capita) as another state. The study neglects to mention that the child firearm accidental death rate is on a long-term decline.

"During the 10-year study period, the annual [child firearm accidental death] rate declined from 0.69 to 0.31 per 100,000. (Based on the same CDC figures used by the study available online.)"[10]

Obviously, my own objections, with which Schlafly also agrees, and which were described for the reader in this two-part critique, are more broad and encompassing and extend not only to flaws in specific assumptions and methodologies but also to the overall design of the study and the misuse of epidemiologic research.

Miller and associates' complex study using an even more complex methodology—e.g., "pooled, cross-sectional, time-series data from the fifty states over a one year period" and the so-called "Cook's Index" as proxy for firearm availability—are yet more colorful examples of what the eminent epidemiologist and physician Dr. Bruce G. Charlton, of the University of Newcastle upon Tyne, calls "statistical malpractice."[11]

The peer review process at the *Journal of Trauma* failed. The reviewers must have become lost, along with the authors, in the concoction of numbers and fecund statistics. Miller and associates used statistical malpractice in their failed effort to blame firearms per se for the tragic loss of children's lives without seriously considering the role of more important variables.

Despite the authors' claim that "state level analyses were adjusted for state urbanization, poverty, and education levels," they actually failed to do so because of the lack of control over the overwhelmingly complex, confounding factors. What about other variables, such as reading and television-watching habits in children, culture and ethnicity, that were not even considered by the investigators?

Errors of this type are referred to as "ecologic fallacy" in epidemiologic studies, whereby complex analytical techniques are combined with large data sets involving general populations extending over long periods of time.

Statistics are not science. They may show correlations, but they cannot prove cause and effect relationships because of the large amounts of variance and myriad numbers of confounding factors.[12]

This type of statistical legerdemain to prove cause and effect relationships in science was indeed exposed years ago by Dr. Charlton, who warned other scientists:

> *Minimization of bias is a matter of controlling and excluding extraneous causes from observation and experiment so that the cause of interest may be isolated and characterized.... Maximization of precision, on the other hand, is the attempt to reveal the true magnitude of a variable which is being obscured by the 'noise' [from the] limitations of measurement.*[11]

Conclusion

The authors of the Miller study failed not only to exclude extraneous causes from their "pooled, cross-sectional, time-series data" but also to incorporate into their analysis and conclusions the "true magnitude of the variables"—poverty, level of education, ethnicity, urbanization, race, broken families, et cetera—among the children in the several states.

In fact, in observing cultural differences, such as juvenile violence, lower socioeconomic and educational standards, impacting most detrimentally the southern states and analyzing the findings of the *Journal of Trauma* study, the thoughtful critic and honest scholar could very well ask himself if indeed the South has fully recovered from the devastation of the Civil War and the Reconstruction that followed more than a century ago.[13]

Try as the authors may have done, statistical adjustments failed to remove the multiple confounding variables. Dr. Charlton's admonition was forsaken in the conception and design of the Miller study.

> *As a result, medicine has been deluged with more or less uninterpretable 'answers' generated by heavyweight statistics operating on big databases of dubious validity. Such numerical manipulations cannot, in principle, do the work of hypothesis testing. Statistical analysis has expanded beyond its legitimate realm of activity. The seductive offer of precision without the need for understanding is a snare to the incautious because exactitude is so often mistaken for explanation.*[11]

In other words, this published gun (control) study is an example of politically driven propaganda, result-oriented research with preordained, biased conclusions, which can only be characterized as junk science.[12,14-16]

Still, if the editors of the *Journal of Trauma* had insisted in publishing it, they should have printed it with an editorial caveat that such "pooled, cross-sectional, timed-series data" studies, involving such large populations over a long period of time, are utterly unreliable, even more so than cohort and case studies analyses, subject to ecologic fallacy limiting their value in science.

The editors of the *Journal of Trauma* have done a disservice to their readers, obfuscating rather than contributing to solving the problem of violence in our society.

CHAPTER 11
DEBUNKING THE TYPICAL ECOLOGIC STUDY LINKING GUN OWNERSHIP WITH VIOLENT CRIME

It's very seldom that the same man knows much of science,
and about the things that were known before science came.

—Lord Dunsany (1878—1957),
Edward Plunkett, 18th Baron of Dunsany, Anglo-Irish writer and dramatist

Ecologic studies are notorious for inherent errors of methodology, confounding variables, and magnifying other sample biases intrinsic to fault-prone, population-based epidemiologic studies. But in the paper, "Firearm Ownership and Violent Crime in the U.S.—An Ecologic Study," published in the *American Journal of Preventive Medicine* in 2015,[1] we find additional problems resulting from the well-known proclivity of many public health researchers of using preordained, result-oriented research to push their personal views favoring gun control and aiming at disarming law-abiding citizens, purportedly to reduce gun crime perpetrated by the not-so-law-abiding felons and career criminals who, as a matter of course, ignore and flout the law.[2-4]

The Obligatory Comparison with
"Other Industrialized Nations"

From the outset the article reveals the authors' biases. The reader should note that Dr. David Hemenway, a well-known anti-gun Professor of Health Policy at the Harvard School of Public Health, was also a coauthor in the study discussed in the previous chapter. Even though more than a decade has passed, the ingrained bias, the error of methodology, and the preordained results persist. This new study begins by listing frightening statistics of gun homicides in the U.S. and making the usual obligatory comparison with other "industrialized nations (mostly Europe)," neglecting world demographics, migrations, socioeconomics, history and geography. To me, as a Hispanic (Cuban-American), this selective obligatory comparison with the "industrialized nations," usually the European social democracies, is irksome and outright offensive. Is this convenient neglect of the rest of the world motivated by more than convenience or is there something else? Are not the citizens of other less developed nations of equal value in terms of life to those of the developed nations and industrialized Europe? Why don't these elitist authors compare gun laws and discuss violent crime, much less express any humanitarian concern for gun violence in our next door neighbor, Mexico, or our comparable in size neighbor to the south Brazil, and most of the Western hemisphere?[5-6]

In fact, when it comes to violence, objectively compared to developed nations, the U.S. is in the middle of the pack, despite high immigration and a large heterogeneous population. When considering the rest of the world, the U.S. is far behind Latin America (including Brazil), Africa, and much of Eastern Europe and Eurasia (including Russia).

The authors' discussion then proceeds with another obligatory phraseology linking, "firearm availability and violent crime." In the international global perception, this phraseology sometimes refers to what has been termed "America's gun culture" by European publications, *The Economist* among them. Considering history and geopolitics, it may be worth mentioning that what has been termed "America's gun culture" may have contributed in part to the mindset and dogged determination of Americans toward the liberation of Europeans from the Nazis during World War II, and subsequently for decades protected all of the indulgent and effete social democracies of Western Europe from the menacing Soviet Red Army and the threat of the T-54/55 Soviet tanks rolling and overrunning the central and western European landscape during the Cold War.[7-9]

Now, let's return to the study. To the authors' credit, a minor effort was made to "capture data" on demographics and socioeconomics, but the information was unfortunately lost in the cocktail of bewilderingly complex analytical techniques and large data sets created by these ecological concoctions.[10-11] The reality is that for these authors, firearm violence was the sole issue under discussion; no other societal causes were remotely considered for the endemic violence in the U.S., such as the decades-long decline in educational level, the influence of the vulgar popular culture, television violence, increasing rates of single parenthood and broken families, drug trafficking and gang-related violence, the permissive criminal justice system, and the state of dependency and alienation fostered by the welfare state—a veritable cultural regression perpetuating immorality and violence[12] that journalist Cal Thomas wrote in a recent column is morally "rotting from within."[13]

In this study, linking homicides to guns was the ultimate objective. No distinction was made to separate criminal homicides from justifiable gun homicides or self-defense shootings. No significant effort was made to delineate the beneficial aspects (preventive or defensive uses) of gun ownership in incidents involving assaults, robberies, and homicides—e.g., the very topics supposedly of interest to the researchers.

Nevertheless, the authors purportedly reached alarming conclusions— namely, that states with higher levels of gun ownership have an increased risk for assaults and robberies perpetrated with firearms.[1] Haven't we heard that before regardless of time, place, population sample or collected data?

Blissfully Ignoring Previous Objections

Although the flaws of the ecologic methodology are evident, the omissions are even more damaging to the study. The seminal work in these areas conducted and published by researcher John Lott is not cited or even mentioned.[3]

The authors cannot see the forest for the trees: The fact is lost that while Americans continue to purchase and possess more private firearms than ever in our history, rates of homicide and violent crimes have steadily diminished for several decades because more guns, at least in the hands of the law-abiding citizens, does not translate into more crime.[3-4] The number of private firearms has in fact increased from approximately 200 million in 1995 to 300 million in 2012, with a concomitant decrease in both homicides and violent crimes since 1993 to the present.[2,14]

Moreover, as shown by the work of Gary Kleck and John Lott, firearms in the hands of law-abiding citizens decrease crime. There is considerable historical evidence that gun ownership in the hands of citizens also protects their property and their freedom.[7-9] The problem with endemic crime is not which states have the most guns but with irresponsible gun ownership and the proportion of illegal guns in the hands of criminal elements.[12,14] Despite laws to the effect, we as a society have not kept guns from falling into the wrong hands because of our broken criminal justice and mental health systems, not to mention an overall deteriorating moral value system, due to the prevailing zeitgeist of our time. This should be obvious to anyone who cares to reflect and evaluate our descent in cultural devolution.[12,13]

This study is subject to similar flaws as those repeatedly found in much of the public health literature dealing with guns and violence, including the one previously analyzed in Chapters 9 and 10 in which senior researcher Hemenway was also one of the authors.[15] No significant effort was made to address some of the objections many of us made regarding bias and politicization of their gun research. Consequently, we can understand why Congress in 1996 after carefully studying the issue defunded and thereafter wisely refused to resume funding "gun [control] research"—or rather, gun control propaganda masquerading as gun violence research.[17-22]

Doctors for Responsible Gun Ownership (DRGO), individual physicians, and independent investigators have been documenting this fact for years.[19,20] Yet if the question is asked about who is responsible for defunding gun research, public health apologists will answer that the NRA is solely responsible![21-22] *Ignored is the fact independent investigators have provided Congress over the years with published articles and confirmatory evidence that much of the gun research conducted by public health researchers was junk science, biased research, promulgated by the ideologically committed as well as self-serving public health officials in cahoots with the very public relations-conscious leaders of the AMA, "organized medicine," and their publications.*[14,16-20,23]

It should also be of interest that private researchers, particularly those associated or sponsored by the pharmaceutical and chemical industries, are frequently disparaged by those in the PHE, as if the fiduciary association of the former immediately taints their integrity, work, and conclusions. But why is this not so the other way around, for those receiving tax money or donations from anti-gun magnates such as George Soros and Michael Bloomberg? Why is this not the case also for research funded by private tax-exempt foundations, such as the Joyce Foundation, which are known to have progressive, socioeconomic agendas to reconstruct society in their image and with ideological axes to grind? Why do those same gun researchers, decade after decade, keep telling us that more studies are needed (and additional funding necessary)—militating for their own financial self-interests as well as subsidizing their ideological agendas? These are good questions whose answers may save taxpayers bundles of money and in the long term, perhaps, even preserve their freedom!

CHAPTER 12

WHO COULD COMPLAIN ABOUT INNOCUOUS PUBLIC DATABASES?

Epidemiology [is a] main culprit, because statistical mal-practice typically occurs when complex analytical tech-niques are combined with large data sets. Indeed, the better the science, the less the need for complex analysis, and big databases are a sign not of rigor but of poor control.

—Bruce G. Charlton, M.D.,
University of Newcastle upon Tyne, from his
article "Statistical Malpractice" (1996)

A much more subtle approach than faulty ecologic studies at promoting gun control, so to speak through the back door, was recently made by Boston University public health researchers, Michael Siegle and Molly Pahn. Their article, titled "New public database reveals striking differences in how guns are regulated from state to state" seems innocuous enough, until one inspects the content of the article.[1]

Biased Compilers, Suspect Databases

Neuroradiologist Tom Vaughan, M.D., a witty writer and an active DRGO member, carefully analyzed the article by Siegle and Pahn. He wrote: "While such a database, constructed impartially, could be very useful, the authors reveal their strong anti-Second Amendment bias. They have salted the article with a few facts, but they have also included several misleading statements as well as blatant lies."[2] Indeed, this was my very own impression.

To begin with, as Dr. Vaughan noted, although there was a small spike in the firearms death in the period between 2014 and 2015, the authors conveniently failed to describe the trend of the previous 35 years, which saw a decrease in firearm deaths despite a tremendous increase in gun purchases. So except for this spike in the last reported two years, an astronomical increase in gun ownership has taken place during those 35 years, with a concomitant impressive reduction in violent crime during the same period![2] The incredible omission of this vital information is simply astonishing negligence or deliberate omission with the researchers simply getting caught red-handed in the act of academic dishonesty!

Dr. Vaughan, commented:

> *Two blatant lies are used in a ham-fisted attempt to discredit pro-gun legislation. The first is a gross mischaracterization of what are generally termed 'stand your ground' laws. Vilifying these has become a cause célèbre with the anti-gun crowd. Siegel claims these laws 'allow people to shoot other people as a first resort in public.' This is of course an outrageous mendacity, and a lie of the sort that should discredit any university professor.[2]*

Dr. Vaughan is of course correct because the statement veers off from colorful hyperbole to overt inflammatory mendacity. The DRGO physician further pointed out:

> *The second outright lie in the article regards the Protection of Lawful Commerce in Arms Act and the protection it affords firearms manufacturers when their legally manufactured products are used in the commission of crimes. After initially admitting that the law simply does exactly that, they falsely claim 'no other consumer product manufacturer enjoys such broad immunity.' As if Lexus could be held liable if one of their cars was deliberately driven into a crowd of people, or Stanley could be successfully sued when one of their hammers is used to bludgeon someone to death.[2]*

I too had my share of criticisms of the Siegel and Pahn article, supposedly announcing the inception of an objective public database. The authors conveniently failed to describe the general trend of the previous 35 years stating only, "From 2014 to 2015, the United States experienced its largest annual increase in firearm deaths over the past 35 years, a 7.8 percent upturn in a single year."[1]

This period witnessed a decrease in firearm deaths despite a tremendous increase in gun purchases. So except for the brief spike of 2014–2015 a tremendous increase in gun ownership took place during which time violent crime also dropped dramatically. Yet, Siegle and Pahn deliberately omitted describing this trend so they could arrive at their predetermined conclusion that more firearms equal more deaths. Simply stated, by neglecting to mention a long and important period of study as to exclude inconvenient data, Siegle and Pahn committed academic dishonesty.

I would be remiss, if I did not inform the reader that the FBI has released the latest 2016 crime statistics that show violent crime rose 4.1 percent, while property crime decreased 1.3 percent in the 2015 to 2016 period. But, as the FBI observes, "taken collectively these offenses declined for the 14th consecutive year." We do not know if this increase in violent crime represents a continuation of the spike (representing a true reversal and an increase in violent crime rates) in the 2014–2016 year period or whether this is a transient aberration. As noted, property crimes continued their downward trend. In either case, the spike or trend does not contravene what has happened in the previous 35 years or the relationship we have established objectively that more guns does not translate into more crime. What needs to be established is whether this recent spike is related to resurgence in violent crime due to increased racial strife and the political incitement that surfaced and intensified during Obama's second term, or whether it's related to homegrown Islamic terrorism, as we will analyze with mass shootings in Chapter 22. It should be noted that this latest rise in violent crime, particularly homicides, according to the Brennan Center was "fueled by just three cities, Chicago, Baltimore, and Washington, D.C." In fact, Chicago accounted for more than half the number. All three cities have strict gun control laws.[3]

Ignoring the Federal System of Law Enforcement

As for common crime and gun violence in the 2014–2015 period, "What did Congress do to confront this problem?" Siegle and Pahn, prejudicially ask.[1] To which I pointedly reply that it is a problem for the states to solve, not the federal government. Common crime, even those perpetrated with firearms, is in the purview of the state governments. Federal policing has resulted in the militarization of local law enforcement,[3] which in turn has been responsible for several high profile police shootings that have then been used, conveniently, by the sensationalist and liberal media to denigrate the local police, foment unrest based on race baiting, and irresponsibly incite further violence, riots, and street crime. Some irresponsible politicians have even sided with the street thugs and blamed the police for the riots and violence.[4] The effect of this denigration and attack on the local police has resulted in a cycle of violence, police shootings and, generally, to yield the streets to the thugs who have been turned lose in the communities, predictably spinning a cycle of more urban disorder and crime.[5]

Moreover, we should stress that centralization of the police force, as Siegle and Pahn subtly yet distinctly propose under their innocent sounding new database announcement, is an authoritarian concept that is foreign to our Constitution. Our founders decried "standing armies" as a feature of tyrannical government. Indeed, the exercise of police powers is a prerogative of the states in our Republican decentralized federalist system of government. The states have been called "the laboratories of democracy," and to be abso- lutely sure that the states preserve their prerogatives, James Madison inserted the Tenth Amendment in the Bill of Rights, which reads: "The powers not delegated to the United States by the Constitution, nor prohibited by it to the states, belong to the states respectively, or to the people." Those powers include local police in crime control, not standing federal armies. Little by little these progressive academicians seek to erode the constitution with such pronouncements, assuming that we dull conservatives will be caught napping!

Law-abiding citizens are not the problem. When it comes to crime, the criminals who by definition do not obey the laws are the culprits.[6] The FBI statistics reveal that 75 percent of all violent crimes for any locality are committed by six percent of hardened criminals and repeat offenders. The typical murderer has had a prior criminal history of at least six years with four felony arrests in his record before he finally commits murder.[7] But it is the lawful citizens who lose more freedom bit by bit and suffer from more gun control laws. Very few crimes are committed by citizens with concealed carry weapons (CCW) licenses. In fact, less than one to two percent of permit holders do so, and the transgressions are usually technicalities. Yet the suggestion by the gun prohibitionists that lawful citizens with firearms are prone to violence and create mayhem, supposedly like in an Old Wild West scenario, is used to demonize gun-owning citizens and concealed carry license holders.

Siegle and Pahn misconstrued the point that "stand your ground" laws instigate killings. With caustic and inflammatory rhetoric, the authors wrote:

"States are increasingly enacting laws that allow people to shoot other people as a first resort in public, instead of retreating when threatened. If a person perceives a threat of serious bodily harm, so-called 'stand your ground' laws, allow them to fire their gun with immunity from prosecution, as long as they are in a place they have a legal right to be." How is that for objective phraseology supposedly coming from unbiased data collectors! The authors, though, are correct when they report that between 2004 and 2017, 24 states enacted "stand your ground" laws. However, the authors failed to mention that following adoption of these laws there was no increase in the rates of criminal homicides or mass shootings in those states. Needless to say, that was not mentioned by the authors because it did not fit with their preconceived notions and was contrary to what they were bent on proving.

Siegle and Pahn also misrepresented the so-called "gun show loophole" by which only licensed firearm dealers are required to do federal background checks. Dr. Vaughan noted that the authors failed to reveal that in the past 10 years those who have committed homicides with a purchased firearm had passed the federal check, a fact acknowledged even by *The New York Times*. And most importantly that "several studies have demonstrated that common criminals obtain their guns almost exclusively through illegal means—between known criminals, theft, etc." Dr. Vaughan also added, "They [criminals] will never subject themselves to background checks."[2]

Dr. Vaughan is again correct. A U.S. Department of Justice study found that for a typical year as in 2004, "among state prison inmates who possessed a gun at the time of the offense, less than two percent bought their firearm at a flea market or gun show and 40 percent obtained their firearm from an illegal source."[8]

In short, how can we trust these so-called public databases, when they are promulgated by such biased public health researchers as evinced by the outlandish irrepressible statements made in announcing the database? The answer is obvious. We can't. Science once again has been subverted by political ideology, and the disarming of lawful Americans is to be planned and conducted at their own [taxpayer] expense.

Other Criticisms of the Public Health Model of Gun Control

Doctors for Responsible Gun Ownership (DRGO) has been very critical of the AMA and "organized medicine" as well as the PHE's gun control agenda. In a three-part series, Dr. Arthur Z. Przebinda, an imaging specialist in Southern California and DRGO's Project Director, explored the "public health" approach to gun control. One of his conclusions is that the PHE in studying gun violence uses faulty epidemiological studies, and in its preconceived obsession with the gun as an evil "talisman" that must be restricted, neglects other important factors. He writes, "The rejection of psychological, sociological and criminological factors as foremost contributors of 'gun violence' is the bedrock on which public health advocacy research rests. That is why all public health work on the matter portrays guns and gun ownership as the determining factor in whatever societal ill we'd all like to see alleviated." He adds, "Public health *must* disregard social, economic, and mental health factors for its advocacy to be coherent."[9] Indeed, as we have observed in previous chapters, much of the work of public health on the issue of guns and violence has neglected criminological, psychosocial and psychiatric factors because their work has been tainted by preconceived ideology and preordained results.

Another illustrative example of a faulty epidemiological study making guns inherently evil was shown in another recent study published in the *American Journal of Public Health* attempting to demonstrate that firearms "drive" rural suicides in the state of Maryland. Dr. Thomas E. Gift, M.D., a child and adolescent psychiatrist and an associate clinical professor of psychiatry at the University of Rochester Medical School, has criticized this study on various points, including geographic and social misrepresentation in that the authors claimed that they were comparing rural and urban areas but, "the counties in Maryland they labeled as 'rural' were largely suburban." Another criticism was the use of complex numerical manipulations, "without any attempt to control for the associations which arose solely by chance, but they called "significant." Yet, they ignored the small level of statistical confidence "by the very low percentage of total suicides that occurred in the counties they label rural."[10]

We have previously shown how public health researchers had tried to promote the view that guns were like viruses causing an epidemic of gun violence in the form of homicides. By now readers may suspect that this new study funded and conducted by the Johns Hopkins Bloomberg School of Public Health would also try to link guns as the causative agent (the virus) for suicides. Indeed, this new study had a preordained goal—that gun availability promotes suicides by demonstrating that "rural" counties in Maryland with higher rates of gun ownership had higher rates of suicides. The study, biased from the outset and riddled with errors of methodology, failed to prove such a cause and effect relationship.

We have also discussed the work of Dr. Timothy Wheeler, founder and past director of DRGO—initially a project of the Claremont Institute, now a project of the Second Amendment Foundation—in the context of the subversion of science and medicine in earlier chapters by both the AMA and the PHE. Wheeler has also been adamant that "organized medicine" has done a disservice to their members for the continued politicization of medicine as to both medical journalism and ethical boundary violations. These are among the issues that we will be discussing in the next chapters when we more deeply explore the politics of the AMA and the major medical journals, sponsored and beholden to the various organizations falling under the umbrella of "organized medicine."

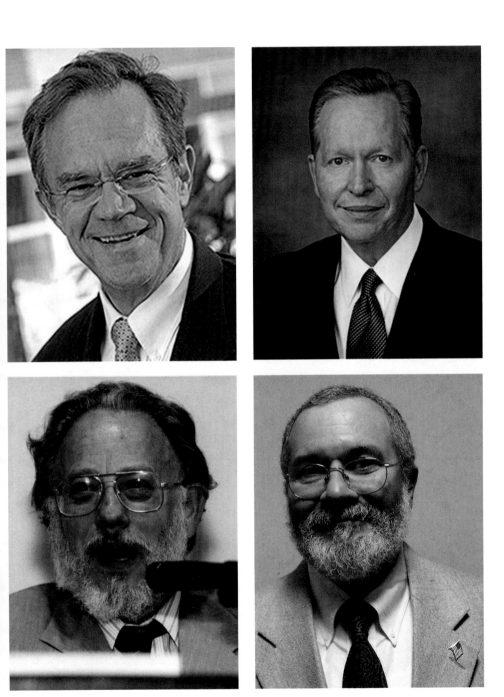

The four witnesses who testified before the U.S. House Appropriations Subcommittee about the misuse of science by public health researchers in the pursuit of a politicized gun control agenda. From left to right: William C. Waters, IV, M.D. (c. 2008); Timothy W. Wheeler, M.D. (c. 2016); Don B. Kates, JD (c. 2008); and Miguel A. Faria, Jr., M.D. (c. 2008). Don B. Kates, courtesy of the Independent Institute.

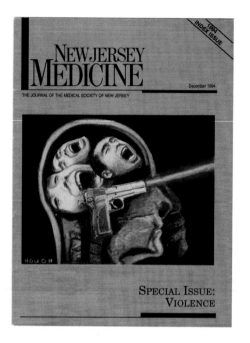

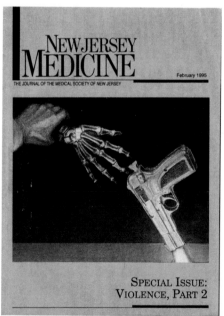

The mainstream media used their publications for gun control propaganda, and so did the public health establishment and the medical journals. From top to bottom: *New Jersey Medicine,* December 1994 and February 1995. Courtesy of the Medical Society of New Jersey. *Injury Prevention Newsletter* of the CDC, Spring 1995, "Women, Guns, and Domestic Violence." Among the many instructions to activists, the newsletter advised picketing gun manufacturing sites, boycotting publications that accept advertising from gun manufacturers, launching programs to indoctrinate pediatricians and the police about guns, et cetera. The Newsletter was entered into evidence in the files of misuse of taxpayers' money intended for public health research used as political propaganda.

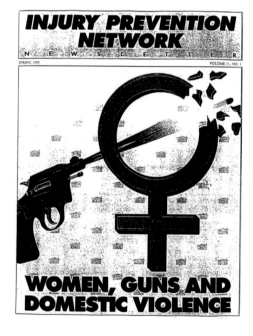

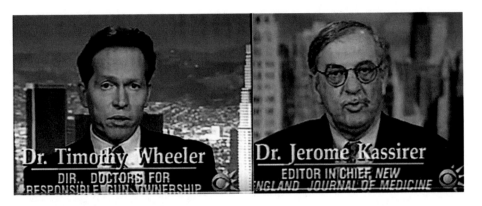

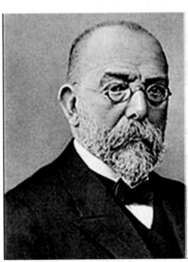

Koch's Postulates

Evidence required to establish etiologic relationship between microorganism and disease:

1. Microorganism must be observed in every case of the disease

2. It must be isolated and grown in pure culture

3. The pure culture, when inoculated in animals, must reproduce the disease

4. Microorganism must be recovered from the diseased animal

Top: Dr. Timothy Wheeler faced Dr. Jerome Kassirer, editor of the *New England Journal of Medicine*, on *CBS This Morning*, September 1995. Dr. Wheeler showed on television a newsletter advocating gun control masquerading as science and published and distributed at taxpayer expense. Courtesy of Doctors for Responsible Gun Ownership (DRGO). Bottom: Robert Koch (1843–1910) German physician, pathologist, and microbiologist with his Postulates of Pathogenicity. (Author's file)

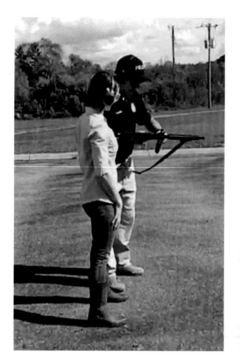
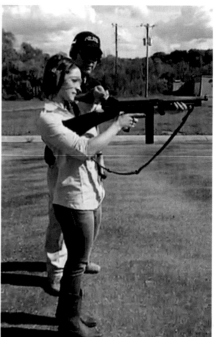
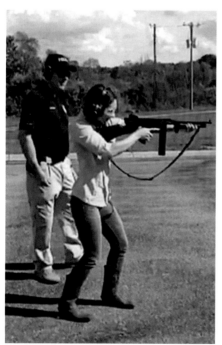
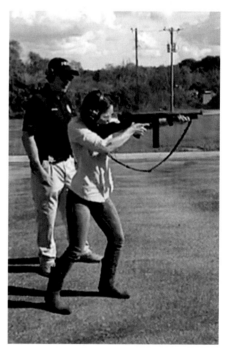

Elena Faria Mitchell, author's daughter and now a practicing attorney, receives firearm training from the local police department just before graduating from the University of Virginia School of Law in 2015. (Author's files)

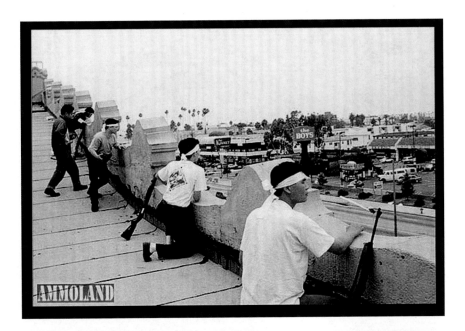

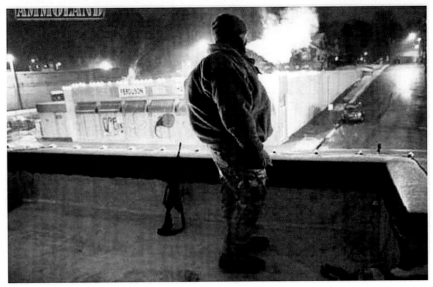

Top: Korean shopkeepers protect their stores from looters on the roof of their buildings during the Rodney King riots in L.A. in the spring of 1992. Bottom: Citizens (Oath Keepers) patrol and guard from rooftops during the Ferguson riots in November 2014 to protect their businesses, despite police opposition. Courtesy of Ammoland & Dean Weingarten (2014) and http://gunwatch.blogspot.com/.

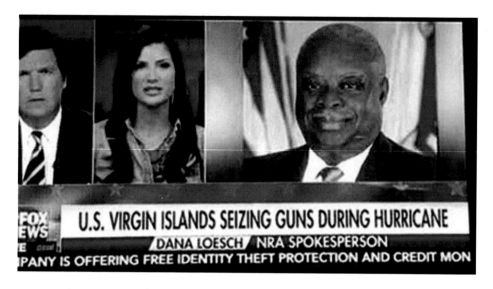

U.S. VIRGIN ISLANDS SEIZING GUNS DURING HURRICANE
DANA LOESCH / NRA SPOKESPERSON
PANY IS OFFERING FREE IDENTITY THEFT PROTECTION AND CREDIT MON

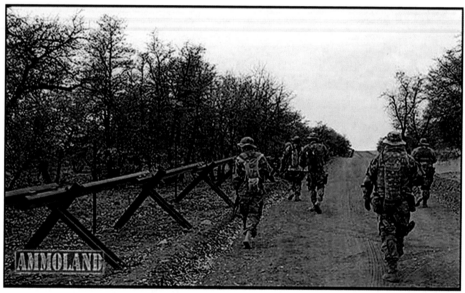

Top: U.S. Virgin Islands planning confiscation of firearms in anticipation of Hurricane Irma in the late summer of 2017. Bottom: As a result of inadequate government response to natural disasters, such as Hurricane Katrina, citizen militia forces are prepared to protect lives and property in the hinterlands of states like Arizona, Florida, and Indiana. "America's Top Militia Forces Prepped for Society's Worst-Case-Scenarios" was a one-hour Discovery Channel Special (October 2012). Courtesy of Ammoland.

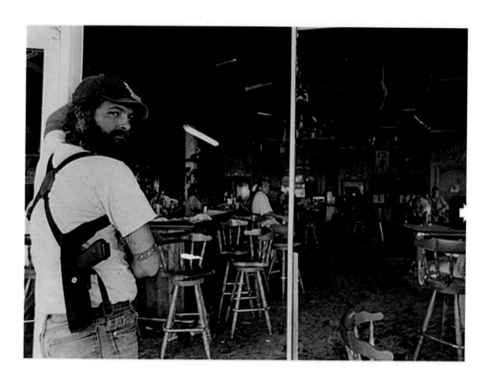

Firearms and "Assault Weapons" during Natural Disasters (I)

Adam "Tad" Verret of Homestead, owner of the Blarney Stone Tavern, protects his business from looters during Hurricane Andrew in 1992. He wrote the author (October 21, 2017):

> *We were without power for months after Hurricane Andrew. We had to protect our property. This was before the widespread use of cell phones. I, personally, used my firearm to protect us twice and got into a gunfight with thieves trying to steal a car, late at night. We got our car back and we didn't get hurt. The Glock model 21 in the shoulder harness I'm wearing was held by Miami-Dade PD until they cleared the shooting. We weren't arrested or charged. Interesting times...Glad I had the right to protect us!*

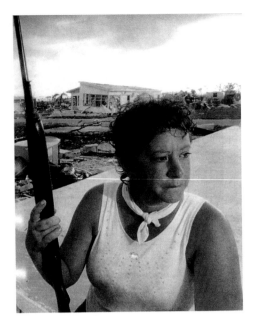
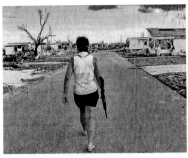
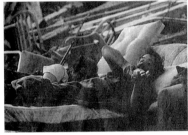

Firearms and "Assault Weapons" during Natural Disasters (II)

Marjorie Conklin Barber of Florida City protected her property and that of her neighbors with a firearm in the aftermath of the devastation of Hurricane Andrew during August 1992. She and her brother Larry (with an M1 rifle) successfully confronted looters and protected what was left of her property. Left: Marjorie Conklin standing guard. Top: Patrolling the neighborhood, rifle in hand. Bottom: Larry Conklin, protecting "what little is left of their property." The photos are reprinted courtesy of Marjorie Conklin Barbie and Larry Conklin. In an interview for this book, Marjorie explained (January 3, 2018):

I was raised in New York in a hunting family, so guns were always a part of my life. I was taught as a young child the damage a gun can do. At the age of 12, I joined a junior NRA gun club and got my first 22 rifle for target practice. I was a member for about four years. Then I got involved with life and growing up and guns took a backstage. After Hurricane Andrew hit, my brother Larry stayed with me at what was left of our house. He has always been an avid gun collector and hunter. We utilized the guns, ammo, and MRE meals to protect and sustain ourselves. During that time I did have one occurrence where I had to draw down on a looter who was stealing from my neighbor's house. As I was preparing to shoot—he backed off and left. It made us so mad that everything we had was destroyed, and yet thugs thought they could just come and take what little we had left. If he had needed food I probably would have shared what we had. But to steal a TV? Bolstered by this experience, I changed occupations and became a correctional officer for the state of Florida prison system and retired after 13 years. I have always been and will always be comfortable with guns, especially to protect myself, my home, and my property.

U.S. Accidental Firearm Deaths

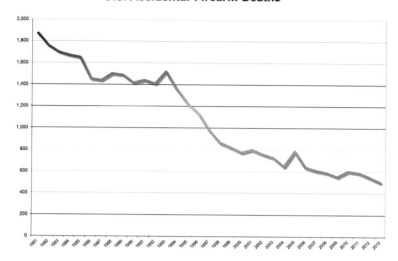

Center for Disease Control, WISQARS

www.GunFacts.info

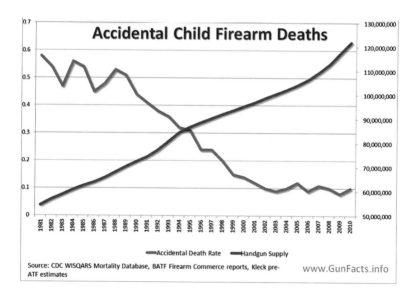

Accidental Child Firearm Deaths

━━Accidental Death Rate   ━━Handgun Supply

Source: CDC WISQARS Mortality Database, BATF Firearm Commerce reports, Kleck pre-ATF estimates

www.GunFacts.info

Top: U.S. Accidental Firearm Deaths have been declining precipitously for more than half a century. Bottom: Likewise, Accidental Child Firearm Deaths have been declining, as related in the text, despite a record number of firearms in the hands of Americans. All graphs, unless otherwise stated, are published courtesy of Guy Smith, from his e-book, *Gun Facts: Version 6.2.*

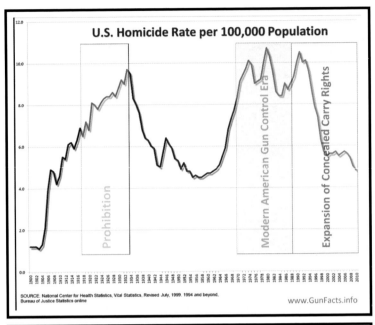

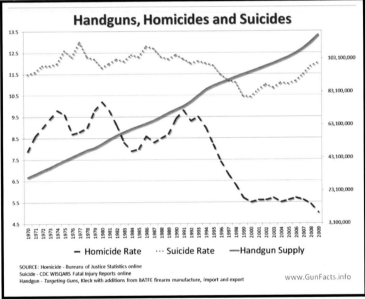

Top: The U.S. Homicide Rate, already on the rise in the modern era of the 20th Century, further increased after alcohol prohibition (XVIII Amendment, 1919) and declined after its repeal (XXI Amendment, 1933), only to increase again after the Gun Control Act of 1968 and the inception of the modern gun control era, remaining so until about 1992 when it drastically declined. Bottom: Handguns, Homicides and Suicides. While the number of handguns increased almost in linear fashion from the 1970s to the present day, suicide rates somewhat stabilized and homicides continued to decline until 2014.

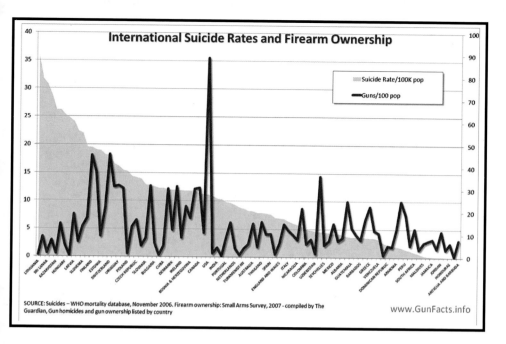

SOURCE: Suicides – WHO mortality database, November 2006. Firearm ownership: Small Arms Survey, 2007 - compiled by The Guardian, Gun homicides and gun ownership listed by country

www.GunFacts.info

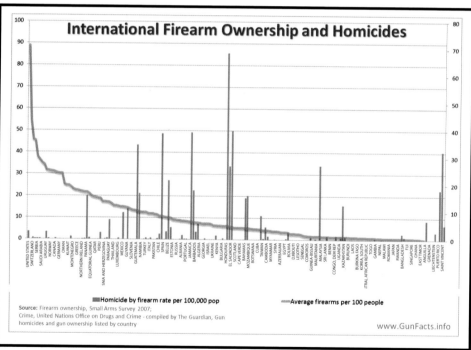

Source: Firearm ownership, Small Arms Survey 2007;
Crime, United Nations Office on Drugs and Crime - compiled by The Guardian, Gun
homicides and gun ownership listed by country

www.GunFacts.info

Top: International Suicide Rates and Firearm Ownership. This graph depicts the position of the U.S. with the grand spike in firearm ownership. Nevertheless, the U.S. occupies a middle position in international suicide rates. Bottom: International Firearm Ownership and Homicides. Despite the extremely high rate of gun ownership, the U.S.—the first blip in this chart—is near the bottom when it comes to homicide rates worldwide. There seems to be no relationship between firearm ownership and international homicide rates because, as with suicide, people use different cultural methods or substitute whatever device they have available to kill themselves or others.

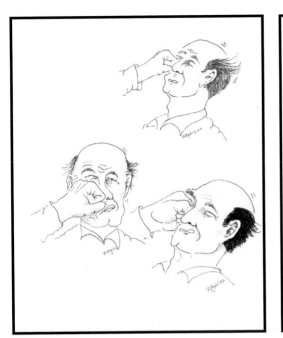

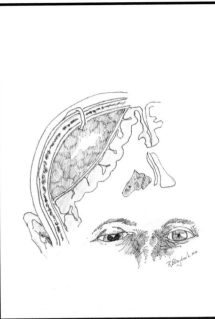

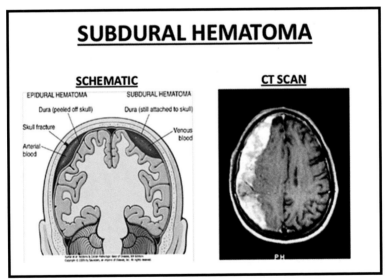

Blunt Head Trauma Causing Brain Damage. Top left: Subdural hematoma can result from blows or even vigorous jerking of the head in an older person during a physical struggle. Top right: Frontal view, subdural hematoma with brain compression and cerebral herniation. Drawings courtesy of Russell L. Blaylock, M.D., Theoretical Neuroscience Research, LLC. Bottom: The schematic and CT scan views of subdural hematoma. This comparative illustration is courtesy of Rozelle Mae Birador, R.N., Laguna State Polytechnic University, Philippines.

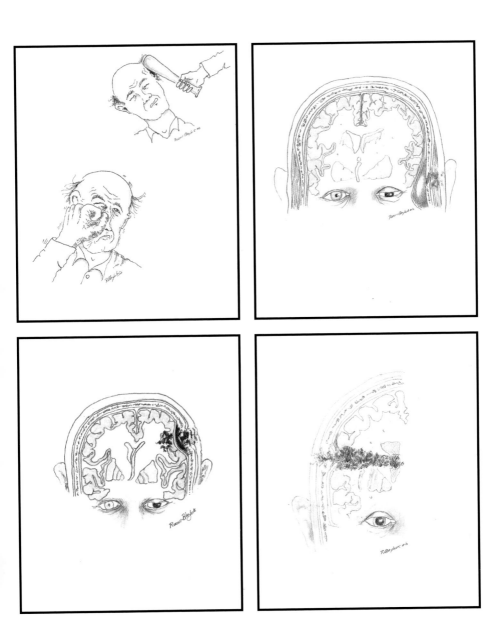

Top left: Head trauma with blunt object may cause subdural hematoma; or Top right: Epidural hematoma with skull fracture; Bottom left: Depressed skull fracture with intracerebral hemorrhage; Bottom right: A sharp object, such as a pair of scissors, a screwdriver, or even a letter opener picked up casually by a burglar can be used for a lethal attack resulting in penetrating brain injury. Drawings courtesy of Russell L. Blaylock, M.D., Theoretical Neuroscience Research, LLC.

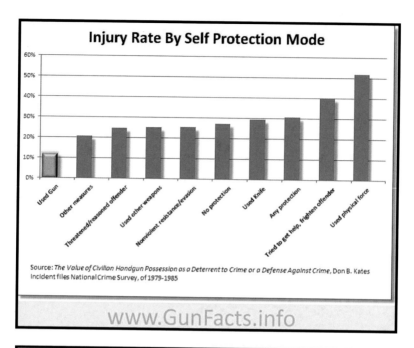

Injury Rate By Self Protection Mode

Source: *The Value of Civilian Handgun Possession as a Deterrent to Crime or a Defense Against Crime*, Don B. Kates Incident files National Crime Survey, of 1979-1985

www.GunFacts.info

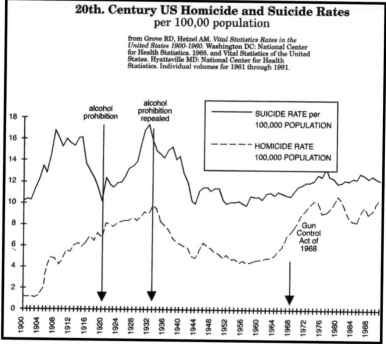

20th. Century US Homicide and Suicide Rates
per 100,00 population

from Grove RD, Hetzel AM. *Vital Statistics Rates in the United States 1900-1960.* Washington DC: National Center for Health Statistics. 1968. and *Vital Statistics of the United States.* Hyattsville MD: National Center for Health Statistics. Individual volumes for 1961 through 1991.

Top: Injury Rate by Self Protection Mode. Using a gun for self-protection is the safest way to avoid injury. Shouting, trying to get help, attempting to frighten the offender, and the use of physical force are the worst methods. Bottom: 20th Century U.S. Homicide and Suicide Rates in Relation to Alcohol Prohibition and the Gun Control Act of 1968.

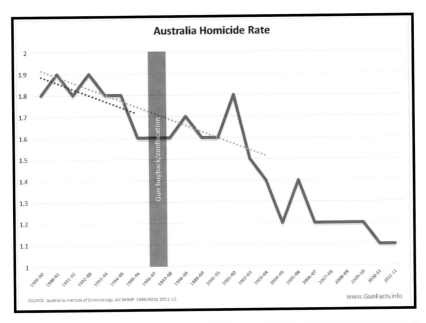

Australia Homicide Rate

Gun buyback/confiscation

SOURCE: Australia Institute of Criminology, AIC NHMP 1989/90 to 2011-12

www.GunFacts.info

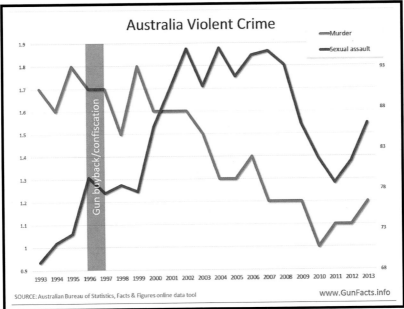

Australia Violent Crime

Murder
Sexual assault

Gun buyback/confiscation

SOURCE: Australian Bureau of Statistics, Facts & Figures online data tool

www.GunFacts.info

Top: Australia's Homicide Rate increased over the next three years following the 1997 Australian Gun Ban, despite the fact the homicide rate had been falling prior to the ban. Repeated gun buyback and confiscation efforts by the Australian government have not resulted in further decreases in crime. Bottom: Australia Violent Crime—i.e., murder and sexual assaults—also increased immediately after the Gun Ban, then decreased, only to increase again after 2010.

British Offenses in 2000	
Offense category	Increase from pre-ban
Armed robbery	170.1%
Kidnapping/abduction	144.0%
Assault	130.9%
Attempted murder	117.6%
Sexual assault	112.6%

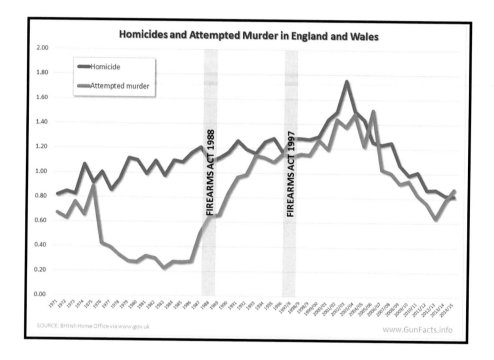

Top: British Offenses in 2000. Armed robbery, kidnapping, assault, attempted murder, and sexual assault all increased more than 100 percent in Great Britain following the Gun Ban of 1997. Bottom: Homicides and attempted murder in England and Wales increased after the Firearm Act of 1988 and even increased more dramatically immediately after the Gun Ban of 1997, only to decline years later but remaining too high, especially for a nation where citizens cannot defend themselves with firearms or any other weapons.

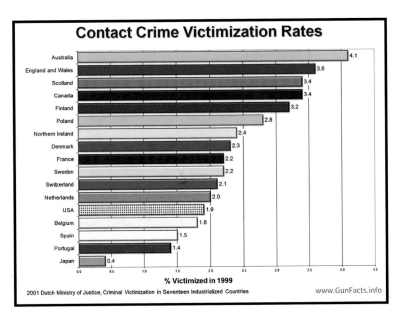

Contact Crime Victimization Rates

Country	% Victimized in 1999
Australia	4.1
England and Wales	3.6
Scotland	3.4
Canada	3.4
Finland	3.2
Poland	2.8
Northern Ireland	2.4
Denmark	2.3
France	2.2
Sweden	2.2
Switzerland	2.1
Netherlands	2.0
USA	1.9
Belgium	1.8
Spain	1.5
Portugal	1.4
Japan	0.4

% Victimized in 1999

2001 Dutch Ministry of Justice, Criminal Victimization in Seventeen Industrialized Countries

www.GunFacts.info

The United States Of America 320,206,000	Compared To Population	England And Wales 53,012,456
3098.6	Offenses per 100,000 Population	24,710
367.9	Violent Crime Rate	1,320
3.9 - 4.5	Murder - Homicide	See Text
25.2	Rape	45.4
109.1	Robbery	99.9
299.1	Aggravated Assault	656.2
2,730.7	Property Crime	3.362.0
610.0	Burglary	804.2
221.3	Auto Theft	140.8

US Data From the FBI Uniform Crime Report, English Data From "Crime in England And Wales, Year Ending September 2014

Top: Contact Crime Victimization Rates are much higher in Australia and Great Britain than in any of the other industrialized nations. The U.S. is near the bottom and Japan, as expected, is at the very bottom of the list. Bottom: England and Wales versus the U.S. As to what has happened in England and Wales compared to the U.S. in other areas of crime, one must look at the FBI Uniform Crime Report for the year, ending in 2014. General offenses in England and Wales are eight times the rate in the U.S.; the violent crime rate is four times; rape is almost twice; aggravated assault, twice; and property crimes and burglaries are, of course, also higher. Only in homicides and auto theft are the crime rates higher in the U.S., but even in those areas the Brits are catching up.

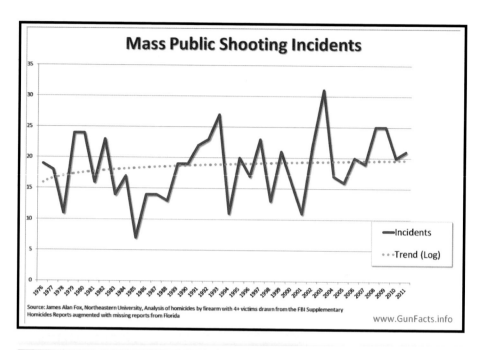

Mass Public Shooting Incidents

Source: James Alan Fox, Northeastern University, Analysis of homicides by firearm with 4+ victims drawn from the FBI Supplementary Homicides Reports augmented with missing reports from Florida

www.GunFacts.info

Legend: —Incidents   •••Trend (Log)

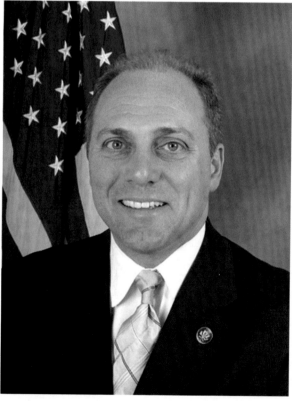

Top: Mass Public Shooting Incidents increased very little between 1976 to 2011, despite various small spikes and dives and a continuous increase in population. I suspect this may have changed for the worse in 2017. We need better ways to predict these deranged killers and detect the terrorists before they strike. Bottom: One voice opposing the chorus calling for gun control was that of U.S. Representative Steve Scalise (R-LA), the Congressman who was shot and seriously wounded at a political mass shooting in 2017. He told Fox News anchor Martha MacCallum that the shooting "fortified" his view on gun rights.

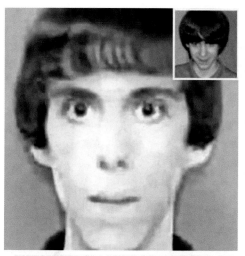

20-year-old Adam Lanza, a loner with a personality disorder, shot 26 people mostly children at Sandy Hook Elementary School in Newtown, Connecticut, on December 14, 2012.

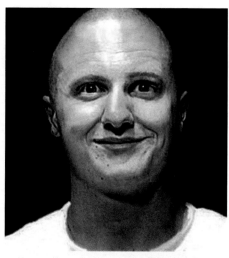

22-year-old Jared Loughner, a disturbed individual, shot and killed 5 people and wounded 15 others, including U.S. Representative Gabrielle Giffords in Arizona in 2011.

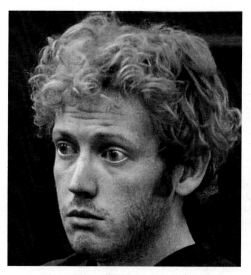

24-year-old James Holmes murdered 12 people and wounded 70 other at a movie theater in Aurora, Colorado, on July 20, 2012.

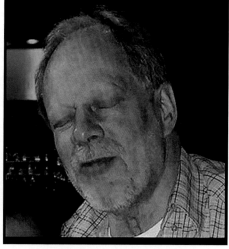

64-year-old Stephen Paddock killed 59 people and wounded 530 others at a Las Vegas outdoor music festival on October 1, 2017.

(Widely circulated photo of Stephen Paddock, allegedly taken the night before the shooting).

Four deranged mass shooters and cold-blooded killers.

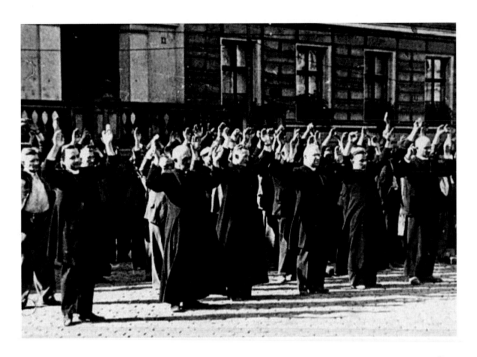

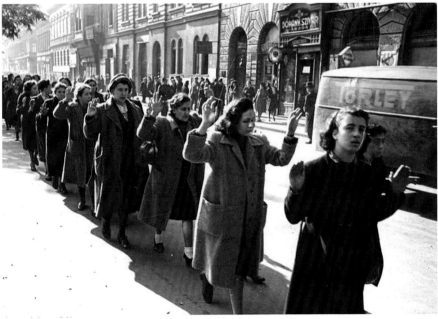

Top: Public execution of unarmed Polish priests and civilians in Bydgoszcz's Old Market Square on September 9, 1939. This photograph is in the public domain in both Poland and the United States. Bottom: Captured Jewish women being deported from Budapest to concentration camps in 1943–1944. Courtesy of German Federal Archives.

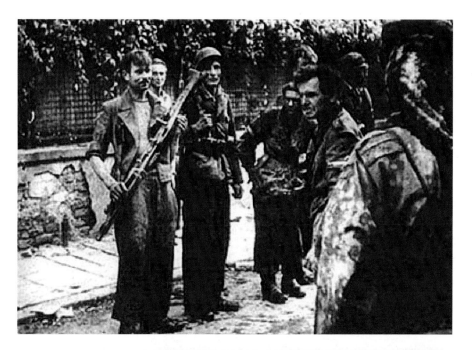

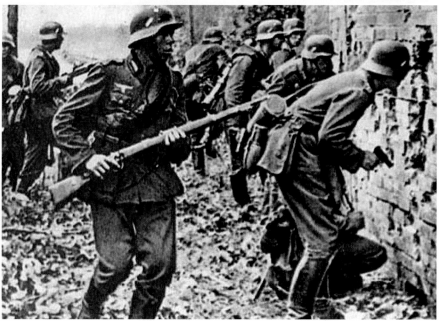

Top: Polish resistant fighters during an uprising in 1944. Courtesy of *Surgical Neurology International*. Bottom: German soldiers in the streets fighting in Poland in 1944. These photos are in the public domain and I first used them in seminal articles in *Surgical Neurology International*.

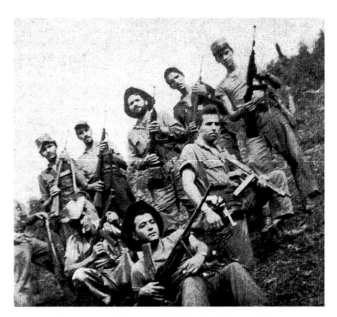

Anti-communist Cuban insurgents fighting against Fidel Castro
(1959–1964). Courtesy of *Surgical Neurology International.*

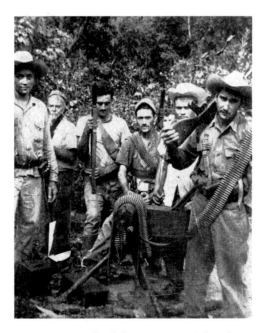

Anti-communist guerrillas fight communist Cuban forces in the
Escambray Mountains (1961–1964). Courtesy of Enrique Encinosa,
from his book *Cuba en Guerra* (1994).

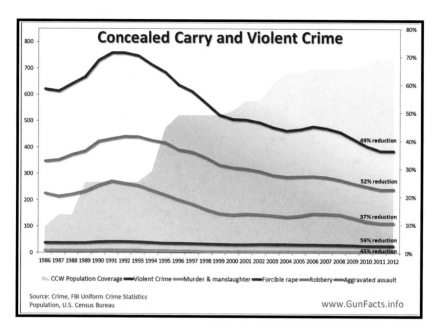

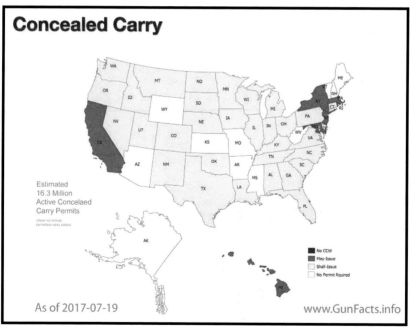

Top: Concealed Carry and Violent Crime. The states that passed concealed carry legislation have experienced a significant reduction in violent crime as noted in the graph from the early 1990s to the present. Bottom: Concealed Carry map of the U.S. The vast majority of states have "shall issue" concealed carry, or "no permit required" legislation in place to the benefit of lawful citizens.

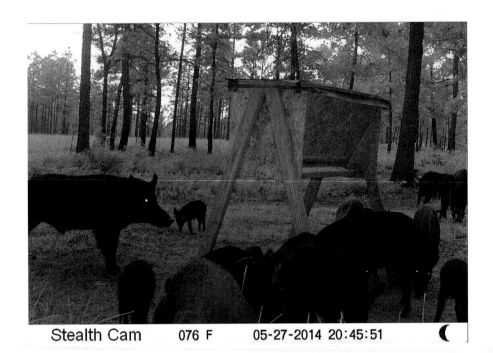

Stealth Cam   076 F   05-27-2014 20:45:51

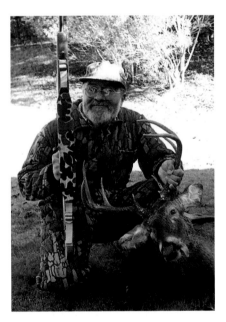

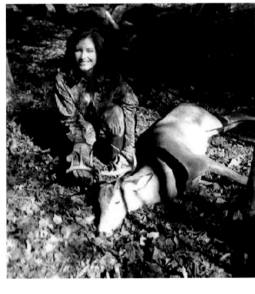

Top: Feral hogs in Taylor County, Georgia, May 27, 2014 caught on Stealth Cam. Courtesy of Dale and Regina Kirkland. Bottom Left: The author with his "trophy" buck, 2008. Bottom Right: The author's wife, Helen, with another buck she tracked and helped pull out of a deep ravine in 2013. Families that hunt together, stay together. The Farias have been married for more than 40 years.

PART 4

THE AMA AND THE MEDICAL POLITICIANS ENTER PARTISAN POLITICS

CHAPTER 13

RE-ENTERS THE AMA WITH DWINDLING MEMBERSHIP BUT WITH LOTS OF MONEY

When any institution becomes large and compartmentalized, with departments and subdepartments, then the conscience of the institution will often become so fragmented and diluted as to be virtually nonexistent, and the organization becomes inherently evil.

—M. Scott Peck, M.D. (1936—2005),
American psychiatrist and best-selling author of *The Road Less Traveled* (1978)

In 1991 when the AMA joined the PHE in the gun control movement, it was under the thinly veiled pretext of "facing head on" the problem of domestic violence. The political move was partly ideological but mostly opportunistic, as to score public relation points. It did not concern the AMA leadership that many American physicians, whom they claimed to represent, owned guns and enjoyed hunting and skeet shooting as recreational sports as well as also partake in their legacy of freedom. In fact, in the doctor's lounge at our hospital, I can testify that after health care issues and local politics, the next major topics of conversation were families, hunting, and fishing.

However, these ramblings apparently did not faze the AMA, and by the year 2000, "organized medicine" had joined the gun prohibitionist movement in full force. At its 2001 annual meeting, led by the long-time Speaker of the AMA House of Delegates who recently had been elected president of the AMA, Richard F. Corlin, M.D., the AMA re-joined the gun control movement full steam ahead by calling for the doctors organization to increase funding to "study data on firearms injuries."[1]

It did not trouble, Dr. Corlin and the AMA that PHE researchers had been conducting "gun research" for several decades and that the studies had been judged to be biased, result-oriented, and based on what was characterized by a number of serious investigators as junk science.[2]

Medical Censorship of Political Incorrectness

The AMA, using its publication empire, has been publishing this "research" in its gamut of journals, including the *Journal of the American Medical Association (JAMA)*, and through the rest of "organized medicine" by the specialty and state medical journals. Unfortunately, only researchers that embraced the politically correct, preordained conclusions that "easy gun availability results in violence and crime" and that "guns and bullets are pathogens that must be eradicated," were published. Contrary views were censored.

The monolithic wall of censorship was only momentarily breached by the *Journal of the Medical Association of Georgia (JMAG)* while I was editor from 1993 to 1995. I have recounted in previous chapters the more successful part

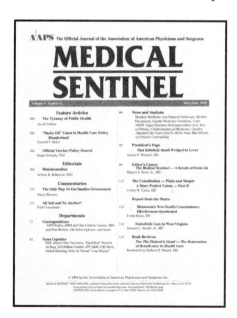

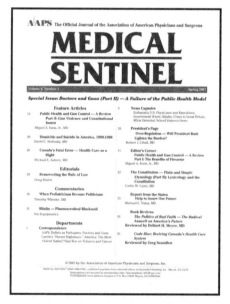

of the story. But I only mentioned in passing the consequences of that momentary breach, the story of my professional travails that I related in a chapter titled, "Censorship and Editorial Lynching in the Deep South," in my second book, *Medical Warrior: Fighting Corporate Socialized Medicine* (1997).[3]

However, the momentum was not completely lost and the wall of censorship was cracked further with my editorship and the advent of the *Medical Sentinel*, which I founded and was the official, peer-reviewed journal of the Association of American Physicians and Surgeons (AAPS).[4] From 1996 to 2002, this medical journal provided a breath of fresh air in medical journalism. I have devoted Chapter 14 in this book to comparing my humble editorship of the *Medical Sentinel* with that of the grandiose Dr. George Lundberg of *JAMA* because the comparison represents stark contrasts in medical journalism.

We have already recounted that in the spring of 1996, Drs. Timothy Wheeler (Doctors for Responsible Gun Ownership), William C. Waters, IV (Doctors for Integrity in Policy Research), myself (as editor of the newly founded *Medical Sentinel*), and the legal scholar Don B. Kates testified before a congressional subcommittee about the biased, result-oriented research conducted by the CDC and its politicized branch, the NCIPC; and as a result, as we described in previous chapters, the latter entity was ordered by Congress not to conduct tainted gun [control] "research."[5,6]

The AMA had been moving steadily to the left in a variety of issues, from the perversion of medical ethics to gun control to score political points, serve opportunism, make profits, as well as to satisfy political correctness.[7] Yet that had not always been the case. In *Medical Warrior* I also described how, over the years, the AMA tried to please everyone but ended up pleasing no one, to be all things to all people, embracing pragmatism and political correctness—whether in discussion of socioeconomic policies or medical ethics.[8]

I had been told, by at least one AMA defender, "It's just politics!" That may be, but when dealing with ethics and constitutional issues, principles should not be compromised by playing politics. There was simply too much at stake in public health for the leading doctors organization to act in that cowardly fashion.

Can the Medical Profession Survive Flexible Ethics?

Thinking of the misguided steps the AMA has taken in the last several decades, both in terms of political and ethical issues, I coined the term "flexible (medical) ethics" to refer to "organized medicine's" systematic abandonment of traditional medical ethics and cynically embracing pragmatism and political expediency.[7] The Hippocratic tradition based on moral principles and the individual patient has been methodically supplanted by the situational ethics of the moment and the exculpatory moral relativism of the times. This has been done, not from an awakening of moral certitudes, but to force medical ethics in pragmatic fashion to fit the political correctness or political expediency of the time, not to mention reaching fiduciary goals. To make the new flexible bioethics fit the progressive objectives of the organization, the AMA has stretched medical ethics in a procrustean bed—from ethically questionable professional endorsement of products to publishing medical procedure code books, the latter self-serving books physicians are obligated to purchase each year in order to comply with government edits. It would be difficult for anyone to come up with a more profitable scheme of public-private partnership, benefitting each partner at the expense of a third party—the physicians.

Nevertheless, while AMA membership remains low, its coffers remain full. The AMA has plenty of money to encourage the various schools of public health to fund gun control efforts, and ingratiate itself with the mainstream liberal media and the progressive camp, which it fully joined. Indeed, the AMA's finances remain in good shape, despite steadily dwindling membership and questionable performance in achieving health care goals benefitting patients and doctors. As a result, the AMA has become irrelevant to both!

Yet, the AMA continued to march to the left. The rump AMA membership, estimated at between 15 to 25 percent of medical doctors, now includes largely, non-private practice physicians and salaried doctors, such as hospitalists and public health workers, representing the liberal left wing of the profession. Along its liberal line, the AMA had been supporting ObamaCare, but a ruckus arose in 2016 when the AMA also supported the appointment of Dr. Tom Price for Secretary of Health and Human Services (HHS). As usual the AMA was trying to walk a tight rope and be all things to all people. An article by the Boston Global Media group gave plenty of space to liberal doctors to vent their anger at the organization's endorsement of Dr. Price, a long time conservative member of "organized medicine" who opposed ObamaCare.

Even former editor of the *New England Journal of Medicine* and a senior lecturer in the department of global health and social medicine at Harvard Medical School, Marcia Angell M.D., opined: "They [AMA] end up being followers rather than leaders because they want to be where the action is."[9] That statement puts it mildly, but points in the right direction in terms of leadership, principles, and lack of moral courage.

Traditional Medical Ethics Superseded by Expediency and Flexible Ethics

The medical writers of antiquity wrote and discussed medical ethics merely as physicians trying to find the best way and the right way to conduct themselves using immutable, self-evident principles and propositions in conducting their professional duties. They considered themselves both moral philosophers and medical practitioners. Ethical principles were considered absolute, and in a benevolent profession were supposed to guide the conduct of its members—dedicated practitioners who had answered a professional calling. The physicians were to stand clearly for the principles stated in the Oath of Hippocrates and the body of his writings, and not just echo what was considered politically expedient, or parrot the rhetoric of demagogic politicians. The new AMA changed all that. It seemed that the organization, seeking fashionable, politically correct ways and self-aggrandizement, in order "to be where the action is," had been disappointing the rank and file members for years—immersing itself in political issues and making professional pronouncements that changed directions like a weathervane.

The leadership positions filled years ago by the old, traditional AMA leaders were once held in great respect. But this is no longer the case. The trappings of power have corrupted the new politically correct leadership, and they are no longer seen as doing devoted professional service; no longer dedicated at preserving and improving the profession; no longer devoted to the well-being of their patients. Instead they are addicted to expedient policies, to playing medical politics, as well as to extravagant and luxuriant travel and excessive expenses—given the disclosed reimbursement figures paid to AMA officers as far back as 1996.

It's not surprising that physicians have become demoralized, many of them thinking of the time when they will retire. Others no longer recommend the profession to their children and medical dynasties are ending. And yet, no one has been in the past a better advocate for patients than their physicians. The State has taken that role away from doctors, and unfortunately this situation is not in the best interest of the public. How can the State be trusted, especially when power-hungry Democrats assume power?

Consider the anti-gun, anti-liberty, and pro-dependency policies of the Clinton and Obama administrations when they held power. Obama, before becoming president, denigrated many working-class Americans, many having lost their jobs in industry, berating them with his callous remark, "They get bitter, they cling to guns or religion or antipathy to people who aren't like them or anti-immigrant sentiment or anti-trade sentiment as a way to explain their frustrations." Yet, given the historic record, what government can be trusted that does not trust its citizens with firearms?

Americans are tolerant and forgiving. Despite the insult, Barack Obama was elected president in 2008 and reelected in 2012. Americans chose better in 2016 and elected Donald Trump, a friend of the Second Amendment. He not only carried Ohio and Pennsylvania, hit hard by the recession, but also Wisconsin and Michigan, states where citizens clung to their voting levers, wanting to regain their jobs and keep their guns.

An Empire of Money but Not of Members

The arrogance of officialdom should be tempered and controlled, and assistance to foreign hands should be curtailed, lest Rome fall.
—**Cicero, 55 B.C.**

Let's return to the service of the medical politicians of the AMA. In the March/April 1998 issue of the *Medical Sentinel*, we reported that in 1996, three AMA officers were paid more than $200,000 for their part-time "playing politics" within "organized medicine." Below are the reported AMA Officers and positions held in 1996 with their reimbursement figures:

Dr. Nancy Dickey, Chairman, $258,790

Dr. Lonnie Bristow, Immediate Past Pres., $229,540

Dr. Daniel Johnson, Jr. President, $221,970

Dr. Percy Wootton, President-elect, $168,720

Dr. Thomas Reardon, Vice-Chairman, $147,929

Dr. Robert McAfee,* Immediate Past President, $135,440

Dr. Yank Coble Jr., Trustee, $105,915

Dr. Randolph Smoak Jr., Secretary-Treasurer, $99,087

Dr. Regina Benjamin, Trustee, $91,716

Dr. Timothy Flaherty, Trustee, $90,792

Dr. John Nelson, Trustee, $90,405

Dr. Donald Lewers, Trustee, $87,521

Dr. Richard Corlin, Speaker, $85,875

Dr. William Jacott, Trustee, $82,369

Dr. Palma Formica, Trustee, $75,492

*Term ended in June 1996

Perhaps the previous publication of these figures[7] had a bit of an impact in restraining the medical politicians. The reimbursement figures have increased since then but only slightly at least up to 2012. Even those figures were very difficult to find.[10]

There is no reason to suppose that since 2012 those reimbursement figures have not increased along with the AMA's operating budget, which had already risen to $247 million by 2001.

AMA finances were so good and its coffers so full that in 1997, Dr. Randolph Smoak Jr., who was then AMA secretary-treasurer and subsequently president, reported that every revenue category had increased except for membership dues. Furthermore, Smoak noted, "This good news should continue to keep the AMA relevant for the physicians of 1997 and the future. Indeed, the AMA is projected to receive an $8.2 million gain in real estate sales. And will end 1997 with $5.9 million in the black ... and robust reserve levels that should exceed $148 million in 1999."[11]

These predictions, for the most part, materialized. As a result, rumors circulated that the AMA no longer needed (and needs) members to remain financially afloat. The rumors were confirmed by the *Chicago Tribune*, which reported in the fall of 1997 in the midst of the AMA-Sunbeam scandal that over 70 percent of the AMA's revenues "came from sources other than membership—including real estate and the publication of coding books, which are revised annually and required for physician compliance with government rules and regulations."[11]

Despite an embarrassingly decreasing membership of American physicians, which was 32 percent in 2001 but now stands between 15 to 25 percent, the AMA still claims to represent the medical profession.

Make no mistake about it, the AMA may not have the membership numbers, but it has ample finances to fund gun control efforts and other leftward leaning projects, such as supporting ObamaCare, which it did during the administration of President Barack Obama and still does.

The source of this wealth is the AMA's publication empire, which rests solidly on a monopolistic pact with the Health Care Financing Administration (HCFA), a secret agreement that was brought to light in an article by the General Counsel of the Association of American Physician and Surgeons (AAPS) Andrew L. Schlafly in the Summer 1998 issue of the *Medical Sentinel*.[12] The AMA leadership even refused to show those documents to the rank-and-file membership. But the Association of American Physicians and Surgeons (AAPS), not so easily thwarted, obtained the documents from a source independent from the AMA and HCFA.

Schlafly revealed that under provisions of this pact, the AMA was given a monopoly over the government-imposed coding standards for physicians. By contractual obligation, HCFA must enforce the coding systems developed by the AMA upon the same physicians the AMA purportedly serves and represents. This contract has been in effect since 1983 when AMA Executive Vice President James H. Sammons, M.D., signed the agreement. The AMA continues to impose these money-making but onerous coding regulations on physicians in the name of HCFA.

Who pays for this government-granted AMA monopoly and regulatory burden? Ultimately, the patient does. Year after year, American physicians must purchase the new coding books in order to bill the government and third-party insurance carriers for medical services rendered to patients. Codes must be current, and physicians must not make billing errors. Coding errors may result in the government accusation of fraud and abuse, prosecution, and jail time.

Schlafly is indeed correct when he asserts:

Virtually every crime has a motive, and the motive here is money. Lots of it. The AMA declared on its website that the AMA 'generates approximately two-thirds of its annual $200 million operating budget from non-dues sources.' Of that $133 million in non-dues revenue, the AMA's publication revenue, including sales of those expensive CPT codebooks, is its most prominent source. The victims of these endlessly complicated revisions to coding are physicians rendering private medical care. Each year physicians pay substantial costs and expend precious hours trying to keep up with the rules imposed by the AMA's CPT moneymaking machine. The time and money lost by physicians due to the AMA could be far better spent in the service of patients.[12]

In subsequent chapters we will discuss other topics which confirm the AMA is moving leftward in the political spectrum, whether it is medical journalism, ethics, unionization, or the corporate practice of medicine,[13] and it's of interest that while the AMA efforts to provide legal relief to physicians via tort reform have failed, it has more successfully promoted litigation against HMOs to the benefit of trial lawyers.[14]

CHAPTER 14

OUTLANDISH AND BIASED MEDICAL JOURNALISM

'There's glory for you!' 'I don't know what you mean by "glory,"'
Alice said. Humpty Dumpty smiled contemptuously. ...'When
I use a word,' Humpty Dumpty said, in rather a scornful
tone, 'it means just what I choose it to mean—neither more
nor less.' 'The question is,' said Alice, 'whether you can make
words mean so many different things.' 'The question is,' said
Humpty Dumpty, 'which is to be MASTER—that's all.'

—Lewis Carroll (1832—1898),
Through the Looking Glass (1871)

I was struck that particular morning when I heard on the radio on January 15, 1999, from the authoritative radio commentator Paul Harvey (and later confirmed by CNN) that the long time editor of the *Journal of the American Medical Association* (*JAMA*), George D. Lundberg, M.D., had been summarily fired by Dr. E. Ratcliffe Anderson, Executive Vice President of the American Medical Association (AMA) for essentially using *JAMA* for his own political purposes. *The chickens had come home to roost*, I thought.

In March 1994, the *Journal of the Medical Association of Georgia* (*JMAG*) published a series of articles debunking many of the fallacies previously published in the medical literature, including *JAMA*, *NEJM* and dozens of the specialty journals. *JMAG* criticized the faulty application of the public health model to the study of guns and violence while documenting the beneficial aspects of gun ownership in the hands of law-abiding citizens.[1] Without having first read the articles, Dr. Lundberg commented, "The Georgia articles are contrary to virtually all recognized, publicly published research regarding firearms in our society. My belief is a careful analysis of their [data] and methods will show it to be flawed."[2] So much for objectivity, the liberalizing thought about the free flow and exchange of ideas, fairness, and the eternal quest for scientific truth!

In 1991 when the AMA launched its campaign against domestic violence, particularly after I became editor of the *Journal of the Medical Association of Georgia (JMAG)*, I came to the shocking realization that the medical literature was biased and prone to exert a leftist political influence on society. Domestic violence was a safe topic that could serve as a springboard to a more controversial issue, which turned out to be gun control.

In gun control, the medical politicians of "organized medicine" used a pincer strategy with the mainstream liberal media to exploit tragedies in the pursuit of their agenda and score public relation points in the process. Leading publications in the press—for example, *U.S News and World Report* (August 13, 1994), *The Economist*, (March 26, 1994 and April 29, 1995) *Newsweek* (August 23, 1999)—all featured graphic covers (and articles) decrying gun violence in America, but saying nothing about the beneficial aspects of gun ownership, or America's legacy of freedom because of the willingness of Americans to sacrifice their lives and treasure to defend that freedom, and even the liberty of other nations, with firearms.

The media campaign came in waves, frequently following mass-shooting incidents; but through the 1990s, it came in a torrent, and the medical politicians of the AMA and "organized medicine" spared no tragedy or statistic, using public health as the vehicle and emotive journal covers in the campaign to help impose gun prohibition in America. The *Journal of the American Medical Association (JAMA;* June 10, 1992), for example, used expressionism with a highly inflammatory picture of a naked man lying on a blood-stained bed, blood dripping and pooling on the floor and splashing a nude woman standing beside him. Numerous state medical journals followed suit, including The *New Jersey Medicine* (December 1994 and February 1995) and the *Wisconsin Medical Journal* (October 1994), just to cite a couple of examples. Of these journals, the AMA and the Medical Association of Georgia flatly denied permission to use their covers for illustration in this book; the AMA representative wrote he was sorry: "We could not be more flexible in this matter." Only the Medical Society of New Jersey stood by their publication and extended us that courtesy.

In succumbing to propaganda, instead of providing a balanced and honest approach, not just to gun violence but almost every other political or socioeconomic issue, the medical literature echoed the emotionalism and parroted the rhetoric and political correctness of the mainstream liberal media. Those issues in the AMA journals were not based on scientific truth or objectivity, as would be expected from professional medical journals, but expounded on liberal clichés. The AMA literature, state medical journals, and even major publications such as The *New England Journal of Medicine (NEJM)* and *JAMA* led, but in some cases were subservient to and followed the popular press, particularly with political and trendy issues, such as guns, AIDS, gender politics, even the socialization of American medicine—topics championed by the progressive media.[3]

The AMA occasionally led the way, and despite the expressed sentiments and wishes of the vast majority of practicing physicians who wanted to preserve the individual-based and traditional medical ethics inherent to the Oath of Hippocrates, AMA leaders assisted by medical journal editors were spearheading efforts in health care reform in the opposite direction, towards population-based, utilitarian ethics and the step-by-step socialization of American medicine.[3] They were also pushing for medical issues in which their political ideology, not science, predominated in medical pronouncements—for example, gun control, sexual lifestyles (in which they should have been at the forefront of discussing the risks and consequences of sexually transmitted diseases), and not promoting divisive gender politics and different sexual lifestyles.

The Story of Dr. Lundberg, Editor of JAMA (1982—1999)

Returning to the case of the fired Dr. George D. Lundberg, there is no question that doctor had had a great deal to do with the leftist turn in the AMA publications. He had been editor of *JAMA* for 17 years, and he had hoped to break the record set by an illustrious and greater predecessor, Morris Fishbein, M.D., the prolific and outspoken, long-time editor of *JAMA* who had been at the editorial helm for 20 years, from 1924 to 1949.

But Dr. Fishbein had himself been ousted because he "outshined" the AMA leadership, and the Board of Trustees simply came to resent his influence.[4]

It was now Dr. Lundberg's turn to be fired, although, he had been promoted by the AMA to be in charge of Scientific Information and Multimedia, and his thinking was in tune with AMA thinking in most issues, such as more government intervention in medicine, gun control, and population-based utilitarian ethics. Incidentally, utilitarian ethics refer to the judgment of a course of action being good (right) or bad (wrong) based on societal consequences, such as cost, and not necessarily on benefits to the individual patient. Physicians have been trained from time immemorial to place the interest of the patient first, rather than society, and never do harm to the patient deliberately under any circumstances.

Supposedly, the AMA leadership was "outraged" with Dr. Lundberg because he had published an article based on a survey of college students that concluded oral sex did not constitute "having sex." Even worse, the article had been given precedence in publication over other articles to coincide with the "scientific" whitewashing of the allegations involving President Bill Clinton and White House intern Monica Lewinsky.

After the 1999 coup, at a press conference, AMA Vice President Ratcliffe Anderson, M.D. said that Dr. Lundberg "inappropriately and inexcusably had interjected *JAMA* into a major political debate that had nothing to do with science and medicine." From AMA headquarters, President Nancy Dickey, M.D. further explained:

> *Because JAMA means so much to us, when sudden change strikes, it sends a ripple of surprise from one end of the medical profession to the other. That certainly occurred with the recent dismissal of George D. Lundberg, M.D., the 14th physician to head the Journal. The dismissal triggered national publicity and many inquiries to the AMA from physicians and JAMA contributors who expressed concern over the future direction of JAMA...*

> *As he said in his public statements, E. Ratcliffe Anderson Jr., M.D., the AMA's executive vice president and CEO, has, over the past several months lost confidence and trust in Dr.*

Lundberg's ability to maintain the Journal's historic integrity. The latest evidence was the decision to publish an article based upon the 1991 Kinsey Institute survey on what constitutes having "had sex" so it coincided with the [presidential] impeachment proceedings in the U.S. Senate.

It was Dr. Anderson's belief—shared by the AMA Board of Trustees—that publishing that survey at that time interjected JAMA into a major political debate that had nothing to do with science or medicine. That was unacceptable...

While the Kinsey article was a factor, Dr. Anderson's decision was reached after several months of observation and was not based solely on any single circumstance. Dr. Anderson has informed the Board that he would not dismiss a subordinate for a single transgression, saying, "this is not a single mistake." The Board believes the decision Dr. Anderson reached was based on principle, was fully justified, and is supported by the Board of Trustees.

We have a responsibility to the medical profession, our patients and the country to ensure that the editorial decisions of JAMA are based on science and the highest standards of medical journalism. The decision to replace Dr. Lundberg was necessary to live up to that responsibility.[5]

Despite this rebuke, Dr. Lundberg had told CNN that adolescent sexual behavior was associated with sexually transmitted diseases, and therefore arguably he was writing within the realm of public health.

Michael Fumento, senior fellow at the Hudson Institute, apparently agreed with Dr. Lundberg's dismissal and used him as only one example of the politicization of science and medicine in medical journalism. In *The Wall Street Journal*, Fumento wrote:

Yet Dr. Lundberg's action was a mere misdemeanor

*compared with the high crimes JAMA and other top medical
and science journals have committed in recent years. These
alleged bulwarks of reason and reality have the power to
make or break drugs, therapies, and careers, and to influence
national and international policy. All, almost certainly quite
intentionally, have helped bring new meaning to the term
'political science.'[6]*

As another example, Fumento cited a case report by Dr. Devra Lee Davis, an environmentalist epidemiologist at the World Resources Institute, whose field of interest according to Fumento is "attempting to prove a link between man-made chemicals and diseases." Her flawed study published in *JAMA*, purportedly linked a declining male birth rate between 1970 and 1990. What Dr. Davis did not mention or the editor of *JAMA* failed to do, or just plainly ignored, was to ask the question of why Dr. Davis "began counting in 1970, when government statistics of sex ratios of newborns go back to 1940?" The inconvenient answer is that the 1940 to 1990 interval shows that "the ratios swing up and down from decade to decade," and, elucidates Fumento, "Ms. Davis simply snipped off years she found inconvenient."[6] Moreover, Dr. Davis did not explain why black male birth rates were not affected and, in fact, were increasing since 1970. We have seen this type of selective omission of data and the truncation of inconvenient periods of study before in medical and public health gun studies. This constitutes pure and simple academic dishonesty that should not be tolerated. The problem of leftist preconceived notions and systematic dishonesty injected into "scientific studies" runs deep.

AMA Leaders Embarrassed at JAMA's Kinky Sex

Another writer who also commented and did not lament the firing of Dr. Lundberg was Timothy Wheeler, M.D., past director of Doctors for Responsible Gun Ownership (DRGO). He wrote:

*To liberals, Journal of the American Medical Association
(JAMA) editor George Lundberg was a knight in shining*

> armor. For years the AMA's scientific journal was the soapbox
> from which he dispensed progressive gospel such as gun pro-
> hibition and race-based preferences in medical school admis-
> sions. But now he's gone too far...He's fired.

Dr. Wheeler then elucidated further on the reason for Dr. Lundberg's fast track publication of the article, to protect the Democrat President Clinton from the sexual misconduct charges, and inoculate him against, "the subsequent lies, and Mr. Clinton's current impeachment trial in the United States Senate on charges of perjury and obstruction of justice."[7]

Dr. Wheeler agreed with my assessment of the AMA marching to the left of the political spectrum. He wrote:

> The AMA has undergone a steady trend from a conservative
> old boys club to a more left-leaning old boys and girls club.
> AMA management has done nothing to discourage JAMA's
> social activist leanings over the years. As a result, a medical
> journal which once had promise as a top peer-reviewed learning
> resource for doctors has become a mouthpiece for political inter-
> ests. As usual, real science has suffered in the process. Lundberg's
> dismissal is a good first step toward rehabilitating JAMA.[7]

Providing a veneer of scientific cover for President Clinton in his presidential hour of need during the Senate impeachment trial was not Dr. Wheeler's only complaint. He also faulted Dr. Lundberg as a "media-savvy editor [who] was known for courting the press and the public with attention-grabbing articles on diets, firearms, and 'alternative' medicine. And he always artfully applied a scientific spin to these media morsels, even when the scientific basis was shaky."[7]

Social embarrassment about kinky sex and lies, perjury, and the appearance that *JAMA* and the AMA were closing ranks behind a disgraced president, forced the AMA leadership to do what standing by ethical principles could not do. Left-wing ideology and political stridency could not do what political expediency and social embarrassment could: Dr. Lundberg was fired in an attempt to get the politically correct and prim house of the AMA and *JAMA* in order.

While I believe that the free flow and exchange of ideas are essential to a free society, organizations should also adhere to their stated missions and pick their editors, men and women, who represent and encapsulate the views of the organization. These editors will then function in the spirit of journalistic freedom.

The AMA was not faultless; while *JAMA's* mission statement read: "To promote the science and art of medicine and the betterment of the public health," *JAMA* also was allowed to function "under a set of goals and objectives" which were outlined by Dr. Lundberg himself in a *JAMA* article[8] and were approved by the AMA Board of Trustees in April 1993. Among these critical objectives we find:

"[Objective] 5. *To foster responsible and balanced debate on controversial issues* that affect medicine and health care.

"[Objective] 6. *To forecast important issues and trends in medicine* and health care.

"[Objective] 7. To inform readers about *nonclinical aspects of medicine and public health, including the political, philosophic, ethical, legal, environmental, economic, historical, and cultural.*

"[Objective] 8. To recognize that, in addition to these specific objectives, *the journal has a social responsibility* to improve the total human condition and to promote the integrity of science.

"[Objective] 10. To achieve the highest level of *ethical medical journalism* and to produce a publication that is timely, credible, and enjoyable to read."[9] [Emphasis added.]

One should question whether it was wise for *JAMA* and the AMA to immerse themselves in some of these objectives, in particular "social responsibility," a liberal buzzword that can become easily a subject of abuse and exploitation for political purposes (as has been relentlessly done over the years by left-wing radicals, liberation theology extremists, and sundry medical editors). While this progressive propaganda has been promulgated, the other side has been censored and nothing stated about the needs for freedom in medicine and the reinstatement of individual-based ethics of Hippocrates that are the moral principles on which patient advocacy and traditional medical ethics are based.

The fact is the AMA had opened itself to the politicization of science and medicine through the type of research it sponsored, the public relations campaigns it funded, and the medical publications it sanctioned. Thus, the AMA leadership set itself up for the Lundberg fiasco, when they allowed politics to enter the picture masquerading as objective, scientific medical journalism. This fiasco now added another item to the long list of AMA scandals, e.g., Sunbeam, CPT code monopoly, Evaluation & Management (E&M) guidelines, which had been accumulating since the late 1990s.

We have mentioned the CPT code monopoly and the E&M guidelines. In the Sunbeam fiasco, the AMA had to pay nearly $10 million to the Sunbeam Corporation in 1998 for breach of contract, not honoring an endorsement of the Sunbeam "health at home" products, after a membership backlash against it because of problems with professional ethics.

Dr. Lundberg did have considerable leeway to publish the articles that he selected under the approved *JAMA* objectives. What some editors in medical journalism, particularly those of us who have been true victims of censorship and political correctness, would question is whether Dr. Lundberg faithfully and honestly executed those objectives, particularly whether or not he fostered "responsible and balanced debate on controversial issues" during his long tenure as editor of *JAMA*.

Because of the politicization of published scientific research, and the corrupting influence of unlimited government funding of public health, medical researchers, more and more, are ignoring traditional research on the basic and clinical sciences (e.g., investigations as to the physiologic and genetic basis for longevity, radiation exposure and hormesis, neuroscience and behavior) and sometimes they even plainly ignore the scientific method altogether, in the quest for the preordained results expected by their sponsors wielding political power, most notably with politicized gun research.

Instead of hard science research, time and resources are spent in the public health arena on "end-of-life care" (so as to give the State moral justification to curtail and stop treatment to the vulnerable and chronically ill in order to save the government money), gun research (always leading to more gun control and justified with the mantra of "gun violence as a public health issue"), domestic violence, and binge drinking—some of these topics belonging more appropriately in the realms of religion, sociology, and criminology.

During his years as editor of *JAMA*, Dr. Lundberg helped move *JAMA*, and with it the AMA leadership, to the left of the political spectrum, towards more government infringement in medical practice and the step-by-step socialization of American medicine by advancing managed care, managed competition, and corporate socialized medicine.[10] More recently the step-by-step process included supporting ObamaCare and preparing the ground for a single payer system—being sold to Americans as just a simple extension of Medicare, e.g., Medicare For All.

The single payer system (fully government-controlled, socialized medicine) remains the biggest threat to the survival of private medical care and medicine as an independent profession. And yet, all these years the AMA had been contemplating the socialization of American medicine and flirting with the idea of universal coverage, while claiming to prefer private sector solutions and insisting that it opposed the single payer system and the complete government takeover of medicine.[11]

When the Republican congressional attempt at repeal of ObamaCare failed in 2017, and the GOP became further disunited and disconnected by its failure—the AMA remained silent. In fact, authoritarian socialist progressives were so sure of victory that they gloated at the thought of winning the health care debate, which seemed to be moving rapidly in their direction, so much so that some of them admitted that Medicare For All was not enough. They were ready for full government control and the single payer system. At this critical juncture, when the organization may have made a difference, the silence from "organized medicine" remained deafening and not a word was heard from the medical politicians of the AMA.[12]

What Dr. Lundberg overwhelmingly selected for publication and what he frequently wrote in the left field of medical politics alienated practicing physicians in the trenches, who, by in large, only wanted the AMA to represent them as a profession, but otherwise to be left alone by the government to practice medicine. Former AMA members, such as myself and countless others, became fed up with *JAMA* and the politicking and power politics of "organized medicine." Many of us left the AMA discouraged, frustrated, and totally convinced most of the AMA leaders just wanted the pomp and circumstance of rubbing shoulders with politicians to obtain a "seat at the [government policymakers] table"—not to argue hard points but to pick up the scraps thrown to them by the politicians, especially from the left. And this is not just a complaint leveled from conservative physicians, but also from journalists on the left—for example, Howard Wolinsky and Tom Brune in their book, *The Serpent on the Staff* (1994) that we cited earlier as a source[4]—as well as from progressive physicians, such as *NEJM* editor Dr. Marcia Angell, who observed: "They [AMA] end up being followers rather than leaders because they want to be where the action is."[13]

Dr. Lundberg not only presided over this professional alienation but also frequently, in sharing the leadership's ideology, carried the water for them and perhaps shared with them the blame for the further hemorrhaging of AMA membership.

National Health Care Reform

From a different perspective, Dr. Lundberg's dismissal was not an issue of journalistic freedom but that of an editor who used *JAMA* to promote left-wing, liberal views—while censoring those views and opinions with which he disagreed. Take for instance, Dr. Lundberg's call for the step-by-step socialization of American medicine (under the disingenuous guise of saving medicine from a complete government takeover) during the health care debate from 1992 to 1994. In a pivotal editorial he wrote:

> As long as we are in a free society with medical pluralism, providing access means that there must be insurance coverage for all, either paid for by individuals (or families), by employers, by government, or by some combination thereof. But, insurance alone is not enough. There must also be education regarding the availability of care, attempts to remove cultural and language barriers that would prevent adequate care, provision of local resources (or transportation to appropriate facilities), and the abolition of racial discrimination as it manifests itself in health care provision. If we retain a system of private health insurance, such insurance must be community-rated and not risk-rated, must be available to all without consideration of preexisting conditions, must be transportable by the insured, available to all US inhabitants (or covered by government), and affordable. If all of these conditions cannot

be met, then private insurance for the general populace should
cease to exist for basic medical care and should be confined to
individually purchased 'boutique' care.[14]

If the foregoing dissertation is not gradualism in the socialization of American medicine, thinly disguised, I don't know what is! Additionally, to control the expenditures that socialized medicine would bring, Dr. Lundberg advised: "Payment for providing access for all can be made available by promptly effecting cost controls that slow the anticipated increase in expenditures for health care."[14]

Keep in mind that Dr. Lundberg insisted his reforms were needed to prevent the complete "government takeover" of medicine. Here are steps he thought absolutely necessary to control health care costs with his socialized program:

- *Clearly futile care should cease.*

- *Unnecessary and inappropriate care should stop.*

- *Self-referral to physician-owned facilities should be eliminated.*

- *The tort system of liability should be reformed.*

- *Managed care and managed competition should be drastically expanded.*

- *All Americans should have a primary care physician to function as caregiver, patient advocate, adviser, and medical manager-gatekeeper for access to specialty care.*

- *We should retain a private-public mix of payers and the health care industry.*

All these points were innocuous enough but they were also deceptive. The bottom line came when Dr. Lundberg added:

Even if all of this is done we still must have some form of
global budget that curtails the flow of new money from

government and insurers. Excess capacity and utilization
must be limited and a ceiling established no matter how
distasteful or politically dangerous that may seem to be. To
fairly set such global budgets (by state or nationally) it will
be necessary to legislate a national health expenditure board,
with independent authority to effect such decisions.[14]

In other words, his prescriptions for reform were cost-containment by rationing medical care, especially to the most vulnerable, and health care dictated by government edict, not the free market. Reform of the tort system and the private-public mix were crumbs thrown to the audience from his editorial table. The fact is Dr. Lundberg's prescription was nothing short of effecting the government takeover of medicine in a more easily digestible and palatable form. This stand on national health reform, not to mention gun control, exemplifies the fact that over the years, when it came to socio-economic and political issues, the AMA, through Dr. Lundberg and *JAMA*, moved to the left or to the politically correct side of the medical fence. Never mind that many of these left-wing political views went, by and large, contrary to the vast majority of practicing physicians.

HIV/AIDS and Gun Control–Inverted Public Health Models

Let us now further take the issue of the politics of HIV/AIDS and the issue of gun control, within the much-ballyhooed context of public health. And once again 1991 was a key year in medical politicking. In that year, the AMA helped defeat legislation (H.R. 2608) allowing physicians to test their patients for HIV without the considerable legal constraints placed on practitioners and thereby hampered the much needed public health policy of universal testing. Incidentally, the public health establishment went along with this policy, contrary to common sense and standard public health practice.

For too many critical years in the 1990s, universal testing remained acutely needed to contain the deadly AIDS epidemic, but it was not implemented because the AMA and PHE caved in to the demands of the homosexual community and gay and gender politics. And yet, inexplicably, at the same time that physicians' hands were tied, *JAMA* and the AMA trampled upon Principle VI of the AMA Code of Ethics about freedom of choice and free association and proclaimed that physicians were legally and "ethically" compelled to treat patients with AIDS, regardless of experience or expertise.[15]

Thus, because of expediency, power politics, and political correctness, *JAMA* and the AMA helped HIV/AIDS become the first politically protected disease, and HIV seropositivity a socioeconomic and political issue, rather than the serious public health menace it posed to a significant segment of the population. Because the proper public health measures to combat this disease, which at the time was 100 percent fatal, were not instituted and because of the politicization of HIV/AIDS, medicine's fight against HIV was extremely difficult.[16] It was dedicated, true scientific research in the basic sciences of virology and biochemistry, and the extensive development of life-saving drugs in the pharmaceutical industry that finally put a dent in the HIV epidemic. It's ironic that it was the pharmaceutical industry—with its free-market incentives for research and development (R&D), as well as humanitarian concerns (free drugs were charitably shipped to the third world), an industry maligned by self-righteous, progressive critics, who so much abhor the odious profit motive—and not the PHE's politicized and ineffective measures—that brought salvation to untold millions.

And yet, as we have seen, while the public health model was not fully applied towards HIV/AIDS containment, a truly public health emergency, public health officials at the CDC and elsewhere, supported by *JAMA* and the AMA, did their utmost to apply the public health model to gun control—where is did not apply.[17] Dr. Lundberg himself was a proponent of gun control as a public health issue, rather than as an aspect of criminology. Along with a large segment of the PHE, Dr. Lundberg espoused the erroneous concept of guns and bullets as virulent pathogens that needed to be stamped out by limiting gun availability and ultimately eradicating firearms.

In an editorial written with former Surgeon General C. Everett Koop, M.D., Dr. Lundberg drew an inappropriate comparison between motor vehicle accidental deaths with gun deaths (including homicides and suicides, by far the largest share of gun deaths). The analogy was faulty as Dr. Edgar Suter, DIPR chairman, astutely pointed out:

The selectivity of the analogy is further apparent when we recognize that licensing and registration of automobiles is necessary only on public roads. No license or registration is required to own and operate a motor vehicle of any kind on private property. The advocates of the automobile model of gun ownership would be forced by their own logic to accept use of any kind of firearm on private property without license or registration. Since any state's automobile and driver license is valid in every state, further extension of the analogy suggests that the licensing of guns and gun owners would allow citizens to 'own and operate' firearms in every U.S. jurisdiction. A national concealed firearms license valid throughout this nation would be a significant enhancement of self-protection, a deterrent to violent crime, and a compromise quite enticing to many gun owners.[18]

In the same editorial, Drs. Lundberg and Koop also made the stupefying and extraordinary claim that "one million U.S. inhabitants die prematurely each year as a result of intentional homicide or suicide,"[19] which as Dr. Suter correctly noted, "is a 35-fold exaggeration or careless distortion of fatality figures. With this grand but erroneous assertion, we questioned the competence of éminences grises in the field of gun violence."[18]

Crime and violence, unlike AIDS, are issues for sociology and criminology, yet with the help of *JAMA,* the AMA, and the power of propaganda of the mainstream liberal media, they have become, erroneously, public health issues to the detriment of public policy.

What is published in such prestigious journals as *JAMA* and the *NEJM,* and then repeated by the mainstream liberal media, is of crucial importance because the medical literature in general and these journals in particular are given great credence by the public and by policy makers. And yet, under such editors as Dr. Lundberg in *JAMA* and Drs. Jerome Kassirer and Marcia Angell (1988—2000) in the *NEJM,* censorship was practiced (although they deny doing so) not only against those who attempted to breach the walls of political correctness and medical orthodoxy but also those who only wanted to express contrarian views and be heard in written commentaries or even letters to the editor. The medical scholar, Dr. David C. Stolinsky, has written many letters to the prestigious medical journals, including *Lancet,* attempting to correct misinformation. He has told me that he has not had a letter published in over a decade. When Dr. Edgar Suter tried to get his work published in the medical journals and failed, he was not alone, and once again, I can speak from personal experience. Most of my letters to *JAMA* and *NEJM* have never been published. In 1999, Garen J. Wintemute and associates wrote an article in the *NEJM* linking recent purchases of guns to violent crime and suicides. I wrote a letter debunking some of their "facts" and logic. Initially, I was informed that my letter would be published, but a month later Deputy Editor Gregory Curfman wrote that after all my letter would not be published. Wintemute and associates "facts" and faulty logic went uncorrected![20] With a few exceptions, the monolithic wall of censorship of mainstream medical journalism has not yet been permanently breached.

"Respectable" Medical Journalism?

The truth is that image-conscious medical politicians, particularly the AMA leadership and medical editors swam with the politically correct current of medical journalism and leftist politics, allowing their journals to become mouthpieces of trendy liberalism, framed in savvy public relation sound bites—e.g., instruments of "social responsibility," vehicles for sexual re-orientation and liberalization, gender politics, and other politically correct terms. The medical journals have forfeited their responsibility to keep "organized medicine" leaders' feet to the fire regarding issues that count the most: freedom in medicine, preservation of the practice of private medicine, and the restoration of the patient-doctor relationship. Most physicians are too busy with their medical practice; others demoralized, acquiesce as to what is happening, expecting their leaders to do the right thing.[21] Instead, their leaders have joined each other in the cult of liberal orthodoxy and those with contrarian views are censored in the medical journals or ridiculed at the conferences.

If gun control and issues of social responsibility are fashionable issues with the mainstream liberal media and the trendsetters, then the inclination of the AMA medical politician is to preserve their aura of respectability and go with the flow, no matter the science or the wishes of their medical constituents.

Those who managed occasionally to breach the monolithic wall of censorship of the medical journals and medical news magazines, or who have been published or been allowed to speak, have been ignored or ostracized for taking a stand for what they know to be true—namely, that medical politics has been headed in the wrong direction, led by the pragmatic medical politicians, led inexorably toward the socialization and regimentation of American medicine and the destruction of a once proud and noble profession.[22]

For the last several decades, the AMA opened itself to denunciation for the overt politicization of science and medicine, both through the type of social and politically correct conferences sponsored, the public relations campaigns funded (e.g., domestic violence, gender politics, and gun control) and the medical publications published and disseminated. Gun control, then, is not the only leftward movement of the AMA. It also perverted medical ethics and even espoused physician unionization.[23]

Because physicians have become dissatisfied with the increasing regimentation and corporatism of American medicine—facets of the same coin that the AMA and "organized medicine" support—the AMA began to consider options to counteract the very problems it had helped to create, medical unionization. That campaign fizzled, physicians could be led to water, but they could not be made to drink.

The medical politicians of the AMA have been caught up in the trappings of power allowing the ethics of the profession to be transmogrified from the Oath and tradition of Hippocrates and individual-based ethics to the heavily government-regulated, population-based ethics and the collectivist corporate practice of medicine.[10]

Salaried physicians who have unionized, encouraged by the AMA's new leftward direction, not only have joined in solidarity with some of the most radical left movements in the political spectrum, such as the labor unions and the National Education Association (NEA), but also have placed themselves in a great ethical dilemma. Will these physicians set on this path eventually refuse to care for their patients, joining the strike and abandoning those with whom they have established a patient-doctor relationship? It goes without saying these actions would go against whatever remains of the grain of medicine, a sacred calling according to the tradition of Hippocrates.

Physicians should do what they have already been doing, and what they should continue to do—quit the AMA and join other associations, such as their specialty organizations for their specialized fields, and if they own fire-arms and love freedom, they should also join Doctors for Responsible Gun Ownership (DRGO). They also need to become more political, quit believing what they read in the one-sided liberal press and their socioeconomics journals, and instead become more aware of what is going on by reading online news and political issues in alternative sources of media, such as GOPUSA. com, *The Washington Times* and *Fox News*. If you are not a physician but a concerned citizen who is reading this book and you believe in gun rights and engage in hunting or sport shooting, then you should join the NRA or Gun Owners of America (GOA).

CHAPTER 15
AMA EXHORTS DOCTORS TO SPY ON PATIENTS' GUN OWNERSHIP

*False is the idea of utility that sacrifices a thousand real
advantages for one imaginary or trifling inconvenience;
that would take fire from men because it burns, and water
because one may drown in it; that has no remedy for evils
except destruction. The laws that forbid the carrying of
arms are laws of such a nature. They disarm only those who
are neither inclined nor determined to commit crimes.*

—Cesare Beccaria (1738—1794),
Italian criminologist, jurist and philosopher, who was admired
and quoted by Thomas Jefferson in his Commonplace book

We have always thought that privacy and confidentiality would be protected
when conversing with a physician or psychiatrist, but we need to think again.[1]
In what was described as an effort to curb handgun violence, a group called
Doctors Against Handgun Injury called for sweeping changes in doctor-pa-
tient confidentiality that would allow physicians, including psychiatrists, to
pry into patient gun ownership.

In the past, the medical community fought strenuously against any
invasion by government or others into the confidentiality of patient records
and information. For example, the American Psychiatric Association (APA)
had, in the past and for obvious reasons, been a bulwark in the defense of
patient privacy and medical record confidentiality.[2] But since the turn of the
millennium events have taken a nefarious course. The APA regrettably joined
Doctors Against Handgun Injury, a gun prohibitionist coalition.

"Organized Medicine" Rallies Doctors to Spy For Gun Control!

In 2001 the coalition—which also included the AMA and, not sur-prisingly, the strident American Academy of Pediatrics (AAP) and 10 other medical organizations reportedly comprising 600,000 doctors—called for a variety of patient privacy-invading measures in the name of gun safety.

Don't be fooled by their innocuous-sounding name. In a revealing article published in the *New York Observer* (March 15, 2001), Doctors Against Handgun Injury went further and announced a campaign to push for increas-ingly more stringent gun control measures and engaging "in what it calls 'upstream intervention'—that is, using regular checkups to ask patients about firearm ownership and storage in their homes."[3]

The article went on, "To promote public safety, health professionals and health systems should ask about firearm ownership when taking a medical history or engaging in preventive counseling. Patients should be provided with information about the risks of having a firearm in the home, as well as methods to reduce the risk, should they continue to choose to keep them."[3]

According to the *New York Observer* article, "The group is also calling for more conventional measures, such as mandatory background checks of purchasers at gun shows, limits on the number of guns that can be purchased by individuals and a waiting period for all gun buyers. This is the first time that such a large group of doctors has taken a position on gun control."[3] This is a regrettable and ill-conceived effort against patient privacy and violating the sanctity of the patient-doctor relationship.

This policy, particularly by psychiatrists, constitutes a breach in medical ethics, a boundary violation in reference to abuse of the patient-doctor rela-tionship, and an egregious invasion of patient privacy.[4]

The AAP, AMA, APA Lead the Pack!

As to the commitment of the AMA and "organized medicine" to sacrifice medical ethics and patient privacy for the long term ideological and political gain of pushing for strict gun control and civilian disarmament, there is no longer any doubt.[5]

In the case of the American Psychiatric Association (APA), one only has to peruse its position statement on homicide prevention and gun control promulgated by its leadership as early as 1993:

> In view of the need to reinforce individual and group sanctions against the use of violence as a social instrument, behavioral mode, or adaptorional [sic] pattern, as psychiatrists have done with drug abuse, suicidal actions, and antisocial behavior, the American Psychiatric Association recommends that strong controls be placed on the availability of all types of firearms to private citizens.[6]

Why would the AMA and "organized medicine" become involved in this politically expedient but potentially explosive issue of gun control and condone the systematic violation of the privacy of vulnerable patients?

The continuous effort by the AMA to increase membership, although expensive, remained highly unproductive. As the AMA became more politicized and vocal and as government became more intrusive in the practice of medicine, things only got worse. Members continued to leave the organization in droves, and membership fell to the bare bones 15 percent membership it holds today.[5]

The gun control effort, as we noted earlier, was also a convenient ploy to get endless, politically correct, praiseworthy media publicity and score public relations points while ingratiating "organized medicine" to the liberal media. The truth, sound scholarship, free inquiry, and the free flow and exchange of information, as it regards the benefits of firearms in the hands of law-abiding citizens, was rejected. Opportunistic politics would supersede the social sciences of sociology and criminology.

Besides, many of the groups in "organized medicine" had become used to receiving money from the government, taxpayers' money, for their medical politicking efforts. For example, during the years of the Clinton administration, groups such as the American Academy of Pediatrics (AAP), the American Public Health Association (APHA), the American Medical Women's Association (AMWA), the American College of Physicians (ACP), and the American Academy of Family Physicians (AAFP) all drank heavily from the government trough to the tune of millions of dollars of taxpayer money.

In the case of the AAP, the amount was a whopping $1.1 million of taxpayer money at the height of the Clinton health care debate of 1993 to 1994![7] One has to wonder if "organized medicine"—the AMA, the APA, and their cohorts—have learned any of the lessons from the recent chronicles of their profession? To our peril, apparently not.

Ethical Boundary Violations Ignored by the Hypocritical "Organized Medicine"

With good professional reasons, Doctors for Responsible Gun Ownership (DRGO) denounced this new intrusion into the patient-doctor relationship as an ethical boundary violation. A boundary violation takes place when a physician breaches the patient's trust and uses his authority to invade the patients' privacy to advance a political agenda. As Dr. Timothy Wheeler explained in an article in the *Medical Sentinel*:

> A patient who seeks medical or psychiatric treatment is often
> in a uniquely dependent, anxious, vulnerable, and exploitable
> state. In seeking help, patients assume positions of relative
> powerlessness in which they expose their dignity, and reveal
> intimacies of body or mind, or both. Thus, compromised,
> the patient relies heavily on the physician to act only in the
> patient's interest and not the physician's.[4]

From time immemorial, patient privacy and confidentiality have been ethical concepts that, up until now, were fundamental to all physicians and to the patient-doctor relationship. The Oath of Hippocrates, in fact, states:

> Whatever, in connection with my professional practice or
> not in connection with it, I may see or hear in the lives of
> men, I will not divulge, as reckoning that all such should be
> kept secret. While I continue to keep this oath inviolate, may
> it be granted to me to enjoy life and the practice of the art,

respected by all men at all times, but should I trespass and
violate this oath, may the reverse be my lot.[8]

For psychiatrists, who of necessity should be able to obtain very personal and confidential information for their patients' mental health evaluation and treatment, trust must be paramount.

Some psychiatrists, again with sound professional and legal reasons, have claimed in their medical practices a patient-doctor privilege, similar to the attorney-client privilege that lawyers legally enjoy in their profession, and which is a notch above what physicians now possess in patient-doctor confidentiality. Thus, both doctors and patients should receive this push by "organized medicine," including the APA, with great concern and trepidation.

With this new incursion by the medical profession into gun politics, it's easy to see why patients may be more reluctant and less candid than ever with their physicians, which may, in turn, be detrimental to their medical care. With good reason, patients may now perceive that their doctors, in asking them about guns in their homes, are acting more as an arm of the government prying into their personal lives, than as their advocates in health care.

I should inform the reader that in response to the difficulties patients encounter finding physicians who will protect their privacy, Doctors for Responsible Gun Ownership (DRGO) has launched 2Adoc.com, a referral service that "will connect patients with gun-friendly healthcare providers who respect their Second Amendment rights and who would not engage in anti-gun activism in the patient exam room."[8]

It will be easy to discern that physicians involved in this intrusion of privacy are placing the "good of society (and the State)" above their ethical obligation to put their individual patients first, as required by the Oath of Hippocrates and traditional medical ethics.

The extensive and more impersonal use of electronic medical records makes this issue of medical privacy more important than ever. Because of the need for physicians to share medical information on mutual patients and for continuity of medical care, information contained in the electronic medical record can fall into the wrong hands to the detriment of patients, particularly about gun ownership information being entered in the government databases.

What can be more private than gun ownership? It is ironic that in an era where privacy is so enforced in other areas, particularly in job applications, whereby employers are very restricted as to the questions they can ask a prospective employee during a job interview, doctors, on the other hand, have become agents of the State, asking their patients about gun ownership with the encouragement of their professional organizations. Yes, guns are dangerous and must be safely handled, but so too are cleaning agents, automobiles, chemicals, pesticides, herbicides, and electrical cords. I can understand asking parents about these items as well as car seats for infants and toddlers, ordinary life-saving items when properly used. But in the case of guns, pediatricians are prying into a constitutional right that must be respected and not broached unless the patient asks. He may advise if asked but inquiring whether the patient has a gun in the home or not is prying and inappropriate. When the physician proceeds to pry, he is acting against the patients' best interest. If parents keep a gun in the home, the physician have no business recording this type of information in a medical record, and when they do, they are acting as agents of the State, facilitating future banning and confiscation, as has happened in Washington, D.C., Detroit, and New York City. Moreover, there might be unsavory individuals working in the doctors' office, given the restrictions employers have in asking questions to applicants, as well as the fact that lawsuits are rampant and have made letters of reference worthless when it comes to describing such questionable persons. In short, recorded information about the presence or absence of guns in the home is accessible by individuals as well as government and may be valuable to criminal elements as well as to the State.

Florida Firearm Owners Privacy Act (FOPA)

To prevent anti-gun doctors from using their ex-cathedra positions of power over their patients when asking them intrusive questions about firearms in their homes, several states recently took action to curb the abuses already taking place. For example, Florida's Firearm Owners' Privacy Act (FOPA) was passed with this intention, but it was almost immediately challenged by zealot anti-gun physicians (the law has been referred as the "Docs versus Glocks"). The plaintiffs were Florida physicians who opposed the law and backed by the AMA and "organized medicine," which managed to turn the issue into a crusade for preserving the "free speech" of physicians. Dr. Robert B. Young, *an associate clinical professor of Psychiatry at the University of Rochester School of Medicine* and editor of DRGO, explains:

> *To review briefly, Florida's FOPA is a law passed in 2011 that forbids physicians from pressing patients to give up their firearms or otherwise propagandize using the doctor-patient relationship. Doctors can be seen as authoritative in any pronouncements that sound health-related, so using that influence to promote giving up an enumerated Constitutional right when they generally have little or no training in firearm use or safety constitutes inappropriate ethical behavior.*[9]

This was an issue of importance to DRGO, which had worked intensely to preserve the intent of the law. In fact, DRGO provided professional and ethical guidance for Florida legislators in their consideration of the law to prevent unethical boundary violations, preserve patient privacy, prevent indoctrination, and protect patients' constitutional rights to keep firearms in their homes. In a recent DRGO article, Dr. Young narrates in detail the legal battles, which, unfortunately, ultimately ended in defeat: "We worked with Second Amendment attorney Joseph Greenlee and the Second Amendment Foundation and the Citizens Committee for the Right to Keep and Bear Arms on an *amicus* brief submitted in support of the State of Florida to the *en banc* 11th Circuit review." Dr. Young learned from Greenlee that the Gentile Balancing Test, which is the appropriate legal test for professional free speech, was ignored by the *en banc* 11th Circuit review.

Dr. Young continued:

> *According to Greenlee, it is 'a balancing test [that] weighs the State's interest in regulating the professional speech against the professional's First Amendment interest . . . [S]ince the [Supreme] Court has established that states have a compelling interest in regulating professions, and that professionals have diminished First Amendment rights, the scale is tipped heavily in favor of the State when conducting the balancing test. The*

*problem with the test is that it hasn't been used in over 20 years
(because the Supreme Court hasn't addressed the issue), which
explains why it is often overlooked."*[9]

Suffice to say, on February 16, 2017, the entire 11th Circuit Court of
Appeals ruled against the constitutionality of the Florida's Firearm Owners'
Privacy Act. This astounding ruling came, notwithstanding that previously
a three-judge panel from the 11th Circuit had upheld the law. Challenged
from its inception, FOPA was actually never implemented because of the
litigation of plaintiffs.

Lessons Unlearned, Medicine & Psychiatry Subverted by the State

That some physicians would align themselves with the State against
their own patients does not bode well for the future. Doctors should know
better from recent history and, in particular, the dire medical experience in
both the former Soviet Union and Nazi Germany in the past century. In the
USSR, the world bore witness to the perversion of psychiatry, which became
a tool of the totalitarian state. In Chapter 3, we previously addressed the case
of Soviet dissident Vladimir Bukobsky, who spent ten years in Soviet hospitals
and psychiatric wards because of his political beliefs.

Bukobsky later testified to the world that Soviet psychiatrists collected
information on their patients, substantiated purported evidence of mental
illness and concocted testimony against their patients to facilitate their intern-
ment in Soviet psychiatric hospitals for their purported "rehabilitation."
Bukobsky survived and, like the great novelist Aleksandr Solzhenitsyn, who
spent years in the gulags, bore witness to the fact that science must remain
divorced from politics.[10] A story that has not yet been told is the withholding
of medical care (in association with physical and psychological torture) to
political prisoners in communist Cuba and the atrocious misuse of psychiatry against Cuban dissidents to lower levels than even in the Soviet Union.[11]

When science, particularly medicine, becomes wedded to partisan politics, history has shown us, the results are as perverse as they are disastrous to

freedom.[10,11,12] In the momentous article "Medical Science Under Dictatorship," Dr. Leo Alexander, the chief U.S. medical consultant at the Nuremberg War Crimes Trials, examined "the process by which the German medical profession became a willing and unquestioning collaborator with the Nazis." He noted the early changes in medical attitudes that predisposed German physicians to first collect data on their patients to conduct what today we call "cost-effective analysis," and then to use the latter information as a vehicle to commit medical genocide under the auspices of the totalitarianism of National Socialism.

Dr. Alexander warns us that "from small beginnings" the values of an entire society may be subverted, leading to the horrors of a police state. The "small beginnings" in Nazi Germany that Dr. Alexander referred to first led the physicians to collect data from their patients and then violate patient privacy and medical record confidentiality by supplying information to the State.[13]

Organizations with humanitarian-sounding names were set up in Nazi Germany to institute "health" programs, under deceptive, euphemistic terms. For example, questionnaires collected by a "Realm's Work Committee of Institutions for Cure and Care" gathered and reported information on patients who had been ill five years or more and who were unable to work.

> On the basis of name, race, marital status, nationality, next
> of kin, whether regularly visited and by whom, who bore
> financial responsibility, and so forth, decisions were ultimately
> made for the patient euthanasia program heralded by the
> Nazi government for the good of the State and the health of
> the nation.

The first steps taken toward barbarism were the result of the willingness of physicians to participate in patient data collection and the violation of medical privacy. "Corrosion," as Dr. Alexander wrote, "begins in microscopic proportions."[13]

German physicians were, more than any other profession, heavily represented in the Nazi Party, which they joined in droves. German psychiatrists were no exception, and they also enthusiastically supported Nazi

Germany's gun control laws of 1938 that disarmed the civilian population and left a monopoly of force in the hands of the German military and the SS.

The rest, as we say, is history.

PART 5

THE SECOND AMENDMENT IN MODERN SOCIETY

CHAPTER 16
WOMEN, GUNS, AND THE NEED FOR SELF-PROTECTION

*How a politician stands on the Second Amendment tells you
how he or she views you as an individual... as a trustworthy
and productive citizen, or as part of an unruly crowd that needs
to be lorded over, controlled, supervised, and taken care of.*

—Dr. Suzanna Gratia Hupp,
who lost both parents in the 1991 Luby's cafeteria massacre

We will be repeating some important points of criminology in this chapter because as Goethe, the greatest German literary figure of his age, warned us over two centuries ago—the truth requires repetition because error and mendacity are being preached all the time by zealot propagandists using not only academia but also the popular press to deceive the multitudes.

It is no secret the mainstream liberal media and the entrenched, political medical establishment, although frequently denying it, support draconian gun control measures that, if unopposed, would lead to the confiscation and banning of firearms. Supported by "organized medicine" and progressive, anti-gun, medical journal editors, vociferous politicians, such as Senator Charles Schumer (D-NY), Dianne Feinstein (D-CA), and Dick Durbin (D-Il), have repeatedly proposed drastic gun control measures justifying it on the concept of "gun violence as a public health issue" and using this faulty paradigm to limit the availability of guns in the U.S. [1] Not surprisingly, these anti-gun politicians have been very successful in their own states—e.g., New York, California, and Illinois—which are very liberal states largely revolving around the large urban centers of New York City, Chicago, Los Angeles, and San Francisco. In addition to the state of California, where confiscation is no longer a threat but a law being fought in the courts, such cities as New York and Chicago, Washington, D.C., and Detroit, have experienced gun confiscation in futile attempts to stem the tide of gun violence in the inner cities. Instead, law-abiding citizens, including working single mothers, were left defenseless. The crime in those cities, particularly in Chicago, is endemic and out of control.

Backed by the public health establishment (PHE), liberal politicians in those states, as well as in New Jersey, Massachusetts, and Maryland, continue to espouse the erroneous concept of guns and bullets as virulent pathogens that need to be stamped out by limiting gun availability and ultimately eradicating guns from the citizenry. As we have previously noted, the problem is that guns and bullets are inanimate objects that do not follow the epidemiologic methodology and do not subscribe to Koch's Postulates of Pathogenicity. So using gun control instead of crime control is futile and destined to failure. And yet anti-gun activists and progressive politicians continue to preach that if a little gun control is ineffective, then more drastic measures are needed.

Gun control, in place of crime control, must be understood as an ongoing campaign orchestrated and kept alive by gun prohibitionists and Democrat politicians, who are willing to exploit our understandable concern for street violence and crime to advance not only their gun prohibitionist agenda but also expand the ever-increasing government, collectivism, and regimentation. At the same time, they know they have the impediment of the Second Amendment that they must neutralize, not by emendation of the U.S. Constitution as would be required by the constitutional process, but by limiting the scope of the Second Amendment per se, by gradual erosion and by enacting "reasonable restrictions" where possible, such as banning certain firearms, challenging concealed carry laws and the Castle Doctrine, and demonizing "stand your ground" legislation—all of which will be discussed in Chapter 25.

Ignoring the Beneficial Aspects of Firearms

We previously discussed how the monolithic wall of the entrenched, anti-gun, medical establishment was temporarily breached in 1994 with the studies published in the *Journal of the Medical Association of Georgia*, which I edited at the time. In the January 1994 issue, criminologist and Florida State University Professor Gary Kleck, author of the influential book *Point Blank: Guns and Violence in America* (1991), further analyzed the study conducted by Arthur Kellermann, M.D. and associates at the Center for Injury Control at Emory University. The study purported to have found that of people killed at home, 76 percent were shot by a family member or an acquaintance, and concluded that people who keep guns in their home are themselves more likely to be victims of homicide than those who don't. In the words of the authors, "Rather than confer protection, guns kept in the home are associated with an increase in the risk of homicide by a family member or intimate acquaintance."[2]

This information is still repeated over and over by the mainstream liberal media as an established fact, and also by the medical journals that should know better, but we must remember that when it comes to the topic of guns and violence, politics and ideology reign supreme over science and criminology. For example, Kleck's analysis disclosed several flaws in Kellermann's methodology. First, "violent households" would be expected "to be more likely to own guns than people in less violent households, even if guns themselves made no contribution at all to the violence." Second, Kleck emphasized that the Kellermann study did not indicate what percentage of gun uses was defensive and what percentage was criminal usage. For example, 63 percent of the "victims" were men; yet we do not know how many of these homicides represent genuine acts of self-defense by women against abusive husbands or lovers, and committed as justifiable homicides. In fact, according to the authors, "a majority of the homicides (50.9 percent) occurred in the context of a quarrel or a romantic triangle."[2] In this regard, it should be pointed out that other critics noted, "About half of the shootings by one spouse or the other are defensive killings of husbands by victimized wives. So it misleadingly characterizes many cases in which guns save innocent lives as gun murders."[3]

Furthermore, only gun uses that resulted in death were analyzed, thus the study ended up excluding the vast majority of gun uses that did not result in death, and which are more likely to be defensive uses by victims of crime to protect themselves.[3,4] In fact, as Kleck pointed out in his critique, "At least three-fourths of all uses of guns in crime-related incidents are defensive uses by the crime victims."[3] In a classic paper published in *The Journal of Criminal Law and Criminology*, Professors Gary Kleck and Marc Gertz found that among the up to 2.5 million defensive uses of firearms, there were as many as 200,000 cases of women defending themselves against sexual abuse. And yet in less than eight percent of cases, the citizen will kill or wound the assailant.[5]

Once again in the 1993 *NEJM* study Kellermann and associates went along with the faulty *post hoc ergo propter hoc* reasoning, "after it therefore because of it," blaming guns for the rise of crime and violence in America by faulty association. As a neurosurgeon who has spent his fair share of hours in the middle of the night treating victims of gunshot wounds, I also deplore the rising violence and crime in America—but the truth needed to be told, politically incorrect and inconvenient as it may be. The floodgates of dissension were opened when I also proposed in the aforementioned issue of the *Journal of the Medical Association of Georgia* that physicians have a professional obligation to base their opinions on objective data and scientific information, rather than on emotionalism or political expediency. After devoting an entire issue to the topic of guns and violence, we concluded that objective cumulative data indicates that indiscriminate gun control disarms the law-abiding citizens, while it does not prevent criminals and street thugs from perpetrating crimes on unwary victims. Moreover, guns in the hands of law-abiding citizens deter crime and clearly afford the benefit of self-protection.[6]

To begin with, less than one to two percent of crimes committed with firearms are carried out by concealed carry weapons (CCW) license holders. The vast majority of criminals obtain their guns illegally, which is not difficult since there are already over 300 million guns in circulation in the U.S., and criminals do what they do best—break the laws and perpetrate crime.[4-6]

Severe limitations on gun ownership would not only be unconstitutional but also difficult to accomplish, especially with those who do not comply with the law: the criminals. Americans know that they not only have a right to self-protection but also understand that the right embodied in the

Second Amendment is the right that secures all the others. In the mid-1990s there were approximately 500,000 police officers in the United States.[7] Thus, assuming three eight-hour shifts and other circumstances, such as vacations, leaves, and sick days, there were only 150,000 police on duty at any given time to protect a population of 250 million. Despite an increase in the number of police today and a general population exceeding 300 million, there is no reason to suppose the ratio has changed significantly and, then as now, the police cannot be in all places at all times.

Moreover, the duty of the police officers is not to prevent crime, but to apprehend criminals and bring them to justice—after a crime has been committed. Contrary to popular belief, the police do not have a legal duty to protect the public against criminals. According to several court opinions including the 1982 ruling *Bowers v. DeVito*, "There is no constitutional right to be protected by the state against being murdered by criminals or madmen. The constitution...does not require the federal government or the states to provide services, even so elementary a service as maintaining law and order."[8]

"Assault Weapons" in the Hands of Citizens

In the final analysis, despite the various beneficent and comforting police mottos, such as "protect and serve," the State has no legal responsibility to protect individual citizens from crime. Because the State only assumes a collective duty to the community, Americans must preserve their natural and constitutional right to keep and bear arms, and must assume some responsibility for self-protection from street thugs and ruffians stalking the streets of America. This was well exemplified during the Los Angeles riots in the spring of 1992, when Korean business owners protected their premises with firearms and saved their businesses from looting and burning. Other businesses that were left undefended were looted or burnt during the two days of civil unrest following the jury acquittal of four Los Angeles police officers of the beating of Rodney G. King. Millions of dollars of property were lost in the conflagration. Similar episodes have taken place in more recent years, such as in Ferguson, Missouri on November 25, 2014, where a riot erupted after a grand jury declined to indict the white police officer that fatally shot Michael Brown, a black youth. Protesters set fire to buildings and cars and plundered businesses in the area. The riot was further incited by the media, which had been adding fuel to the combustible mixture with incendiary, nonstop coverage since the shooting incident the previous August. As in previous riots, businesses that were protected with firearms were saved.[9]

The much maligned and mischaracterized "assault weapons" have been used quite effectively by private citizens to protect themselves and their property during urban crises as well as during and in the aftermath of natural disasters. We have already mentioned Ferguson, Missouri, in 2014 and the Korean shopkeepers during the 1992 Rodney King L.A. riots more than two decades ago, who protected their property not only with pistols but also with high capacity "assault weapons." Sadly, another shameful cause for plundering and looting are natural disasters.

After Hurricane Hugo assailed South Carolina in September 1989—devastating Isle of Palms, Sullivan's Island, and the city of Charleston—Governor Carroll Campbell Jr. issued "shoot on sight" orders to the National Guard. The National Guard, in some cases assisted by armed citizens, deterred some of the looters. Other South Carolina residents, a journalist reported, "Left nothing to chance. M.R. Thomas stood on his James Island lawn with a Smith & Wesson .357 revolver strapped over his shorts." He protected his property and kept watch, "There's been looting in the neighborhood, and I'm just trying to give looters the message that if they come back, I'm ready."[10] There were 89 looting arrests in South Carolina in the wake of Hurricane Hugo. Despite the number, looting was limited throughout South Carolina because citizens like Mr. Thomas were armed while defending their property. Many had "assault weapons" that acted as deterrent to crime.

Consider the catastrophic Hurricane Andrew in the late summer of 1992 that smashed into Florida causing $30 billion in damage and killing 43 people. The powerful hurricane devastated homes, businesses, and the southeastern Florida coastline. It also demolished government defense installations, like Homestead Air Force Base, where every building was damaged or destroyed and base personnel evacuated and told to stay away for days. Scattered looting took place. A 2015 article recapitulating the incident neglected to inform the readers that looting was limited because citizens used high capacity magazine "assault weapons"[11]—just as the Korean shopkeepers in Los Angeles in spring 1992 had done to protect their property. It's a sad chapter in the chronicles of humanity that after these horrific natural disasters, good citizens need to be armed to protect themselves, their families, and their property from the usual parasitic thugs marauding the land bent on capitalizing on the suffering of others.[12]

And in the wake of Hurricane Irma (September, 10-13, 2017), ignoring the property damage and human suffering in Florida and other locales in Georgia, like the city of Macon, thugs once again seized the opportunity to burn a store and loot businesses after the heavy winds and rains caused widespread loss of electrical power and burglar alarm outages leaving unattended businesses helpless.[13]

In such cases of tragic mayhem, suffering citizens are forced to assume some responsibility for protecting their lives and property. As intimated earlier, it seems all in all that the year 1992 was instructive in demonstrating the need for firearms, including high-magazine "assault weapons" in the lawful civilian population as well as in recognizing the harm that civilian disarmament can inflict on citizens during times of civil disorders or natural disasters.

Besides preventing and repelling crime, firearms (including handguns) are used 215,000 times each year by citizens to defend themselves against dangerous animals, such as poisonous snakes, alligators, feral hogs, and rabid animals.[7] In fact, speaking of Florida, where strange encounters with dangerous animals (many of them aggressive and not native to this country) are reported with increasing frequency—e.g., attacks by bands of wild rhesus macaque monkeys in a state park in Ocala, alligator attacks everywhere, and even encounters with pythons in the Florida Everglades—Floridians would be fortunate if they happen to carry a so-called "assault weapon" for self-protection.

According to the Bureau of Justice Statistics, despite all the media discussion about "assault weapons," less than one percent of gun crimes are committed with "assault weapons" nationwide. Many sport and hunting semi-automatic rifles that have a paramilitary appearance are erroneously referred to as either assault weapons or assault rifles. These are misnomers that only reflect the mainstream liberal media's ignorance or deliberate mischaracterization and mislabeling of firearms by gun prohibitionists in promoting their agenda.

There are major differences between assault weapons and assault rifles. "Assault weapon" is really a legislative term that arose in 1989 with the Clinton administration's gun control agenda. It refers to the efforts of the Democrat administration and their confreres in Congress to pass a ban on certain types of firearms that were deemed to be very dangerous and used by criminals to commit crimes. The so-called "assault weapons" included 19 specific types of rifles, such as the Chinese or Russian AK-47 and the Colt AR-15 Sporter rifle. Additionally, there were other characteristics of these "assault weapons," such as large capacity magazines, a pistol-type grip to the stock, and mean-looking external paramilitary appearance. These characteristics led to a list that encompassed over 200 types of rifles, including hunting and recreational sporting rifles, handguns, and shotguns.

On the other hand, "assault rifles" are true military weapons, fully automatic, capable of producing bursts of automatic fire and designed so that in war, they are more likely to wound than to kill, thus tying up more enemy troops and resources. Assault rifles fire in semi-automatic or automatic mode as selected by the shooter. But the fact remains that assault rifles, as fully automatic rifles, have been strictly regulated since passage of the National Firearm Act of 1934 (updated in 1968 and 1986), and they have nothing to do with "assault weapons," which are semi-automatic civilian firearms. The mainstream liberal media has contributed to the confusion in their drive to promote gun control, linking the two types of firearms as one and the same, and they have been quite successful. The term assault rifle is hardly mentioned today, and the discussion revolves around "assault weapons," the ferocious looking, civilian firearms that many people still erroneously think are fully automatic, military weapons and more dangerous than other firearms.

As prominent firearm expert, Edward Ezell, Curator of the Smithsonian Institute and National Firearm Collection, testified to the Senate Judiciary Committee in 1989 at the outset of the debate, handguns and 12-gauge shotguns were the primary firearms used in common crimes. That is still the case today, despite the notoriety of "assault weapons." The anti-gun activists have promulgated the myth that 16 percent of homicides are perpetrated with the "dangerous" assault weapons. The fact is that less than 6 percent of criminals use any firearm that can even be mischaracterized as an "assault weapon." Criminals are five times more likely to use a handgun in crime than a paramilitary weapon.[14]

"Assault weapons" have not been under attack just at the federal level. Several states have passed assault weapons bans, despite the usefulness of these semi-automatic weapons for sports shooting as well as life-saving tools during natural catastrophes, civil unrest, and individual acts of self-defense against multiple criminal assailants (as we will see in Chapter 22). These firearms have been so mischaracterized and maligned that some legislatures and courts are yet to assess favorably. On November 27, 2017, the U.S. Supreme Court refused to take up Maryland's assault weapons ban. The 4th Circuit Court of Appeals upheld Maryland's Firearm Safety Act of 2013 banning, "the AR-15 and other military-style rifles and shotguns, often referred to as 'assault weapons,' and detachable large-capacity magazines." Again, "assault weapons" were confused with "assault rifles" and characterized as military weapons and thus excluded from Second Amendment protection by the Circuit Court. Interestingly, the judge who wrote the majority decision stated, "Put simply, we have no power to extend Second Amendment protection to the weapons of war that the Heller decision [2008] explicitly excluded from such coverage."[14]

Curiously, it was precisely in *Miller v. U.S.* (1938), the last federal ruling on the Second Amendment until the Heller decision, that ownership of military-style weapons (firearms) were specifically protected as a pre-existent individual right by the Second Amendment.[14]

Women and Guns

Guns, including semi-automatic firearms and "assault weapons," are useful for self, family, and property protection. So it is not surprising that in a survey of 1,800 prison inmates, 81 percent agreed that a smart criminal tried to find out if his potential victim is armed, 74 percent said that burglars avoid houses when people are home because they fear being shot, and 34 percent admit to having been scared off, shot at, wounded, or even captured by armed citizens.[15]

Professor Gary Kleck noted that citizens acting in self-defense kill at least twice and up to three times more assailants and robbers than do the police.[5] In his scholarly compiled books, Kleck garners statistics evincing the fact that the defensive uses of handguns by citizens surpass criminal uses because in America many citizens own guns for self and family protection. Yes, firearms are used more frequently by law-abiding citizens to repel crime than by criminals to perpetrate crime.[2,5] Moreover, criminologist Don B.

Kates and medical editor Patricia T. Harris maintain that "...by focusing on homes the statistics exclude the numerous instances in which shopkeepers kill robbers. When the number of abused wives and shopkeepers who shoot criminals is accounted, the figure for defensive killing increases by about 1,000 percent..."[4]

Data gathered by Professor Kleck therefore concluded that given the relative use of guns for self-protection versus criminal uses: *"[The] life-saving uses of guns annually...would dwarf the nearly 37,000 lives taken with guns."*[3] As Edgar Suter, M.D., pointed out years ago from his review of the available literature, *"as many as 75 lives are potentially saved for every life lost to a gun."* In our estimation, the beneficial uses of guns have not been properly portrayed in the medical literature or the popular press.[5,16]

National Victims Data suggests that "while victims resisting with knives, clubs, or bare hands are about twice as likely to be injured as those who submit, victims who resist with a gun are only half as likely to be injured as those who put up no defense."[5]Similarly, regarding women and self-defense, "among those victims using handguns in self-defense, 66 percent of them were successful in warding off the attack and keeping their property. Among those victims using non-gun weapons, only 40 percent were successful. Among those victims fleeing the scene, only 35 percent were successful. Among those victims invoking physical force, only 22 percent were successful. Among those using verbal shouting only 20 percent were successful..."[5] The gun is the great equalizer for women when they are accosted in the street or when they are defending themselves and their children at home.

In the U.S., women who do not know how to protect themselves continue to be targets of crime. According to a survey by William Barnhill of *The Washington Post*, "73 percent of all women now over the age of 12 will be victimized, more than a third of them raped, robbed, or assaulted at some point in their lives." But women are beginning to fight back. In the U.S., at least 12 million women now own handguns. Thus, according to Tracey Martin, former manager of the National Rifle Association's Education and Training Division, "a gun can make the difference between being the victim or the victor in a confrontation with a criminal."[17] Paxton Quigley, who once advocated gun control but now recommends that women learn to protect themselves with handguns, stated, "Guns in the hands of women who know how to use them do deter crime."[17] Indeed, civil rights attorney

David Kopel has also observed: "The U.S. Census Bureau conducts in-person interviews with several thousand persons annually, for the National Crime Victimization Survey (NCVS). In 1992–2002, over 2,000 of the persons interviewed disclosed they had been raped or sexually assaulted. Of them, only 26 volunteered that they used a weapon to resist. In none of those 26 cases was the rape completed; in none of the cases did the victim suffer additional injury after she deployed her weapon."[18] Robert J. Kukla wrote in his book, *Gun Control*, "Today...a dainty and delicate woman, with courage and determination, is more than the equal of any brute who ever trampled the sand of a Roman arena. The difference is the firearm."[18]

Firearm safety training is essential for citizens not familiar with guns, particularly for women who have been victimized and suddenly recognize the need for self-protection. They need firearm training and gun safety instruction. And such training reduces victimization and crime completion. Robert W. Lee recounted that some years back "in the wake of a rampage of robberies and rapes, more than 2500 women were trained to use firearms in Orlando, Florida. Within nine months, robberies and attacks plummeted 90 percent; rapes, 25 percent; and aggravated assaults and burglaries, 24 percent."[18] In 1979, a Justice Department study conducted during the Carter administration found that of more than 32,000 attempted rapes, 32 percent were actually completed. The big difference was the possession of a firearm by an intended victim. Of those armed only three percent of the attempts were successful. *When a trained woman is armed with a gun, 97 percent of the time she will be successful at preventing rape, and only half as likely of being injured in the process.*[19]

Domestic Violence and Intimate Partner Abuse

The reader will recall Kellermann and associates first propounded the 43 times fallacy (1986); then in 1993, the 2.7 times fallacy—namely that a gun in the home is more likely to injure the homeowner than an intruder. A more recent claim propounded by the PHE takes a slightly different twist, claiming that if there is a gun in the home at the time of a domestic violence incident, it increases a woman's chance of being killed by 500 percent. As with the previous fallacies that we have thoroughly debunked, this figure is suspect for a number of reasons.[20] First, a school of public health notorious for its anti-gun bias conducted the study, and this bias is immediately obvious in the wording and design of their study. For example, we cannot be certain if the gun was already present in the home or brought to the house specifically by the criminal partner to commit the homicide. Second, instead of empowering the abused and victimized women, who are the innocent parties in this scenario, the PHE researchers want to categorically disarm them while leaving the abusive (criminal) partner potentially armed.[21] Third, the study glosses over the fact that federal and state laws already exist that should have prevented individuals convicted of domestic violence from owning and possessing firearms. We are talking about dysfunctional families, and these domiciles are usually well known to the police because of repeated episodes of domestic violence. Murders in this setting do not happen out of the blue, as we shall see shortly.

Fourth, restraining orders against abusive husbands, intimate partners, or stalkers are very effective and if they are violated, the police should take action. Frequently, the abused partner refuses to press charges and returns to the abusive relationship. Education about how to end this cycle of violence and information regarding resources available in the community should be mandatory in counseling in police departments and shelters. Failing all those measures, the victimized partner should be allowed to own a gun for self-protection and encouraged to undergo firearm training and gun safety instruction. If a woman who has been victimized and who is not familiar with firearms decides to obtain a gun for self-protection, she should undergo training. Firearms can be dangerous to the uninitiated, and in addition to the proper psychological attitude towards armed self-defense, as will be discussed in Chapter 18, five basic rules should always be followed: 1. Treat all guns as if they were loaded; 2. Never point your firearm at anything you don't want to harm; 3. Keep your finger off the trigger until you target is sighted and you are ready to shoot; 4. Always be sure of your target and what lies beyond; 5. Know how to operate and maintain control of your firearm at all times.[22] Remember, training is essential for the uninitiated.

We have described the benefit of armed self-defense measures, when and if all else fails. Even so, the gun prohibitionists want more laws and insist on disarming and preventing the potential victim from being able to defend herself from a criminal predator, who by definition does not obey the law. Moreover, if the criminal were arrested, the revolving prison door system would throw him back out in the street before the ink had dried on his arrest record.

The shortcomings of the permissive criminal justice system and the lack of crime control are the problems. There are more than 20,000 gun laws on the books. We certainly do not need more legislation that disarms the innocent victim and does nothing to deter the abusive partner in domestic violence. Although domestic violence laws may vary by state, federal law is uniform and would be effective if violators were prosecuted to the full extent of the law and incarcerated—recognizing that some hardened criminal elements, once released via the revolving prison door system, will resume their cycle of violence.

These scenarios bring us to the much-ballyhooed "crimes of passion" (briefly mentioned in Chapter 2), that take place impulsively and in the heat of a domestic squabble; but criminologists have pointed out that homicides in this setting are the culmination of a long simmering cycle of violence. One study of the police records in Detroit and Kansas City revealed that, "in 90 percent of domestic homicides, the police had responded at least once before during the prior two years to a disturbance, and in over 50 percent of cases, the police had been called five times or more."[22]

Surely, these are not crimes of passion consummated impulsively in the heat of the moment, but the result of violence in highly dysfunctional families in a setting of alcohol or illicit drug use; abusive husbands who after a long history of spousal abuse finally commit murder; and increasingly, wives defending themselves against abusive husbands. Yes, in many cases, domestic shootings represent acts of self-defense by women from abusive husbands, boyfriends, or intimate acquaintances even if they are recorded in police files as "homicides." In one of his many critiques of Kellermann and associates, Dr. Edgar Suter wrote, "No effort was made by the authors to assess the protective uses of guns by women. In fact, the authors attempted to portray legitimate self-defense as murder."[16]

Women are abused 2 million to 4 million times per year. Their children are similarly abused, even fatally. Almost all the "spouses and domestic partners killed by women each year are the very same men, well known to the police, often with substance abuse histories, who have been brutalizing their wives, girlfriends, and children."[16]

Twenty percent of homicides are self-defense or justifiable in the final analysis. FBI data, because it is based on "preliminary determination rather than final determination," dramatically underreports justifiable homicides. Dr. Suter further commented, "The FBI's definition of 'acquaintance' includes the maniac in one's apartment building and dueling drug dealers."[16]

It should be of interest to note that the pattern of domestic homicides in Australia is similar to that of the United States, and in his 1992 book, *The Samurai, the Mountie, and the Cowboy: Should America Adopt the Gun Controls of Other Democracies?* David Kopel has cited some interesting statistics about women and guns that apply to the U.S. as well as Australia:

> *Twenty-five percent of all homicides are spousal killings with 75 percent of men doing the killing. Although guns are used in many of these homicides, men are less likely to use them because physical force with hands, feet, or any handy object within his reach, frequently suffice for the ultimate crime of passion. In fact, almost 25 percent of men use no weapon at all. On the other hand, women most frequently use a weapon, usually a gun. As in the U.S. experience, the Australian National Committee on Violence (NCV) assessed the situation: "Murders committed by wives are usually desperate, last ditch responses after receiving years of brutal violence."[18]*

Gun control then could reduce the last ditch use of guns by women defending themselves from homicidal husbands, but it would not reduce the killing of wives by husbands, who do not need guns to kill because of their superior physical strength. Kopel suggests gun control then, "may not be a step forward for social justice."[18] I concur.

Data from the Australian National Committee on Violence (NCV) also noted that 35 percent of women killed by husbands had been previously physically assaulted by them. Thus, victims of domestic violence are frequently advised to leave their abusive relationships. Yet, we should not take solace in women following this advice because the converse is not always true: Leaving a bad relationship may not prevent violence towards, or the homicide, of victimized women. Almost 50 percent of women killed by their husbands had already been separated from them.[18]

It is highly ironic that American PHE officials, who are so bent upon saddling Americans with stringent gun control laws and ultimately disarming them, are part and parcel of the same progressive liberal elites that coddle repeat offenders—namely, the abusive husbands, the predatory boyfriends (or "intimate partners" in their vocabulary), dangerous stalkers, and other criminal elements—and make excuses for their crimes. At the same time, they want to disarm and leave the victims defenseless.

As we shall read about in later chapters, these common criminal elements were the cultural equivalent of the "socially friendly" elements that cooperated with the State in the gulag system of the former Soviet Union.

Reaching a Consensus of an Individual Right

If draconian gun control measures (e.g., beginning with step-by-step restrictions, followed by banning and confiscation of particular firearms and/or semi-automatic weapons) are instituted, law-abiding citizens will be certain to feel the impact. They will be the ones with the most to lose, including their constitutionally-protected right to own guns, whether for hunting or for personal protection. This has already happened in some cities, such as Chicago, New Orleans, Los Angeles, Baltimore, and New York, where lawful citizens have been disarmed and left to the mercy of criminals.

The Founding Fathers held that man's constitutional rights were God-given and inalienable. Although the government was, and remains, the guarantor of those rights, it was ultimately on the people themselves that those inalienable rights rested. The informed citizenry were to be the ultimate enforcers, and the Second Amendment itself was to be the vehicle by which that right was to safeguard and secure all others. As if to underscore this fact, the same Congress that passed the Bill of Rights (with the Second Amendment) also passed the Militia Act of 1790, which defined the militia as "every able-bodied man" of military age.[23]

In the *U.S. v. Verdugo-Urquidez* decision of 1990, the Supreme Court held that when the phrase, "the people" is used in the context of the Second Amendment, it means "individuals"—as to mean "the right of the people to keep and bear arms shall not be infringed." Like it or not, to assert that the phrase, "the people" implied a collective right which, when coupled with the locution "well-regulated militia" restricted the meaning of the Second Amendment to a state "militia" of citizen-soldiers, as in the National Guard, is preposterous. If that were the case, the Second Amendment would stand out, alone, as the only amendment in the Bill of Rights that does not stand for individual liberties and as a bulwark against government power—in stark contrast to the other nine amendments, all of which limit the scope and power of government, and protect and enhance the individual rights of citizens. In short, gun control activists want to implement unconstitutional gun control measures, step by step, until they reach their true and ultimate goal: prohibition of civilian gun ownership.

It should be noted that in the *U.S. v. Miller* (1938) decision, the U.S. explicitly protected an individual's right "to keep and bear arms" especially and explicitly the ownership of military-style weapons or so-called "assault weapons," as "part of the ordinary military equipment."[23] It was again in the *Journal of the Medical Association of Georgia* (*JMAG*; this time the June 1995 issue) that legal scholarship on the Second Amendment was reviewed specifically for physicians and public health officials.[24] This article, which I co-authored and published was signed by 37 Second Amendment supporters, including legal and constitutional scholars. It pointed out, "Since 1980, of 39 law review articles, 35 noted the Supreme Court's acknowledgment of the individual right to keep and bear arms,[23] and only four claimed the right was only a collective right of the states."[25]

So, as we wrote in that 1995 article: "In the last decade, constitutional scholars 'from across the political spectrum' have concluded that the Second Amendment protects an individual right, a view that is referred to as the 'Standard Model' by University of Tennessee Professor Glenn Harlan Reynolds."[24] The nation's leading legal and constitutional scholars—including Laurence Tribe of Harvard, Akil Reed Amar of Yale, William Van Alstyne of Duke University, Sanford Levinson of University of Texas Law School, Don B. Kates of the Pacific Institute for Public Policy Research, attorney David Kopel of the Independence Institute, and noted Fairfax, Virginia, attorneys Jeffrey Snyder and Stephen P. Halbrook—all subscribe to the "Standard Model" or individual right view.[23,24,26]

Though the gun control debate has focused on the Second Amendment, legal scholarship also finds support for the Right to Keep and Bear Arms in Ninth Amendment "un-enumerated" rights, Fourteenth Amendment "due process" and "equal protection," and natural rights theory. Also, in the absence of explicit delegated powers, the Tenth Amendment guarantees that the powers not delegated to the federal government are reserved to the states and the people.[27] This latter fact was spelled out in two major Supreme Court cases. In *U.S. v. Lopez* (1995), in striking down the Gun Free Schools Zones Act, U.S. Chief Justice William Rehnquist wrote that the law was unconstitutional because it would otherwise convert the Commerce Clause of the Constitution to a general police power it does not possess. In *Printz et al v. U.S.* (1997), the Court went a step further and, to the chagrin of the gun control lobby, struck down a major section of the federal Brady Law. Associate Justice Antonin Scalia quoted a passage from James Madison (*The Federalist* No. 51): "Just as the separation and independence of the coordinate branches of the federal Government serve to prevent the accumulation of excessive power in any one branch, a healthy balance of power between the States and the Federal Government will reduce the risk of tyranny and abuse from either front." Attorney Elizabeth Swasey, Director of NRA/ILA Crime Strike, noted this was the same passage Chief Justice Rehnquist cited in the *Lopez* case.[27]

It was also in 1999 that we had the momentous court ruling of the *Northern District of Texas, U.S. v. Emerson*, in which U.S. District Court Judge Sam Cummings overturned a federal gun law on Second Amendment grounds stating, "The right of the Second Amendment should be as zealously guarded as the other individual liberties enshrined in the Bill of Rights."[28]

We finally reached a consensus at least legally, constitutionally and morally—a consensus at least between the majority of the citizens, and the greatest legal minds, and the Supreme Court agrees—even if the progressive and rabid anti-gun politicians still do not.

And yet it would take two landmark decisions rendered more than 70 years after *U.S. v. Miller* (1938) for the Supreme Court to definitely rule and affirm that the Second Amendment is an inalienable individual right of all Americans, and those rulings were decided by razor-thin majorities of five to four. Most disturbingly, if Hillary Clinton had won the 2016 presidential election that razor-thin majority on the Supreme Court would have vanished and the decisions reversed or modified out of existence with the appointment of the next Supreme Court Justice to be made by the new president in 2017! We will have more to say about these two landmark

Supreme Court decisions in a later chapter.

Ineffective Background Checks & Dangerous Waiting Periods

The proper approach to gun violence and street crime should not involve penalizing law-abiding citizens and infringing on their right to keep and bear arms. Serious attempts to decrease gun violence should involve preventing accidental shootings, particularly keeping guns away from minors, and most importantly, from convicted felons and criminals, who by their criminal offenses have legally forfeited their right to possess guns. In fact, the vast majority of murderers are career criminals with long criminal records.

The reality is that the typical murderer has a prior criminal history of at least six years with four felony arrests in his record.[29] There are more than 20,000 gun laws on the books throughout the states and many of them need to be enforced; while others penalizing lawful citizens, should be rescinded.

But more restrictive gun laws are not the answer—for example, the Brady Bill passed in several states enforcing waiting periods for gun purchases. These delays have endangered lawful citizens needing a gun quickly for self-protection; yet the law has not kept guns away from criminals, nor reduced crime. Instead, there have been lurid tales of victims killed by attackers, who had previously threatened them, while waiting to pick up newly purchased and badly needed guns for self-protection.

Gun Owners of America (GOA) keeps useful data available for study. Their research shows that waiting periods "threaten the safety of people in imminent danger." One case described was that of Bonnie Elmasri. Mrs. Elmasri tried to obtain a gun for self-protection from an abusive husband, who had repeatedly threatened to kill her. She was informed there was a 48-hour waiting period to buy a handgun. Unfortunately, Bonnie did not get her gun in time. The next day, her abusive husband, a man well known to the police, killed her and her two sons.[30]

Another case described was that of Marine Corporal Rayna Ross. She was able to purchase a gun in a state without a waiting period and was forced to use it in self-defense only two days later, killing her assailant. If Corporal Ross had been subjected to a waiting period, like Bonnie Elmasri, she would have been defenseless against the man stalking her.[30]

In yet another tragic case, Carol Bowne of New Jersey tried to buy a gun for self-protection but was forced to wait several weeks for her background check. While fearfully waiting, the man who had been stalking her and who she was afraid would kill her, stabbed her to death.[31]

A solution that gun prohibitionists have proposed as a cure all for domestic violence and gun crime is the establishment of strict background checks with no time limit or deadline for the FBI to issue an approval. Before the National Instant Criminal Background Check System (NICS) was instituted in 1998, the Brady Handgun Violence Prevention Act or the Brady Law (1994–1998) was in effect. It mandated a federal background check on all firearms purchases and imposed a five-day waiting period before the transfer of the purchased firearm. It was ineffective and did not keep guns out of the hands of criminals.

The National Instant Criminal Background Check System (NICS)

Since 1998, the NICS has been in effect but it has not lived up to the expectations of saving lives by keeping guns away from criminals. Gun Owners of America (GOA) calls background checks ineffective and dangerous and to back up that claim has shown that 95 percent of NICS denials were false positives, which means that lawful citizens were denied purchase of a firearm because of a bureaucratic snafu, such as the person's name was confused with another's, the presence of a traffic violation, or a single transgression that took place decades earlier. In 2010, the NICS processed over 6 million background checks of which 95 percent of the denials issued were incorrect; 72,569 people were denied firearm purchases by the FBI, but just 44 people were prosecuted and only 13 people were convicted and prohibited from buying firearms in the future. And according to the Inspector General Report of 2016, an average of only 32 people are prosecuted each year under the Brady Law.[31]

At initial inspection of the NICS-FBI data, the numbers seem to suggest that the FBI was indeed stopping the bad guys, and many people prohibited from having guns were stopped, but they were not necessarily criminals; they were mostly citizens who had committed non-violent offenses or decades-old misdemeanors. Erich Pratt, executive director of GOA, admits that some criminals are stopped, but stresses that the majority of violent criminals are savvy enough to know their names are in the NICS system and that they cannot pass a background check; therefore, they don't try getting guns that route. Pratt asserts that the denials refer to non-violent people who did not realize they were in the NICS database. As an example, Pratt noted:

> *The FBI chart lists the biggest number of stops relating to those who are 'Convicted of a Crime Punishable by More Than One Year or a Misdemeanor Punishable by More Than Two Years.'[32] The problem with this is that it can cover the military veteran who plea-bargained to a misdemeanor offense for fighting in a bar several decades ago. Such was the case of Jeff Schrader of Georgia, who was convicted of a misdemeanor for fighting against a gang member when he was 19 years old. He went on to serve honorably in the U.S. Navy, but 45 years after his misdemeanor conviction, he tried to buy a gun and was denied![32,33]*

The above category represents 62 percent of the denials. It is of further interest, as we will see in Chapter 19, how laws can change affecting gun rights, as well as the life and liberty of citizens. Pratt added, "By the way, in 1969, Schrader's misdemeanor from Maryland did not qualify as a two-year offense. But it does today, given changes in the law."[32]

Next, Pratt analyzed the FBI data at the second highest category that represented 11 percent of the denials, "Misdemeanor Crime of Domestic Violence Conviction." Here he points out, "The problem with this category is that a mere misdemeanor can disqualify both men and women from ever again exercising their Second Amendment rights." He refers as examples to those of "a wife tearing her husband's pocket during an argument and a daughter throwing the keys at her mom, and missing"—both situations as domestic violence misdemeanors were subject to the ban.[34]

The third highest FBI category with 8 percent of denials was "Unlawful User/Addicted to a Controlled Substance." Pratt observed, "Similar to the previous categories, real abusers typically know they're disqualified. But people in this category can be disqualified because they legally use marijuana with a prescription from a doctor, a class of people who are generally not violent."

The fourth category with eight percent of denials included "Fugitive from Justice." Pratt commented, "Again, this category might sound like it's stopping real bad guys, until you consider that one of the most frequent causes of bench warrants being issued is unpaid traffic tickets where the offender fails to appear before the court."[32,35]

In some particularly egregious cases, no reason for denial is given. Take for instance, John Lopey, a California sheriff who had served 33 years as a state trooper and former U.S. Army Colonel with a top secret clearance, was flagged by the NICS and denied a firearm without cause or notification. Pratt noted that "if he can be denied a gun, then the purpose of the NICS becomes clear—to slowly eliminate private gun ownership."[32]

Pratt concluded:

> *Just because there are people who legitimately fall into the FBI's categories and are legitimately denied doesn't mean that most of these people were truly violent. If truly violent people are getting stopped at gun stores in droves, then why aren't they being prosecuted? When you compare the few people who are incarcerated for purchasing firearms to the billions of dollars— and multiple thousands of man hours—that have been spent running the NICS system, one can argue that such resources would have been more 'effectively' used elsewhere.*[32,36]

Constitutionally, there is also a problem with background checks. Every name submitted by a firearm dealer for NICS check is potentially retained illegally by either the FBI or worse, the ATF. Data retention may be a prelude for illegal and unconstitutional registration. In fact, the General Accounting Office found in 2016 that the ATF had violated the rights of lawful citizens by retaining their names and registering them as gun owners in violation of previous court rulings. Governments, as we will discuss in Chapter 21, have historically used registration as a prelude to banning and confiscation.[31]

Despite this, background checks have not made us safer in preventing some mass-shooting incidents in which the deranged individual or mass terrorist passed the background check. In the 2015 San Bernardino shooting, which will be discussed along with other major mass-shooting incidents in Chapter 22, there was nothing that would have popped up in the background check that could have been used to deny the gun purchases to the planner-terrorist, Syed Farook. Moreover, the neighbor Enrique Marquez, who was implicated in the purchase of two additional assault weapons for the terrorist Farook family, was charged with falsifying information, and then supplying firearms to the homegrown jihadists.

In another Islamic terrorist incident, the Orlando attack, the two guns were also bought legally.[37] Of the reported 73 mass shootings, defined by *Mother Jones* magazine as the killing of four or more victims that have allegedly taken place since 1982, 82 percent of the purchasers passed the background check.[38] About half of the shooters had a mental health history that didn't impede obtaining the weapons for themselves, or their crime guns were bought legally by friends or family members. The NRA agrees that the majority of mass shooters, including those inspired by terrorism or the result of undiagnosed mental illness, pass the background check. We must keep in mind that mass shootings represent a minuscule number of homicide gun deaths. According to the FBI, for the year 2010, mass shootings represent less than one percent of the reported U.S. gun homicides.[39] The NRA opposes the expansion of background checks because they don't stop criminal elements from obtaining guns. Criminals obtain their guns illegally through theft or through straw purchases. The NRA agrees with GOA that background check information has been used illegally for firearm registration.[40]

Towards Viable Solutions?

Nevertheless, shooting rampages are shocking and tragic incidents that the mainstream liberal media sensationalizes, not necessarily to expose the inefficiencies of background checks and to propose constructive solutions in terms of promoting citizen defense initiatives, crime control, better parenting, and better mental health initiatives, but instead to capitalize on the tragedy to push for and try to pass more restrictive but ineffective gun control laws.[20,37]

There is a perfidious and progressively instigated trend to absolve the guilty individual of personal responsibility and accountability, and instead, to blame society at large for every contemporary social affliction. The public health/epidemiologic model of gun control, which we discussed at length in previous chapters, is also flawed in this regard—namely, it deflects accountability from individual transgressors to society at large and even worse to inanimate objects, e.g., guns and bullets. In the one case, it blames an abstraction that becomes everyone but the perpetrator; in the other, it blames inanimate objects. Thus the criminal becomes "the victim" of circumstances. It is in this atmosphere that draconian gun control measures that penalize the law-abiding citizens are repeatedly proposed. Drastic gun control measures have been instituted in cities, such as Washington, D.C. and Chicago, and in states, such as New York, California, and Maryland, to no avail. Draconian gun control measures are always unfair, unproductive, and frequently criminal, as we have seen. We should oppose any gun control measure that would in any way disarm law-abiding citizens and leave them at the mercy of criminals who will continue to obtain guns. Giving lip service to political correctness and joining the bandwagon of political expediency, as the PHE, the AMA and "organized medicine" have done, are not the answers.

A larger dose of individual responsibility and accountability, and more firearm training and gun safety courses are needed. The real culprits behind the violence and crime in America are societal decay, moral disintegration, and failures of America's criminal justice and mental health systems—not inanimate guns and bullets. Strongly needed are principles of moral and spiritual guidance, better child rearing, parenting, and family cohesiveness, along with a tougher criminal justice system without revolving prison doors.

CHAPTER 17

CHILDREN, SHOOTINGS, AND JUVENILE DELINQUENCY

*Boys who own legal firearms have much lower rates
of delinquency and drug use and are even slightly
less delinquent than non-owners of guns.*

—U.S. Department of Justice,

National Institute of Justice, Office of Juvenile Justice
and Delinquency Prevention, NCJ-143454, "Urban
Delinquency and Substance Abuse," August 1995

A Crime Perspective at Odds with Reality

A favorite view of the public health establishment (PHE) is the myth propounded by Dr. Mark Rosenberg, former head of the NCIPC of the CDC, who wrote, "Most of the perpetrators of violence are not criminals by trade or profession. Indeed, in the area of domestic violence, most of the perpetrators are never accused of any crime. The victims and perpetrators are ourselves—ordinary citizens, students, professionals, and even public health workers."[1] That statement is contradicted by available data, government data. The fact, as we have seen, is that the typical murderer has had a prior criminal history of at least six years with four felony arrests in his record before he finally commits murder.[2] The FBI statistics reveal that 75 percent of all violent crimes for any locality are committed by six percent of hardened criminals and repeat offenders.[3] Less than one to two percent of crimes committed with firearms are carried out by licensed (e.g., concealed carry permit holders) law-abiding citizens.[4]

Violent crimes continue to be a problem in medium and large cities with gangs of juvenile delinquents and inner city youth involved in the drug trade. Crimes in rural areas for both blacks and whites, despite the preponderance of guns in this setting, remain low.[4,5] Gun availability does not cause crime. Prohibitionist government policies and gun control (rather than crime control) exacerbate the problem by making it more difficult for law-abiding citizens to defend themselves, their families, and their property. In fact, there was a modest increase in both homicide and suicide following prohibition after ratification of the XVIII Amendment (1919) and passage of the Gun Control Act of 1968.[6] Unreasonable social controls and prohibitions transmogrify innocuous habits and customs into vices and crime that become as forbidden fruit.

Children and Guns

Recall John Lott's finding that children 14 to 15 years of age are 14.5 times more likely to die from automobile injuries, five times more likely to die from drowning or fire and burns, and three times more likely to die from bicycle accidents than they are to die from gun accidents.[7]

A child's death from any cause is a tragedy. In 1991, 145 children between the ages of one and 14 years died of accidental gunshot wounds, 310 children died from suffocation (choking), 1,075 children died from burns, 1,104 died of drowning, and 3,271 died in motor vehicle accidents.[8,9] Yet, these figures have improved. Dr. Tom Vaughan researched this topic and wrote:

> *According to the CDC, during the 15 years from 2001 to 2015, 697 children 12 and under were killed by accidental gunshot wounds—an average of 47 each year. I can't imagine the anguish of losing a child by a firearm or hunting accident and the profound loss those parents must suffer for the rest of their lives. Unfortunately we do not live in a risk free society, and during that same period, 61,407 children died from all accidental causes, including 21,727 who died in motor*

vehicle accidents, 16,049 who suffocated, 10,182 children who drowned, 5,341 who died in fires, and 1,097 who died of accidental poisoning.[7]

These are all tragedies, but we cannot ban food, matches, swimming pools, and automobiles. Life is not risk free; and the risks we assume with those necessities and amenities of life, and luxuries in the case of swimming pools, are calculated risks. In the case of firearms, we are dealing not only with sporting and self-defense tools but also with constitutionally protected and required appurtenances of freedom. Fortunately, gun accident rates in the United States (including those for children) have been declining steadily since the turn of the century, particularly since 1975,[10] because of the emphasis that has been placed on gun safety education courses, including the NRA's Eddie Eagle *GunSafe®* program which by the year 2000 had already touched providentially over nine million youngsters in the U.S.

We are aware that some studies have criticized the Eddie Eagle *GunSafe®* program as ineffective, suggesting that children parrot the slogan but do not necessarily follow through with the instructions. That may be so in some instances, but the dramatic drop in accidental child deaths since the inception of the program suggests otherwise, and the NRA is expanding the program. The same critical *Forbes* magazine article also made the claim we have been hearing from various anti-gun sources—namely, that the increase in gun ownership has been concentrated in fewer households. This is a preposterous claim made and repeated by anti-gun activists and misinformed people, who have not read the work of Professor Gary Kleck cited previously. Kleck has shown, and even *JAMA* corroborated, that heads of household frequently deny having guns in the home in one-third of cases and for reasons previously discussed. Returning to the issue of the dramatic decrease in accidental child deaths, we must add that it's obvious more parents are practicing better storage of firearms, instructing their children about gun safety, and very definitely more Americans are attending firearm training and gun safety courses. The result is that accidental child (as well as adult) firearm deaths have fallen dramatically in the last 75 years, as we have shown in the preceding paragraphs.[11]

Juvenile Delinquency and Mass Shootings

As far as teenage violence is concerned, we previously asserted that more than 20,000 gun laws are already on the books for adults as well as juveniles, including a sizable number pertaining to the proscription of handgun possession by minors and banning guns on school grounds.[12] Some of these laws need to be enforced, others rescinded. Despite all the media hype regarding guns and violence, the naked truth is that the latest available FBI statistics show that, like the little known drop in gun accident rates, there has been a steady decline in homicide rates for every segment of American society, except for a small glitch in 2014 and 2015, which as we have seen, was immediately used by PHE researchers to make a preposterous claim using truncated data. The larger picture remains that by the end of the millennium, murder and violent crimes reached 30 and 25-year low rates, respectively.[13]

Despite what you have been led to believe and contrary to sensationalized reporting, mass shootings are not more frequent today, only more publicized and propagandized. Northeastern University Criminal Justice Professor James Fox reported that the highest casualty rate for mass murders in the past three decades occurred in 1977! In that year, 38 criminals killed 141 victims. Compare this to 1994, which had the lowest number of mass murders: 31 criminals murdered 74 people. Professor Fox wrote:

> *According to a careful analysis of data on mass shootings (using the widely accepted definition of at least four killed), the Congressional Research Service found that there are, on average, just over 20 incidents annually. More important, the increase in cases, if there was one at all, is negligible. Indeed, the only genuine increase is in hype and hysteria.*[14]

From 2000 to 2013 the FBI, which tracks mass shootings as "active shooter incidents," has found even a lower average of 11.4 incidents occurring per year. One problem is that the definition of what constitutes a mass-shooting incident varies from one publication or organization to the next. What is clearly evident is that the incidents are not increasing, despite media hype and sensationalization.

Yet, obfuscating for political purposes and obviously to increase their numbers, anti-gun activists have now tried to label any incident with two or more casualties as a mass shooting, and public health officials have even attempted to lump murder-suicides as mass shootings! A *Washington Post* report in a moment of clarity summarizes the problem as follows:

> *Similarly, Northeastern University Professor of Criminologist James Alan Fox has said that the inclusion of statistics from the FBI's 'active shooter' report gives the false impression that incidents are rising when they are not. 'A majority of active shooters are not mass shooters,' Fox told Time. 'A majority kills fewer than three.' On Friday, Fox wrote in USA Today that 'media folks reminded us of the unforgettable, high profile shootings that have taken place over the past few months, hinting of a problem that has grown out of control... as if there is a pattern emerging.'[15]*

Incidentally, mass killings are not unique to the United States because of wide gun availability. France, for example had more mass killings in one single year, 2015, than there were mass shootings in the United States in all of Obama's two terms (eight years).[16] And at home, California, one of the states with the strictest gun control laws, including background checks, has the highest number of mass-shooting incidents at 21 cases, counting from 1966 to 2017.[17] We must keep in mind, though, that despite the tragic nature and sensationalism accompanying these heinous crimes, mass shootings represent a miniscule number, one percent or less of homicides, in the U.S.

In the aftermath of the tragic 2018 Valentine's Day high school shooting in Parkland, Florida—where 17 students were massacred by criminal gunman Nikolas Cruz—dramatic calls for drastic gun control measures and exaggerated claims about the number of mass shootings in the U.S. were made. For instance, Democrat Senator Chris Murphy of Connecticut made the mendacious claim, "This happens nowhere else other than the United States of America." The colluding American media did not take Senator Murphy to task, as they do with President Trump's every pronouncement.

In fact, America is not the worst country for mass shootings and does not even make it to the top ten, despite the record number of guns in the hands of Americans. France, Norway, Belgium, Finland, and the Czech Republic, for example, all have more deaths from mass shootings than the U.S., and in fact, from 2009 to 2015, the European Union had 27 percent more casualties per mass shooting incidents than the U.S.[16]

Allow me to digress briefly and once again point out there were plenty of signs that Cruz was criminally deranged and a danger to his community, and nothing was done except dismiss him from school. His violent threats and abnormal behavior were even reported to the FBI. The agency dropped the ball and Cruz was not investigated. The FBI, a politicized shadow of its former self, was too busy, it seems, investigating Russian interference in the U.S. presidential election of 2016—an outcome the FBI along with the mainstream media still refuse to acknowledge.

Again, despite orchestrated perception, violence in school is down. Of the more than 2,000 unfortunate children who die in acts of violence each year, only 34 died in school-related violence during the 1997–1998 school year, according to the Department of Education Annual Report on School Safety. The difference between perception and reality is more reporting, saturation coverage, more gun control hype and sensationalism—all of which may, in fact, result in more copycat killings by deranged predators craving media attention. With that said and notwithstanding the confusing data and despite the assurances of Professor Fox, I am becoming concerned that there might actually be a cluster of increased mass killings not only rampage shootings but also vehicular homicides, plowing into crowds, accumulating for the year 2017 and perhaps thereafter, given a confluence of factors to be discussed in Chapter 22.

Israeli anti-terrorist expert and editor of the European magazine *Visier*, David Th. Schiller, commenting on the U.S. school shootings, wrote: "Schools/kindergartens make for very attractive targets for the deranged gunman as well as for the profit-oriented hostage gangsters or terrorist group. [I]f you crave media attention, as for instance the PLO did [in Israel] in the '70s, nothing will catch the headlines better than an attack on a school full of kids." Mr. Schiller concludes: "We in the terrorism research field have argued for decades that it was exactly the media coverage that spurred more and each time more violent and extreme terrorist incidents. Could we stop the media from advertising the terrorist message? Certainly not."[16] Given what we know now about the psychology of these shootings and Hollywood's excesses with movie violence, perhaps, the question should be rephrased: Is it time to regulate Hollywood and the media?[18] Again, we will have more to say about this in Chapter 22.

Moral Societal Decline

In a 2017 study published in *Pediatrics*, the authors disingenuously claimed 1,300 "children" deaths from firearms by including 17-year-old juvenile delinquents and all types of gun deaths—homicides, gun accidents, and suicides—in the study. (We wonder if 19 year olds might have been included surreptitiously, as in previous studies.)

However, we must give the authors some credit for admitting several important facts that have eluded public health researchers for years. *Reason* magazine summarized the findings as follow:

1. *78 percent of the deaths occurred among 13 to 17 year olds; 53 percent were homicides; and 38 percent were suicides. Less than four percent were accidents involving children 12 or younger.*

2. *40 percent of the homicides involved teenagers and stemmed from "arguments," most likely black-market disputes involving the illegal drug trade; 31 percent were "precipitated by another crime;" 21 percent were gang-related; nine percent were senseless drive-by shootings; and seven percent bystanders. Obviously some of the categories overlap.[19]*

"There isn't a single issue in isolation that increases the likelihood of gun death," the lead author, CDC researcher Katherine Fowler, told *The New York Times*. "Children are at a higher risk of violence if they have academic problems, encouragements to be aggressive, and limited adult supervision. The likelihood of violence is also higher in communities with high levels of instability, gang activity, drug sales, unemployment, or poverty."[19] It is obvious the restrictions that Congress placed on the CDC on gun control activities and junk science research in 1996 have had a beneficial effect at least on some public health researchers.

There is no argument that the death of any child by any cause is a tragedy. Yet, in the case of juvenile violence and crime we must be honest and lay the blame where it belongs: At the feet of a popular culture that has wrought increasing vulgarity, crudity, irresponsibility, permissiveness, violence, and immediate self-gratification, guided by the establishment elite and the intoxicating liberal progressivism of over half a century. Thus, what can we expect of youth devoid of intellectual guidance and lacking a moral compass? Consider some of the characteristics of the postmodern progressivist ethos embraced by the ruling liberal establishment:

1. *Moral relativism. Schools no longer teach traditional morality, the discernment between right and wrong and moral absolutes, factors leading to situational ethics and a society without fixed human values. Building the self-esteem of children is placed ahead of personal morality and teaching them moral absolutes. Sadly, parents are also shirking this responsibility, accepting their children's errant behavior, seeking not to make judgments about situations or people. Following the advice of the education experts and progressive academicians, parents want to be "tolerant," friends to their children rather than parents.*

2. *Lack of discipline. Consider the fact parents and teachers in today's environment are afraid of reprimanding the young for fear of being charged with child abuse and prosecuted. Often, parents are not at home (both working, frequently one of them working solely to pay taxes to Uncle Sam) so children, lacking parental guidance at home and discipline in schools, do as they please.*

3. *Lack of accountability. There is a persistent crisis of responsibility in our society. There is a trend to absolve individuals of personal responsibility and a penchant for blaming abstract or inanimate objects, such as injustice, inequality, or guns for the level of violence in our society. This lack of personal responsibility and accountability trickles down to the children and impressionable youth, who learn very early not to accept responsibility for their actions and to blame others for their shortcomings.*

With this background, anti-gun activists posit that more gun control in American society is needed rather than crime control and making the criminal elements pay dearly for their crimes. The lawful citizens then should be disarmed, whereas the criminals, who by definition do not obey the laws, get to keep their illegal guns. As early as 1991, data from the FBI Uniform Crime Report showed that states with permissive gun laws have lower homicide rates than states with restrictive gun control laws. This trend persists according to the most recent data.[5] More gun control surely is not the answer. As stated previously, there is already a surplus of gun laws on the books, including illegal possession of firearms by minors. These laws should be enforced on the young criminal offenders before they become hard-core criminals. And when inner city teenagers or juvenile delinquents from suburbia act as criminals, they should all be tried as adults.

In a study that was not given the attention it deserved, the U.S. Department of Justice's Office of Juvenile Justice and Delinquency Prevention under the Clinton administration tracked 4,000 juveniles ages six to 15 years in Denver, Colorado; Pittsburgh, Pennsylvania; and Rochester, New York, from 1993 to 1995, and contrary to what was expected by the conventional wisdom of the ruling elite, the investigators reached the following unexpected conclusions:

> *Children who get firearms from their parents are less likely to commit acts of violence and street crimes (14 percent) than children who have no guns in their homes (24 percent), whereas children who obtain guns illegally do so at the whopping rate of 74 percent. The study also found that "boys who own legal firearms have much lower rates of delinquency and drug use (than boys who own illegal guns) and are even slightly less delinquent than non-owners of guns."*[20]

This study also provided more evidence that in close nuclear families, where children learn from their parents, youngsters can be taught to use guns responsibly. These youngsters, in fact, become more responsible in their conduct and more civil in their behavior. Children should be taught moral absolutes and universal truths, so that as they journey through life they will exercise their free will, distinguishing right from wrong and fulfilling their destinies imbued with the spirit of goodness.

Sociological studies support the common sense adage that time must be found to spend with children to properly rear them. Parental involvement in academic instruction is an excellent way to do so. It allows parents to debunk left-wing or politically correct public school propaganda and biased instruction. And as we have seen, gun training and safety instruction by parents lead to parenting better children. Some of us even take time to mentor adolescents seeking professions in the medical and other health care fields. A few of us go the extra mile. John Wipfler, M.D., clinical professor of surgery, emergency room physician, and DRGO member, teaches firearm safety to medical students at the University of Illinois College of Medicine. With colleagues, Dr. Wipfler mentors students as part of the course of Emergency Medicine Interest Group, and he uses his farm each autumn as the training facility. The dean of the medical school is supportive, and under Dr. Wipfler's mentorship, medical students spend a six-hour weekend learning about firearm safety, shooting guns, emergency trauma first aid, the treatment of wounds, and the philosophical basis for rightful self-defense. Despite the anti-gun propaganda of the medical politicians, Dr. Wipfler found that the medical students have been "receptive after realizing that firearms are not the 'scary and dreaded guns' that the media makes them out to be." He adds, "They see and witness safe use, and realize that with proper education and carefully-guided instruction, it's not only safe, but fun."[21]

The course has been a great success that needs duplicating. Unfortunately, we are not aware of any other medical school engaged in any type of firearm education program.

CHAPTER 18

SELF-DEFENSE: LETHAL THREAT MAY REQUIRE PROTECTIVE LETHAL FORCE

The act of self-defense can have a double effect: The preservation of one's life; and the killing of the aggressor... The one is intended, the other is not.

—Saint Thomas Aquinas (1225—1274),
Summa Theologica, II, Ch. 64, Art. 7

Violence is a global problem, and each of us must be aware that the day may come when we could be placed in a situation where we or our loved ones could become hapless victims of crime. On the other hand, some of us may have accepted the moral duty to mount an armed defense to protect our families and ourselves if the need arose.

The Ethics of Armed Self-Protection

Western civilization stands on the twin pillars of Judeo-Christian morality and Graeco-Roman ethics; this legacy has stood the test of time as the two traditions became inextricably entwined over the centuries.[1] Among its distilled teachings we find that the individual has the right to life and a moral duty for armed self-defense and for the protection of the family.

In his book, *Safeguarding Liberty: The Constitution and Citizens Militias (1995),* Larry Pratt, executive director emeritus of Gun Owners of America (GOA) explained what is written in both the Old and New Testaments about armed self-defense and the moral principles involved. In the Judeo-Christian tradition, the Bible's first murder, that of Cain killing his brother Abel, illustrates the first point. Cain is not right with God and possessed of evil in his heart killed his brother. For the iniquity of murder, God instituted capital punishment (Genesis 9:5–6; "I will require satisfaction for the death of his fellow-man"). God did not ban the knife or rock that Cain might have used to kill his brother. In fact, it is not clear which one he used to commit fratricide. Nevertheless, it is clear that evil is in the heart of wicked persons who commit murder, and when they do, the guilty are to be punished by the civil magistrates.

There is a big difference between armed self-defense and taking revenge on a transgressor when our lives are not immediately in danger. In Exodus 22:2–3, God affirms: "If the thief is found breaking in, and he is struck so that he dies, there should be no guilt for his bloodshed. If the sun has risen on him, there shall be guilt for his bloodshed." It is clear that in break-ins and robberies, where innocent lives are in danger, good people have the right, even the duty, to protect themselves and their homes using lethal force. Furthermore, in Proverbs 25:26, "A righteous man who falters before the wicked is like a murky spring and a polluted well." Citizens fail as human beings, if they find themselves unarmed and unable to protect their families during life-threatening circumstances.

Both the Old and New Testaments affirm the right to self-defense. In the New Testament, Timothy 5:8, says, "But if anyone does not provide for his own, and especially for those of his household, he has denied the faith and is worse than an unbeliever." Citizens should not only provide sustenance and shelter for their families but also should provide for their protection and defense. Yet, there is a common passage that has been misunderstood in the New Testament, when during the Sermon on the Mount, Jesus commands, "But I tell you not to resist an evil person. But whoever slaps you on your right cheek, turn the other to him also." Pratt denies any intent on pacifism on this passage. As in the Old Testament, when our lives are not in danger, Jesus admonished us not to take revenge. I believe that this passage also exhorts us not to be angry and not to react with violence, when provoked by an attack in which our lives are not in peril. But for a serious attack, Pratt writes: "Resisting an attack is not to be confused with taking vengeance which is the exclusive domain of God (Romans 12:19). This function has been delegated to the civil magistrates." He points out Romans 13:4 that explains that a government official, "is God's minister to you for good. But if you do evil, be afraid; for he does not bear the sword in vain; for he is God's minister, an avenger to execute wrath on him who practices evil."[2]

This brings us to Western civilization's Graeco-Roman legacy, where the ancient Greeks and Romans also dealt with the issue of evil men, assailants and armed self-defense. In fact, the English political philosopher Thomas Hobbes (1588—1679) had posited that before government had been instituted among men, there was a state of nature in which man lived in "continual fear, and danger of violent death; and the life of man was solitary, poor, nasty, brutish, and short."[3] Aristotle (384—322 B.C.) affirmed that there are wicked men who act and do evil for their own sake. Those "brutish persons lacking self-control," the intemperate, and the wicked, posited Aristotle, must be made to behave properly and punished for their crimes by the force of law. Thus, "[The] legislators....punish and take vengeance on those who do wicked acts."[4] And with this erudition it is no wonder Saint Thomas Aquinas (1225—1274) reconciled the teachings of Aristotle to the Christian Church. We have read what the Angelic Doctor and theologian wrote in *Summa Theologica* under this chapter's heading—namely that in stopping an aggressor the intention is to preserve life; the killing of the aggressor is a justified byproduct of his own malevolent action.[4]

The Roman statesman and philosopher Cicero (106—43 B.C.), influenced by Aristotle and the Stoic philosophers discussed the tenets of Natural Law—universal, just, and eternal laws—derived from Nature's God. On self-defense, he wrote, "Civilized people are taught by logic, barbarians by necessity, communities by tradition; and the lesson is inculcated even in wild beasts by nature itself. They learn that they have to defend their own bodies and persons and lives from violence of any and every kind by all means within their power."[5]

Most religions agree on the right to self-defense. The Catholic catechism states: "Legitimate defense can be not only a right but also a grave duty for one who is responsible for the lives of others. The defense of the common good requires that an unjust aggressor be rendered unable to cause harm." Pope John Paul II further expounded on the natural right to self-defense, incorporating the thought of Saint Thomas Aquinas, "Unfortunately, it happens that the need to render the aggressor incapable of causing harm sometimes involves taking his life. In this case, the fatal outcome is attributable to the aggressor whose actions brought it about, even though he may not be morally responsible because of a lack of the use of reason."[6]

From these twin pillars of traditions derive the Anglo-American legacy of ethics, jurisprudence and liberty. The English philosopher John Locke (1632—1704) posited that natural rights were self-evident and gave man the power "to pursue life, health, liberty and possessions." Locke influenced the American founders greatly. In the Declaration of Independence, Thomas Jefferson invoked "the Laws of Nature and of Nature's God" to justify separation from England and then held that "men were endowed by their Creator with certain unalienable Rights, that among these are Life, Liberty, and the pursuit of Happiness."

Locke had already asserted that to preserve life, citizens had the right to armed self-defense with the killing of an aggressor if their lives were in danger. When one's life is threatened, "the law of Nature gave me a right to destroy him who had put himself into a state of war with me, and threatened my destruction."[7] In Chapter 25, we will also discuss the Anglo-American tradition and intent of the law, as it regards a man's home as his castle, where no one can enter without his consent (the Castle Doctrine), and the concept of "stand your ground," the duty not to retreat before a criminal assailant.

Despite our moral and ethical legacy, not everybody sees the problem of crime and self-protection in the same way. Some citizens rely on dialing 911 and believe the police will always be there in a matter of only a few minutes to "protect and serve." We have already discussed the erroneous legality of that in Chapter 16 and, besides, serious injury and even death may be only seconds, not minutes, away. Others do not even want to consider the remote possibility of physically defending themselves and their families or friends. Dr. Michael S. Brown is a Doctors for Responsible Gun Ownership (DRGO) member "who has been studying the gun debate for three decades and considers it a fascinating way to learn about human nature and politics." In a DRGO article titled "The Ethics of Armed Self Defense," he wrote, "It is easy to find people who say they would never use potentially lethal force against another person, even to save their own lives from a criminal assault." This is a dangerous proposition for the potential victims and those around them, and I agree with Dr. Brown when he added, "Under this principle, the life of a violent sociopath is more valuable than theirs… If you won't save your own life by using lethal force, what about your spouse, children, or co-workers?[8]

Dr. Brown further explained that people should be aware that in today's world, they may need to protect themselves or their loved ones: "The thought of being in a violent, self-defense situation and possibly using lethal force, is too stressful for many people to deal with. Due to their upbringing, their religion or their conditioning by the media, they just can't or won't think about it."[7] This attitude could be dangerous and deadly.

Dr. Robert A. Margulies, another DRGO member and emergency medicine physician, is a retired Navy Medical Corps captain and firearm trainer with multiple certifications from the NRA and the Massad Ayoob Group. He agrees with Dr. Brown. In an interview for the Armed Citizens Legal Defense Network ejournal, Dr. Margulies wrote that a victim injured in terms of being unable to mount a reasonable defense would be left unable to seek medical assistance after the attacker has left the scene: "The unprovoked attack puts one in a very dangerous situation. In a dark alleyway, or a subway station after the train has pulled out and very few people are there; that initial impact can produce injuries that without immediate care can be fatal."[9] He is correct that prompt medical attention is sometimes urgently needed because of the development of secondary injuries at both the tissue and cellular levels that are so common in neurosurgical emergencies. For example, at the tissue level a partial or complete laceration of a major artery or vein can result in acute or delayed external or internal hemorrhage. At the cellular level, lack of oxygen (hypoxia) due to severe contusion (bruise) or edema (swelling) with neural compression can cause secondary damage to the brain or spinal cord.

The Problem of Physical Violence

In the context of this chapter we are dealing with interpersonal violence, which relates to intentional force by one or more assailants against another person or persons with the potential to cause injury or bodily harm that may result in disability or death.

From the outset, let's state that despite what we have been led to believe, America is not the most violent nation. When it comes to violence, objectively compared to developed nations, the U.S. is in the middle of the pack; when considering the rest of the world, the U.S is far behind Latin America (including Brazil), Africa, and much of Eastern Europe, Eurasia (Russia and some of the former Soviet Republics), and most of Asia.[10]

Nevertheless, we must admit that we have an endemic problem that needs addressing.[11] Violence perpetrated by assailants carrying (or having the opportunity to rapidly be able to pick up and use) a blunt object to attack another person may result in severe bodily harm and/or head injury.

In the body, severe blunt trauma may result in long bone fractures and external or internal injuries and bleeding—complications requiring urgent surgery by a trauma surgeon. As a neurosurgeon, I'm most familiar with spinal and head injuries, and will reserve my narrative in this chapter to the consequences of assaults resulting in severe blunt trauma to the head of the victim.

Before we proceed with the discussion on the pathophysiology of blunt head trauma, we should briefly remark on the seriousness of a physical assault of one or more assailants upon an unwary victim. The media and the legal system, unfortunately, have not considered the sociological aspects and the seriousness of this type of crime. The burgeoning of criminal gangs in the inner cities and the inability of law enforcement to control them have facilitated the perpetration of this type of crime, which in some cases amount to gratuitous violence and unprovoked aggression. Our permissive society in general and the politics of the Democratic Party in particular, have successfully militated for an excessively lenient criminal justice system, which through plea bargaining, early paroling, and reduced sentences, have become a revolving prison door system, refusing to keep dangerous criminals behind bars. As a result, the most vulnerable in our society suffer and in most cases need guns for self-protection.

Although in this chapter we refer frequently to the more vulnerable and older individuals as frequent victims of crime, young people can also become victims and suffer devastating injuries from blunt trauma to the head. In the escalating violence of the "knockout game," for example, a gang member with or without accomplices attempts to knock out an innocent victim with a single punch to the face or head. This malicious "game" has resulted in serious injuries and death even in young people. One can only imagine such a blow in an older individual with decreased reflexes, decrease muscle mass, stiffer joints, and other underlying disorders of ageing. But imagination is not needed; fatal cases are being reported with increasing frequency. On New Year's Day (2018), a 70-year-old motorist, a retired sheriff's deputy, braked suddenly on a San Bernardino street to avoid hitting a dog. The man who rear-ended him, a violent career criminal and gang member of the Inland Empire, suddenly single punched him in the face. The retired deputy was probably knocked out even before he hit the pavement and never regained consciousness. Fortunately, a Good Samaritan rammed the puncher's vehicle with his truck as the criminal was trying to escape and facilitated his arrest. The deputy sheriff died a few days later.[11]

After a hard punch, knockout or not, a victim can sustain further injuries hitting the head on the pavement. Indeed this secondary trauma is common in someone already dazed and falling down helplessly, but it does not matter whether the fatal blow comes from the fist or the pavement. In the eyes of the law, the attacker is responsible for both. It must also be noted that even if a one-punch injury does not cause death, it frequently causes further head trauma or bodily harm on the fall, which is a level of threat that justifies lethal defensive force with or without a firearm.

In short, criminal lawyers, judges, police, and the public need to recognize that blunt force with bare hands can be lethal, especially when used against a weaker person or the elderly. Legislators need to be aware of this so that laws may be passed, codified into statute, and used for jury instruction, as to provide for armed defense in such dangerous situations. We will reiterate this important point towards the end of the chapter.

The Pathology of Blunt Head Trauma

Penetrating head injuries occur with sharp objects forced into the head, such as knives and screwdrivers, both types of tools I have had to remove surgically in the emergency room under urgent and life-saving circumstances or less urgently in the operating room. In my neurosurgical practice I found that blunt trauma to the head of the victim was more common than penetrating knife injuries, which along with gunshot wounds to the head, we will have to leave for another occasion.

A stick, bludgeon, or some other solid object can be used against another person. If the head is the target, as it frequently is because of its vulnerability to incapacitation following concussion (loss of consciousness), serious trauma to the head may result. Blunt head trauma may result in specific injuries, such as a linear or depressed skull fracture, and additionally can be associated with a traumatic intracerebral hematoma (blood clot within the brain), a brain contusion (brain bruise), or a life-threatening epidural hematoma (laceration of an artery with hemorrhage just under the skull, usually near the temple area causing compression of the brain).

Most depressed (and all open depressed) skull fractures require immediate intervention by the neurosurgeon. The trauma may also cause primary brain damage in the form of a cerebral contusion, or laceration (tearing of the brain), or an expanding hematoma compressing the brain and causing further secondary injury. All of these injuries can be caused by sudden blunt trauma to the head by a criminal assailant, who might have carried or picked up a nearby object to use as a weapon.

Serious blunt trauma to the head in an unexpected altercation or assault, then, may result in an expanding brain hematoma requiring emergency surgery. These lesions result in death when carried out with sufficient lethal force, and if the patients live, such injuries may leave them with serious sequelae, such as brain damage, seizure disorders, or incapacitated in a chronic vegetative state.

Brain hemorrhages can take the form of subdural or epidural hematomas, depending on whether they occur over or under the dura mater, the membrane covering the brain. They can be equally lethal by exerting pressure on the brain, causing swelling and cerebral herniation (a pressure-induced brain shift), that result in compression of vital deep brain structures leading to coma and death.

Acute subdural and epidural hematomas then frequently require emergency surgery to prevent the development of a chronic vegetative state or death. Even when successfully treated, they may leave the patients disabled or incapacitated.

Fatality depends on the force of the injury and on how soon the victim-patient makes it to the operating table. The mortality of acute subdural hematomas (ASH) ranges from 30 to 75 percent.[12] Admittedly, much of the lethality with ASH at the high end of the spectrum occurs with motor vehicle accidents, but it also occurs with severe beatings during assaults and the commission of crimes.

Subacute or chronic subdural hematomas (CSH), on the other hand, occur in older people, as a result of blunt head trauma, and are very common even after relatively minor injuries. This occurs because as we age the brain sags, the subdural space enlarges, predisposing older folks to the tearing of the bridging veins at the top of the head inside the skull. Chronic subdural hematomas can occur after relatively minor injuries or even after a vigorous struggle or simply the shaking or bumping of the head during a scuffle with an assailant.

What all this means is that a potential injury, such as I've described: an acute subdural hematoma (ASH) from a major beating; acute epidural hematoma (AEH) from a single pipe or bludgeon blow to the side of the head; or a chronic subdural hematoma (CSH) from just a vigorous struggle or simple shaking of the head during an altercation—can be potential lethal force that may be prevented by countering with preventive, protective deadly force to avoid serious injury and irreversible brain damage to the innocent victim.

Sometimes difficult to diagnose, subacute and chronic subdural hematomas usually present in older victims days or weeks after an assault. Yet these hematomas can also cause severe brain damage, incapacitation, or death. In other words, a serious or mortal injury can occur when weaker persons are attacked by assailants intent on injuring and incapacitating their target, male or female, in order to rob or sexually assault them. It can only be countered successfully and most reliably with a firearm.[13,14]

It's worth emphasizing that in the case of preventing a chronic subdural hematoma in an older person, say an individual over 50 years of age, the blunt trauma or jerking of the head may result from an assailant just using his hands as the offensive weapon, and yet for that potential victim only a firearm would be invariably effective in stopping the attacker.

The Case for Defensive Lethal Force

Violence is rampant and endemic. Assault in the streets or during home invasions, whether the object is robbery or rape, frequently takes defenseless persons by surprise. The best defense is ready, armed defense. The firearm must be immediately available, usually concealed for self-defense when one is outside the home, or kept in a secure place but readily accessible when inside the home. Criminologists have determined that a firearm is the most effective weapon of defense against violent assailants.[13-16]

In dealing with assault cases, one must also keep in mind that a person bent on attacking and victimizing another person carries the advantages of timing, selection, and purposeful intent.[9] They are intent on hurting, robbing, raping, or killing their victims. Thus they have the advantage of having selected the time, place, and the victims themselves. Moreover, the victims do not expect the attack and are often taken by surprise. Frequently, assailants are younger, more agile, and stronger than their victims (whom they have picked as suitable targets). Smart unarmed assailants might hesitate to physically assault an Arnold Schwarzenegger or a Jesse Ventura when they were in their prime, but not frail individuals they believe they could successfully victimize such as women, the handicapped, and the elderly.

Most importantly, an unarmed predator can wield deadly force with his hands, feet, or other simple objects easily carried. A stolen candle stick in the hands of a determined assailant should be considered a lethal weapon and treated as conveying deadly force, especially when the assailant has entered or broken into a home and the victim, male or female, reasonably feels threatened and in mortal danger.

As stated previously, criminologists have noted the advantage of armed self-defense. National Victims Data suggests that "while victims resisting with knives, clubs, or bare hands are about twice as likely to be injured as those who submit, victims who resist with a gun are only half as likely to be injured as those who put up no defense."

Similarly, regarding women and self-defense, "among those victims using handguns in self-defense, 66 percent of them were successful in warding off the attack and keeping their property. Among those victims using non-gun weapons, only 40 percent were successful.[14] Among those victims fleeing the scene, only 35 percent were successful. Among those victims invoking physical force, only 22 percent were successful. Among those using verbal shouting only 20 percent were successful..."[15] The gun is the great equalizer for women, the elderly, the physically weaker, and the handicapped, when they are accosted in the street or when they are defending themselves and their children at home.

When severe bodily injury and blunt head trauma are a possibility, deadly force used in self-defense is warranted and morally justified.[2-7] And the safest and most effective defense is with the use of firearms by the intended victims, that is, by citizens who know how to use firearms and are determined beforehand to protect themselves and their families from predators.

Unpredictable violence with blunt head trauma should be considered capable of causing severe bodily harm. Neurosurgical complications of head injuries may include seizure disorders, paralysis, blindness, and mental and emotional problems that result as sequelae of brain injuries, not to mention the death of the victim.

In short, guns are the great equalizer for both men and women assaulted by criminal predators, who hold the advantage in acts of violence, and who purposely or unintentionally inflict bodily harm in the commission of their crimes. Thus, whenever a person or persons break into and enter a home, a hostile intent must be presupposed, the potential for serious injuries should be anticipated, and the victims are justified in using deadly force for self-defense and family protection.

Business establishments that forbid the carrying of firearms by persons possessing valid concealed carry licenses (CCW) should be legally liable for injuries that those customers may suffer because they are rendered defenseless as a result of the establishments' policies.

It's time that the public, prosecutors, defense attorneys, juries, legislators, and the police understand that blunt trauma to the head can be potentially crippling or lethal during a scuffle with a criminal, and that the use of deadly force by the intended victim is often needed and almost always justified for self-defense and family protection. Legislation at the state and federal levels needs to be passed and laws codified so that juries can be properly instructed as to the legality of armed defense because blunt head trauma can be lethal.

PART 6

TYRANNY AND THE EUROPEAN SOCIAL DEMOCRACIES

THE NAÏVETÉ OF AMERICANS AND THE GUN CONTROL FALLACIES OF THE EUROPEAN SOCIAL DEMOCRACIES

If ye love wealth better than liberty, the tranquility of servitude better than the animating contest of freedom, go home from us in peace. We ask not your counsels or arms. Crouch down and lick the hands, which feed you. May your chains set lightly upon you, and may posterity forget that ye were our countrymen.

—Samuel Adams (1722—1803),
American patriot, in *The Writings of Samuel Adams (1773–1802)*

Frequently I'm inspired to write commentaries and letters to the editor based on articles and opinion pieces published in a local newspaper, *The Telegraph*, (Macon). The newspaper keeps me abreast of the tempo of life in the community and informed about the thinking of the citizens. Over the years I observed a disturbing trend, the often-repeated naïve expression, "If you don't have anything to hide, then you don't have anything to fear!" Really?

There seems to be an interesting dichotomy about citizens' mistrusting and trusting government in different spheres. For instance, with great judgment, they mistrust the economic acumen of government and with good sense, don't trust it with their wallets; yet, they play a different, more cavalier and acquiescent tune when it comes to guarding the jewel of personal freedom.

In one fell swoop many letter writers and liberal commentators would gloss over and discard the constitutional protections guaranteed by the Fourth and Fifth Amendments, crafted by the Founders precisely to preserve liberty and limit the power of government. When the Soviet KGB needed culprits, their motto was, "Show me the man and I will show you his crime." Thus, Soviet citizens were arrested under a variety of charges as "enemies of the State."

Even in the United States, the last bastion of freedom, individuals are not immune to the power of the State. Charges can be brought against anyone once the federal government has zeroed in on the individual it deems dangerous or against political opponents of the administration in office—as both the Democratic Clinton and Obama administrations did by using the power of the Internal Revenue Service (IRS) against conservatives or by charging citizens with tax evasion that would take years to defend against and lead to their financial ruin. The law enforcement power of the State can also be used against individual citizens as has happened in the past with the Bureau of Alcohol, Tobacco, Firearms, and Explosives (ATF) that has been used to conduct raids and dynamic entries into homes, sometimes even getting the address wrong! In short, despite the Bill of Rights, the power of the State can be used against a citizen to take away his liberty and his property.

If You Have Nothing to Hide…Really?

Yet, we continue to hear the expression, "If you have nothing to hide, you have nothing to fear." The fact is that many Americans have lived in freedom for so long, they have become too trusting with their liberty; or like the proverbial frog in a warming pot, don't even seem to notice when their freedoms are being eroded piecemeal.

One letter writer in *The Telegraph* (Macon) received an avalanche of verbal reprimands, and had heaps of derision thrown at her from both liberals and conservatives for her temerity to express emotional fears and concerns about government invasion of her personal privacy. One of the *Telegraph* chastisers, in turn, received his own journalistic reprobation from an irate reader, who defending the woman, wrote:

*The Patriot Act and the War on Drugs have gutted the 4th
Amendment. Our government and law enforcement monitor
our phone calls, internet, mail, what books you read, all
without a warrant signed by a judge. Roadblocks take place
daily under which we can be searched without a warrant.
Under the 'sneak and peek' provision of the Patriot Act, our
homes can be searched without our even knowing about it. It's
easy to see that you are one of the sheep who won't even bleat
as you are led to be fleeced or slaughtered.[1]*

These are strong words but the irate citizen has several valid points
regarding the loss of valuable individual liberty in the guise of providing for
State security. Consider the revelations that have come to light on domestic surveillance; the political abuses of the IRS targeting conservatives and
political opponents in both the Clinton and the Obama administrations; and
abuses by the ATF and other federal agencies. If still in doubt, try to exit the
country or even fly outside the U.S., not with a gun, but with your hard-earned
money in your travel bag and see what happens!

All of this loss of freedom has taken place in the name of security and
safety, with little resistance from the general public and despite Ben Franklin's
admonition, "Those who would give up essential Liberty, to purchase a little
temporary Safety, deserve neither Liberty nor Safety." The chronicles of human
progress are replete with, and history confirms, the danger of government
run amok, exercising excessive or not clearly delineated power in procuring
State security.

"But Dr. Faria," I have been told, "such cruelty and tyranny can happen
in third-world countries, Cuba and the former Soviet Union, but it cannot
happen here. This is America." Really? Ask, or rather read, the story of David
Koresh and the Waco incident—since the victims, men, women and children,
and Mr. Koresh himself, are all dead by the hands of the federal police—to
ascertain the deathly naïveté of just such an attitude. Or research the cases
of Vicky Weaver and Ruby Ridge, and all those little known Americans, such
as Carl Drega, who himself was driven to criminal insanity and murder by
government and bureaucratic injustice; the totally innocent, John Gerald
Quinn, whose home was subjected to a "no-knock" raid (once referred to

as "dynamic entries"), and likewise Bruce Abramski; and the many other lawful American gun owners, who over the years have been victimized by the errors or excesses of the ATF or for technicalities. Tell them, they need no such constitutional protections because they have supposedly done nothing wrong. The judicious adage that a man's home is his castle that not even a king can violate has been thrown out the window, so that the government has arrogated to itself the right to burst into a citizen's home based solely on the suspicion or a tip from an informer working with the police (usually ruffians looking for reduced sentences for their own crimes) and alleging that there is an illegal gun, such as a sawed-off shotgun, in the house.[2]

The Laws, So Voluminous That No Man Can Know Them

The powerful French Minister Cardinal Richelieu stated, "If one would give me six lines written by the hand of the most honest man, I would find something in them to have him hanged." What Richelieu's statement means is that a government can prosecute or blackmail and force anyone to do its bidding, once the person has been targeted by the State, for any offense, imagined or fabricated. The Founding Fathers understood privacy as the right to be left alone by government, and that is why they inserted individual protections in the Bill of Rights, the first ten amendments to the U.S. Constitution, which in this particular instance we refer to the Fourth and Fifth Amendments. The Founders almost did not include the Bill of Rights in the Constitution because for some of them these protections were self-evident and redundant! I'm glad more prescient Anti-Federalist heads from Virginia prevailed on that account and insisted they be written before ratification.

Consequently, many defense attorneys advise their clients not to even talk to police unless legal counsel is present. This is perhaps lamentable, but the fact remains the U.S. government has grown to gargantuan proportions and so have the number of laws on the books and abuses against citizens. A recent article reported, "The Congressional Research Service cannot even count the current number of federal crimes. These laws are scattered in over 50 titles of the United States Code, encompassing roughly 27,000 pages."[3]

Moreover, there might be an excess of over 10,000 additional administrative laws and regulations on the books. James Madison, the master builder of the U. S. Constitution noted in *Federalist Paper #62*:

> *It will be of little avail to the people that the laws are made by men of their choice, if the laws be so voluminous that they cannot be read, or so incoherent that they cannot be understood; if they be repealed or revised before they are promulgated, or undergo such incessant changes that no man, who knows what the law is today, can guess what it will be tomorrow.*

Yes, voluminous they are; and in this labyrinth of laws, government can find incriminating information in the life of any citizen and with the threat of prosecution can blackmail persons to do its bidding, become informants, infringe on their liberties, and confiscate their property, as in asset forfeiture proceedings and outright extralegal confiscations. As if that was not enough, with the government's inexhaustible public funds, defense proceedings can bankrupt intransigent citizens attempting to preserve their liberty and property.

As things now stand, the federal government has the capability to access every email written and phone call made by every citizen. Moreover, today almost everyone uses mobile phones that track location. Reportedly telecommunication companies are required by law to provide tracking information to the government. So lawful but naïve citizen, have you ever said, done something, or gone somewhere that may cause you embarrassment, or worse, done something unknowingly that violated a provision in the 27,000 pages of federal statues or the 10,000 administrative regulations? Unless you are a saint, you could be guilty of some peccadillo or indiscretion that might have gone unrecognized or forgotten. Furthermore, activities that may be legal today may be illegal tomorrow or vice-versa. There is no way to know how information against citizens may be used by government (especially bureaucracy and law enforcement) at different points in time; this can be reinforced by the likes and dislikes of our trendy popular culture, the fickleness of the people (jurors), the incitement and demagoguery of the legislators (who represent them), or the fastidiousness and tenacity of the bureaucrat, who finds the offending transgression.

In communist countries, minor indiscretions were used to force citizens to spy on their neighbors, and foreign dignitaries (caught in "love nests" or trapped in homosexual encounters) were blackmailed to force them to spy on their countries and commit treason.

What about medical or genetic information that may affect your life, the lives of your children and grandchildren in the private or public (government) sector? In the private sector, if a genetic aberration is uncovered, one may have difficulty with health insurance coverage; in the government sector with socialized medicine of the future, a citizen (adult or child) may be subject to rationing or denial of care with the assignation of "futile care" decisions. Such medical care is considered an economic liability to the State, a financial burden that can be dispensed with. So, you still believe you have nothing to hide from the prying eyes of the State and nothing to fear? Think again!

Ignoring the lessons of history and the tragic chronicles of other nations overtaken both by tyranny and democide, as alluded to earlier, we also frequently hear: "Well, it cannot happen here."

Following the shooting rampage at Fort Hood, Texas, where on April 2, 2014, Ivan Lopez, a U.S. Army specialist who served a tour of duty in Iraq, used a .45 caliber semi-automatic handgun to kill three innocent people, for example, I heard: "I see nothing wrong with some restrictions...We have to do something; there are just too many guns out there in the wrong hands." This cliché neglects the fact Fort Hood is a gun-free zone, where an armed madman can shoot innocent victims who are disarmed and unable to defend themselves. In fact, the rampage ended when a female MP drew her weapon, causing Lopez to stop the shooting and take his own life. This is similar to the December 11, 2012 case at the Clackamas Town Center near Portland, Oregon, which had a posted policy prohibiting firearms on the premises. Here another deranged killer with a stolen AR-15 shot two people. The shooter, realizing that another shopper (a concealed carry permit holder) was armed with a handgun, ran into a storage corridor and turned the gun on himself.[4]

Naïve attitudes also ignore the penchant for politicians to take advantage of tragedies, ostensibly with good intentions but in reality to assume more power and institute "socialism with a human face." I read an assertion by a letter writer who insisted, "We owe an apology to the Europeans for the gun violence in America!" And that is not all. I read another letter by a writer who, neglecting history and instead taking a simple snapshot of the moment, claimed: "Countries in Western Europe, like Britain, France, or Sweden, which regulate gun ownership closely, are not in any danger of sliding into tyranny and they don't have the crime."

Those letter writers ignored inconvenient facts, such as the high crime rate in Britain (particularly burglaries ignoring whether the homeowners are present or not) that exceeds that in the U.S., and where citizens are not permitted to defend themselves in their own homes! In Chapter 20 we will be reading about the case of Tony Martin that epitomizes the absurdity and injustice of the European situation on gun control.[5] The Europeans live in confiscatory social democracies, where citizens don't have many of the protections afforded by our Bill of Rights. Most importantly, the Western Europeans were rescued by our armies from the Nazis in World War II, and protected from the Soviet T-54/55 tanks during the Cold War. Since that time, despite NATO, the Europeans remain largely dependent on the U.S. for their security. Ironically, witnessing the resurgent bullying and roaring of the Russian Bear in Georgia, the Caucasus, and invading the Eastern part and usurping the Crimea from the Ukraine, the Europeans are hinting they may require further protection from the U.S.[6]

Western European nations has been free to pursue pacifism and social-ism only because the U.S. protected (and still protects) them with our nuclear deterrent, our military bases, our presence, our defense expenditures, and our guns! It is fair to say that reminiscent of the H.G. Wells classic, *The Time Machine*, the cannibalistic Morlocks (Nazis and Russians) would have long ago devoured the pusillanimous Elois (Western Europeans, including the liberal darling Scandinavians), had it not been for the goodwill of the U.S., the magnanimity of American taxpayers, the sacrifices of American boys in Normandy, the presence of our troops today, and our guns![7, 8] I say the world owes the U.S.—Americans, guns and all—a great debt of gratitude for preserving their freedom and allowing them to make the choice of pursuing their social and economic goals with the pusillanimity they desire!

The American "Gun Culture" That Saved Europe

An interesting conversation with a European neurosurgical colleague, who decries the "gun culture" of America, took place that may be of interest to the readers. The dialogue began with a difference of opinion on an unrelated topic, but in the course of that exchange, I happened to innocently use a figure of speech that offended the colleague, and the conversation below ensued.

What I wrote was, "Although only three paragraphs long, Dr. Ludvic Zrinzo's letter is a loaded gun of criticism with serious implications that require considerable historic and philosophic discussion and cannot possibly be answered fully in a few paragraphs."

Dr Zrinzo: "Dr Faria's comment tries to rewrite my letter but does not succeed. Certainly, my letter was no 'loaded gun'—it caused none of the physical injuries, death and human misery inflicted by the 'loaded gun' culture that some choose to celebrate."

And with that retort, one may say, therein lies the rub. It happens that I had written a two-part comprehensive editorial titled, "America, Guns, and Freedom," which had upset not only Dr. Zrinzo but also his mentor Professor Hariz at a prestigious institution in Europe. Both of them deplore America's "gun culture."[9] A long correspondence had ensued on that occasion with Professor Hariz, who seemed to blame America for most of the evils in the world. Thinking he was naïve, I gently tried to dissuade him from such an erroneous opinion.

I also responded to Dr. Zrinzo cordially that he obviously referred to my two-part editorial, "America, Guns and Freedom," when he made the remark, as they had been published in the medical journal in question. I reminded him that totalitarianism was not just a mere curiosity of the past, but history [10] that should serve as lessons for avoiding erroneous repetition in the future. It was a "gun culture" of free citizens that preserved freedom in the 20th century—and hopefully will do so in the 21st![11,12]

It was the American "gun culture" that liberated Western Europeans from the Nazis during World War II and subsequently also protected all of free Europe from the Red Army and the rolling Soviet tanks during the Cold War. Moreover, witnessing the renewed roaring of the Russian Bear in the Caucasus and the Ukraine, I reminded him the Europeans may require further protection from the U.S. "gun culture" in the near future!

I went on explaining that it had been because of the protection afforded by the American "gun culture" that Europeans, including our cousins in Great Britain, were able to create and sustain in peace the social and economic "safety nets" of which they are so proud.

I was not putting down our Europeans friends to offend them. I stated

Europe was worth defending, as per our treaty obligations, being the birth-place of Western civilization and consequently the midwife of American culture! His derogatory statement, though, required a response.

Then I brought up a little history. Dr. Zrinzo, who practices neuro-surgery in the British National Health Service (NHS) but is not a native Briton, I admitted, may also not have been aware that the celebrated British Home Guard (1940–1944) was short of guns during World War II because of England's gun control tendencies. The Home Guard required guns urgently for the defense of the homeland as the Germans prepared for the invasion of Britain after their victory at Dunkirk. In near panic, some Home Guard units were even issued home-made Croft's pikes (after Lord Croft, the Under-Secretary of State for War), which Prime Minister Winston Churchill had to promote as "effective and silent" weapons to fight the invading Nazis!

But in another hour of need, the "gun culture" of America came to the rescue. Private American citizens and the much hated National Rifle Association (NRA) collected and shipped large numbers of privately donated guns for use by the Home Guard.[13]

Winston Churchill stated eloquently in his book, *Their Finest Hour*, "When the ships from America approached our shores with their priceless arms, special trains were waiting in all ports to receive their cargoes. The Home Guard in every county, in every village, sat up through the night to receive them....By the end of July we were an armed nation...."[13]

Most of the guns were never returned. They were melted down after the war when Britain resumed her gun control policies and social programs—sheltered by the *Pax Americana* as was the rest of Europe.[13]

Dr. Zrinzo, apparently not a bit annoyed by the embarrassing histori-cal facts, then concluded: "I will not engage you further on 'gun culture' or geopolitics save to say that—thankfully—many would disagree with your views on both matters." To which I responded that my historical details were referenced, verifiable facts, and that of course many geopolitical discussions result in disagreements. At the height of the Cold War, for example, there were many Europeans (and some Americans, no doubt) chanting "Better Red than Dead," preferring communist slavery to freedom. I'm thankful that those so chanting did not prevail, instead those of us in the "gun culture" with the contrary opinion won in the Cold War. That ended our discussion at least on the topic of America's "gun culture" with my European colleague.[8,9]

Another concept that progressive gun prohibitionists are unable to grasp about America's "gun culture" is that while it's true that many Americans, particularly in rural areas and most of the South, grow up around guns and hunting—that salutary tradition of the outdoors reinforces Americans inherent patriotism, a patriotism and outlook that Americans inherited from a legacy of freedom. This will be further expounded in Chapter 22 under the subheading, "Revising American History and the 'Gun Culture.'"

The story of Sergeant Alvin York is illustrative of how America's experience in the outdoors, self-sufficiency, hunting, individualism, and cultivation of the "gun culture" can forge character. York grew up in a large and poor family in the Appalachian Mountains of Tennessee. Because they depended on hunting for food, York got very adept in shooting wild animals, such as turkeys and squirrels, with precise shots to the head as to save the rest of the animal for eating.

At age 27 to gain the heart of his sweetheart, a deeply religious girl, York joined a fundamentalist-Methodist sect and made a pacifist commitment to Jesus. In 1917, as World War I raged, York was drafted and because his church was not officially pacifist, he was denied conscientious objector status. He went through basic training but continued to object to war. Because of his obvious sincerity, the major general in command of his unit, George E. Buxton, spoke with him, cited Scripture, and pointed out that Jesus commanded his apostles to carry swords, reminding York that "earthly kingdoms do fight wars and that Christians should render to government the things that are Caesars." Buxton also cited Ezekiel 33:1–6 in which God exhorted the Prophets to command the people to listen to the watchman's trumpet warning of an approaching enemy.[14]

After much soul searching and not completely convinced, Alvin York was sent to France in October 1918. Promptly, his division, already separated from the rest of the army, was sent to rescue a Lost Battalion (the 1st battalion of the 308 Infantry Regiment) that was surrounded by German units. Pvt. York, leading a patrol, surprised the enemy camp, killed one German, and the rest surrendered. Another German unit opened machine gun fire from a nearby hill, killing or wounding nine Americans. With his Enfield rifle, York picked off the German gunners one by one. Before he could reload the rest of the Germans, out of ammunition, attacked with a bayonet charge. York stopped them with the lethal fire of his .45 caliber pistol, ordering them to surrender, which they did. York, with the seven Americans still alive, rounded up several dozen German prisoners. On the way back to American lines, he captured two other groups of Germans, who he "bluffed into surrendering." In all, Alvin York had captured 132 Germans, including four officers.

In his book, *The Morality of Self-Defense and Military Action: The Judeo-Christian Tradition* (2017), David B. Kopel summarized York's additional personal achievements: "Almost single handed, York with his one rifle and one pistol, had killed 25 Germans, and knocked 35 German machine guns out of action. The next day, he returned to the site of the battle, to pray for the soul of the slain Germans. Pvt. York was promoted to sergeant. The French commander Marshall Foch called York's feat the greatest accomplishment of any soldier in Europe." From the Great War, Sergeant York returned to the U.S. an American hero, "representing the simple, honest, and faithful ideas of the old America."[14]

Many Americans in the 21st century still cling to their guns and their Bibles, and it stands to reason that the alleged "gun culture" mentality and patriotic outlook may not be gained solely by an 8-week army basic training boot camp. Life experience, patriotism and the attitude to fight along your fellow soldiers in a just cause—such as freedom and a country's way of life—do not appear in a vacuum. If that were the case, European democrats would have been a more formidable force against Hitler and Nazi Germany, and had not been so easily conquered in World War II. Belgians, Danes, Dutchmen, and even Frenchmen, may have had weapons and adequate training, but the Germans in World War II had no difficulty in conquering and taming them. The Swiss with a similar outlook as Americans and with their own gun culture were left alone.

America's gun culture gave the Allies the edge, just as Stalin's "Patriotic War" stimulated Russians to fight for their motherland, and to make sure they did so the NKVD's SMERCH units (Soviet military police and counter-intelligence units) were everywhere behind the front lines to stiffen Soviet fighting resolve if their morale lapsed. Americans did not need such units to make sure they fought.

And yet, progressive anti-gun zealots want to disarm Americans, feminize our culture and turn us into vacillating pusillanimous Europeans like the Dutch and the Belgians. If one wishes to see the decadence and collapse of Western civilization and the direction it's headed in Europe towards cultural suicide, visit the Netherlands.

Nations of Elois?

As we will show in the next two subheadings, not all Americans subscribe to the "gun culture," but first, let's discuss a science fiction classic. In
the 1960 film classic, *The Time Machine*, based on the H.G. Wells 1895 novel
similarly titled, the protagonist "George," played by Rod Taylor, travels in a
time machine to a distant future, which, at first sight, seems to be a utopia. But
first appearances are deceiving, and a disconcerting reality is soon evident.
George observes that the inhabitants of the distant future, the Elois, are
effeminate and shallow beings, devoid of feelings or high intelligence, and
they neither work nor read books.

Civilization has collapsed and books have decayed. The Elois live a
halcyon and apathetic existence with no cares, duties or concerns, except
for shallow self-indulgence. Food and leisure are provided miraculously.
During the day the Elois, oblivious of their existence, pass the time in care-
free activities—that is until nighttime. At dusk, a siren blares and the Elois,
conditioned by the sound, are herded like sheep to the slaughterhouse to be
cannibalized by the underground predatory Morlocks, a mutant, primordial,
and cannibalistic species in the apocalyptic future.[7]

Returning to the 21st century, we find the civilized world in general
and our nation in particular assailed by economic and security problems.
The United States (and much of the Western world) is at war with a relentless
and savage enemy that, at this point in the conflict, calls itself the Islamic
State (IS). But we have been at war, lest we forget, since September 11, 2001,
when nearly 3,000 innocent Americans were incinerated in a brutal and
unprovoked attack that destroyed the Twin Towers, symbol of American
finance, and damaged the Pentagon, symbol of U.S. military power. It has
been 16 years of war against Islamic terrorism, and as many years of economic woes, not to mention eight years of geopolitical decline during the
Obama administration from which President Trump is trying to pick up the
pieces. Economic competition has intensified with China's trade surpluses
and Russia's military resurgence against Georgia, annexation of the Crimea,
and dangerous instigation of civil war in Eastern Ukraine—events revealing
the weaknesses of America and her allies. It is a dangerous world out there.[6]

Notwithstanding the seriousness of world events, the United States
continues its descent into socialism, and insidious and insipid political
correctness. The prevailing liberal establishment incarnated in the mass

media, the halls of academia, and the popular culture, continue to hold sway in America.

Despite the dangers to the nation and the possibility of Islamic terrorist attacks, the media remain preoccupied with the fatuous issues they continue to espouse, such as "zero tolerance" to guns in schools or banning Christian expressions in public places, so that children who take toy guns or express Christian beliefs are severely censored or suspended from schools. Christian insignias are not permitted anywhere in public. Yet, school bullies are permitted to disrupt and victimize fellow students, as long as they toe politically correct lines. Frankly, political correctness—e.g., the disguised or overt systematic promotion of thoughts desired by the intelligentsia and the censorship of the political causes they oppose—has reached the level of dangerous ludicrousness in American society.

The epitome of absurdity has been reached, when, in the face of a determined and barbarous enemy, who brutally kidnaps, shoots, or beheads journalists, soldiers, and the completely innocent abroad, and more recently uses vehicles to plow into crowds killing innocent bystanders both here and abroad, we remain mired in utter vacuity. Consider the situation of the mainstream media, including the evening news spending an inordinate amount of time editorializing, discussing sexual lifestyles, gender politics, and the life and romantic interests of celebrities, instead of doing more thorough reporting about an increasingly dangerous world.

Hogs Gone Wild

In tandem with this vacuity of the press, consider the decline in American education as standards continue to drop to the lowest common denominator. During the Obama years, more Americans received food stamps than ever before and felt helpless and dependent on the government for every need, from housing to cell phones. The level of dependence reached a point that not only individual Americans but also whole communities felt helpless and dependent on others for everyday living.

Some Americans have become prisoners in their own homes, afraid not only of home break-ins and thugs in their neighborhoods but also of being victimized by wild animals in their own yards. Yes, victimized and terrorized by feral hogs, hogs gone wild roaming their farms and neighborhoods!

This is not a joke. There is an excellent documentary by the Discovery Channel, *Hogs Gone Wild,* that is quite disturbing, not necessarily because of the ferocity and the damage caused by these feral hogs in the United States, but more importantly in my view because of the degree of unexpected helplessness expressed by those terrorized Americans![15]

In many communities in the United States, most notably in this documentary in the Hawaiian Islands, citizens are terrorized, finding themselves under siege by the feral hogs tearing up their property and landscape. The hogs that have gone wild destroy lawns and gardens, scare children and adults, and kill pets. Americans interviewed feel there is nothing they can do. Really? So dependent and helpless some of these Americans have become that they are afraid to venture outside their homes at night—for fear of hog attacks!

And this is at a time when the price of beef and pork remains sky high! Have guns and rugged individualism become so demonized and hunting so politically incorrect that Americans are afraid to even protect their private property, while at the same time failing to utilize a natural resource roaming wild on their private property? Hogs could be an excellent source of meat for the family. Where has the legendary American sense of self-sufficiency and rugged individualism gone?

Wallace Schwam, M.D., is a retired internist and DRGO member, who is rated expert in marksmanship in the Army. He has come to believe that this extreme passivity is related also to the phobia and bias against guns in a segment of the population. He considers it a passivity disorder akin to the Dependent Personality Disorder listed in the American Psychiatric Association Diagnostic and Statistical Manual of Mental Disorders. It is true that not so long ago, Americans strove to be self-reliant, but this attitude has gradually changed in our modern stressful society. Besides the feminizing propaganda of the mainstream liberal media, American culture has drifted towards achieving a society without risk. Unfortunately, life is not without risk. Dr Schwam opines this cultural transformation "seems to relate to a maladaptive quest to achieve absolute safety. When safety concerns block normal risk taking, excessively passive and dependent behavior results."[16] Those are valid psychosocial explanations, and having lived under communism, I also don't underestimate the power of unrelenting media propaganda. The media has been successful in demonizing guns within an ardent community of progressive, anti-gun activists who, although still a very small minority, have been a vociferous one with access to the major media outlets that support them. On top of that, many Americans have fallen into a cycle of dependency, looking for government to solve all their problems.

Trapping Wild Hogs

In the winter of 2015–2016, a prominent local attorney and popular former state legislator, Larry Walker of Perry, Georgia, wrote an article in *The Telegraph* (Macon) on wild hogs and described the increasing destruction of flora, fauna, and property, a scourge in more than 40 states. Wild hogs are a problem for farmers and even terrified homeowners as we have related, but in truth Americans with their firearms should turn the feral wild hogs and boars into an opportunity, as would have been done in times past. My friends and I still do. We hunt them and trap them. But attorney Walker warned us, "…trapping is difficult, if done properly, and shooting is not very effective." I asked: Are there any challenging tasks or arduous sports worth pursuing that are not difficult?

While trapping feral hogs is vastly superior, hunting them is not impossible, and the sport is not devoid of value and excitement: The hog population can be culled, or at least the sounders can be forced out of valuable pasture and agricultural land and chased to more natural habitats in swamps and low-lying brush by hunting and trapping. Farmers should invite hunters with specially trained dogs if necessary to do so. But there is no need to bring more government agencies to do a job that we can do as private hunters. A legendary story, that took place along the banks of the Ocmulgee River, "Whose bread I eat, his song I must sing," told many years ago by the late Dr. J.G. McDaniel of Fulton County, Georgia, illustrates the tale, conveying meanings at several levels:

> *Years ago in the great Horse-Shoe Bend down the river, there lived a drove of wild hogs. Where they came from no one knew, but they survived floods, fire, freezes, droughts and hunters. The greatest compliment a man could pay to a dog was to say that it had fought the hogs in Horse-Shoe Bend and returned alive…Finally a one-gallused man came by the*

*country store on the river road and asked the whereabouts
of these wild hogs. He drove a one-horse wagon, had an ax,
some quilts, a lantern, some corn, and a single barrel shotgun.
He was a slender, slow moving patient man—he chewed his
tobacco deliberately and spat very seldom.*

*Several months later he came back to the same store and
asked for help to bring out the wild hogs…he had them all in a
pen over in the swamp. Bewildered farmers, dubious hunters,
and storekeepers all gathered in the heart of Horse-Shoe
Bend to view the captive hogs. 'It was all very simple, said
the one-gallused man, 'First I put some corn. For three weeks
they would not eat it. Then some of the young grabbed an ear
and ran off in the thicket. Soon they were all eating it; then
I commenced building a pen around the corn, a little higher
each day. When I noticed that they were all waiting for me to
bring the corn and had stopped grubbing for acorns and roots.
I built the trap door. Naturally,' said the patient man, 'they
raised quite a ruckus when they seen they was trapped, but I
can pen any animal on the face of this earth if I can just get
him to depend on me for a free-handout.'[17]*

The story is instructive on several levels: Wild hogs, like men, can be trapped if they can be made dependent on a free-handout!

And so like "the one-gallused man" of Horse-Shoe Bend, we also baited large sturdily constructed traps with corn and successfully trapped the ferocious wild hogs rampaging the farms of friends in Taylor County, Georgia, thereby ending their ruination of crops, sod, and hay farms. Other hunters more effectively use dogs; we didn't. But for three years, the hogs haven't come back! We're ready for them if they do return! It is open season on feral hogs year round in Georgia.

From the pork, we had sausage, pork chops, and ribs stored in our freezer for a couple of years. The meat can also be donated to the needy. It is the most consumed meat in the world. (Wild hog is lower in fat than regular pork.) My friend and butcher, Ernest Thomas of Bolingbroke, does a magnificent job of preparing our favorite cuts. So let's turn this problem into an opportunity, while protecting our property, the environment, and exploiting a natural resource that sorely needs exploiting! A note of caution to the reader: Wild hogs are ferocious and dangerous. They should be handled carefully even when dead. The meat should only be butchered and processed by qualified personnel with special gloves. Pork must be cooked thoroughly like all wild animal meat to prevent contracting diseases, such as trichinosis or salmonellosis (the latter can also be contracted from poultry).

CHAPTER 20
GUN CONTROL IN AUSTRALIA AND GREAT BRITAIN

Et domus sua cuique est tutissimum refu-
gium ("a man's home is his castle")

—Sir Edward Coke (1552—1634)

So long as those [liberties of Englishmen] remain inviolate, the
subject is perfectly free; for every species of compulsive tyranny and
oppression must act in opposition to one or other of those rights.

—Sir William Blackstone (1723—1780),
describing the fifth and last auxiliary right of a citizen, the God-
given right of a person to keep and bear arms for his basic and
natural right of resistance to oppression and for self-preservation. *Commentaries on the Laws of England* (1765)

We're subjects. You're citizens.

—James Atlas (1989),
expression an American heard often from his British cousins

Gun prohibitionists frequently compare gun violence in America to other
"industrialized" or "wealthy" nations, and then condemn the U.S. for its
violent crime rate. First, this is systematic racial and ethnic, as well as economic, discrimination against the less industrialized and less wealthy nations
on a large scale by dismissing the suffering, the injuries, and the lives of the

citizens of those nations, who apparently are not worth comparing. The U.S. should be compared to all nations of the world because, if the ultimate goal is to prevent loss of human life, the study and comparison of crime statistics should include all nations, as men and women of the world belong to the same human species. The lives of people in Latin America, Asia, and Africa count as much as Western Europeans and Scandinavians. (We discussed this shortsightedness in Chapter 11, "The Obligatory Comparison with 'Other Industrialized Nations.'")

From the outset, let us state that cultural differences are important in determining why citizens of different nations may approve of their country's harsh gun control policies. Historical development and cultural differences are frequently ignored in one-size-fits-all pronouncements. Canadian and Australian gun control measures are touted for reducing firearm homicides and suicides, but not the overall percentage of homicides by all causes, as if men and women killed by strangulation, beaten or bludgeoned to death or killed with knives do not count, and violent deaths by other means makes for a less violent society. Is a society less violent because people are killed regularly with knives as in China or with bombs as in Spain and France? Is a society less violent because people kill themselves by jumping off buildings, hanging, and poisoning as is done throughout the world, or by jumping in front of trains or stabbing with swords as in done more specifically in Japan? (We will answer some of these questions in this Chapter, as they refer especially to Australia and the United Kingdom, and we will take another look at suicide in various countries in Chapter 24.)

The Land of the Rising Sun and the British Commonwealth—An Introduction

Great Britain and Canada, part of the British Commonwealth, and Japan, an important island nation in the Far East, share something in common: They are nations in which citizens greatly respect government authority and de-emphasize individualism and personal freedom. The Japanese are not only respectful but are actually submissive to government authority. Americans, for example, would not tolerate home visits by intrusive government officials, insufficient due process in arresting and interrogating suspects, and lack of privacy, as in Japan; nor would they accept the restrictions on freedom of speech as in Britain and Canada, or the class stratification in England and Scotland.

The historical development of these nations should also not be ignored. Canada's colonial history rested on loyalty to the British Crown, and the Canadians fought the Americans both in the American Revolution and the War of 1812 to preserve their ties to England. Canadian loyalists were joined by 200,000 American loyalists, who fled the American colonies to reinforce the Canadians in preserving their ties to the mother country. They accepted British taxation and other restrictions to liberty—preferring British law and order to American rebellion in the latter's pursuit of liberty and independence.

The Japanese stratification of society—e.g., between government officials in positions of authority and the rest of the population who obey and respect them as the modern "samurai"—began in the Middle Ages. The unifiers of Japan—Oda Nobunaga, Toyotomi Hideyoshi, and Tokugawa Ieyasu—following the late 16th and early 17th century, not only established the superiority of the samurai (warrior) and daimyo (feudal lord) classes over the peasants, but also disarmed them and forced them to submit to their authority. The subjugation of the peasants and the rest of the population continued during the Tokugawa Shogunate (1600—1867) and even after the Meiji Restoration of the Mikado in 1867. The samurai class then was not extinguished in modern Japan. The warrior class became the important government officials, the police, and the military, and they continue to be greatly respected in Japanese society.

Thus, despite the advent of democracy in the wake of World War II, Japan has remained an authoritarian and collectivist society, a submissive society, culturally very different from American society in terms of individualism and the exercise of personal freedom. For example, Japanese government officials make home visits to citizens to obtain personal data, collect social and economic data on families, inspect domiciles, and even give parental advice and matrimonial counseling, as does the local police. Moreover, restrictions in freedom of speech (and of the press), suspension of habeas corpus protection and other civil liberty guarantees, while expected from the Japanese, would not be tolerated by the individualist and privacy-conscious Americans. (We also briefly compare cultural and gun perspective differences between Japan and Switzerland in Chapter 24.)

It is no wonder then that given this historical and cultural background, the British and Japanese have acquiesced to draconian gun control, while the Canadians have accepted more moderate gun restrictions. The Australians did resent the erosion of their liberties and fought the step-by-step gun control policies that became draconian, as we shall discuss later in this chapter, after the mass shooting in Port Arthur, Tasmania, in 1996. Still they were not capable of opposing the government with the intensity of the Americans.

We must remember that the Australians, like the Canadians, did not rebel against the British Crown but were granted autonomy and independence gradually. The Australian tradition of liberty and gun rights came from the British common law (e.g., armed citizens for the defense of the realm) and subsequently codified in the English Bill of Rights of 1689 that also established parliamentary supremacy over the king and a constitutional monarchy, events that took place as a result of the Glorious Revolution of 1688. Nevertheless, the English Bill of Rights was not enshrined in a written constitution but qualified as a law ensuring the right of Protestants to possess arms but with the caveat, "suitable to their condition as allowed by law," which in effect could be, and was actually, superseded by more and more restrictive laws that came to negate the rights. The American Bill of Rights, on the other hand, forbid violation of those rights, stating, "Congress should make no laws respecting..." as in the First Amendment, and "...the right of the people to keep and bear arms, shall not be infringed," as in the Second Amendment.

The British, Canadians, and Australians, then never had a Second Amendment in their constitutions, nor a strong gun lobby that could fight the gun-prohibitionist forces arrayed against them. The Australian police, the moralistic academicians, and the liberal press pushed for gun control at every turn and after every mass shooting. Without a strong national gun lobby—as we have in America with the NRA, Gun Owners of America (GOA), supported by myriad sports shooting organizations—the Australians were not able to stop the onslaught against their gun rights or privacy. Under the pretext of possible illegal gun possession, as we shall see in this chapter, the Australian police now can enter any home, search, arrest, and confiscate guns or incriminating information—all without a legal warrant and probable cause. Moreover, as in the rest of the British Commonwealth and Japan, illegally seized evidence, coercive interrogations and confessions are allowed and entered as evidence.[1]

In this chapter we explore in more detail the gun control experience in Australia and Great Britain—two countries to which the United States is frequently compared on that issue as well as in health care. Australia has always been to me a large expansive country, an entire continent that in many ways resembled America, such as its colonization and settlement by a steady stream of penitent Englishmen. Australians expanded the frontiers of British civilization. Americans in turn had Manifest Destiny and westward expansion unmatched in history. Both countries had gold rushes. Australia had ringers and Aborigines. America had cowboys and Indians. Both countries had bold, rugged individualists who conquered a vast territory. Great Britain was the mother country to both along with up to that time the legacy of freedom and justice for all. At one time all three countries loved guns. What happened?

Crocodile Dundee and Gun Control Down Under

In August 1999, the rugged Aussie survivalist whose real life exploits inspired the "Crocodile Dundee" movies died in what appeared to be a mysterious shootout with an Australian law enforcement unit in which a police sergeant was also killed. It was reported that Rodney William Ansell, the 44-year-old, blond haired Aussie, uncannily resembled Paul Hogan, the actor who portrayed him in the movie and the sequel. Although Ansell was admittedly no angel and had previous run-ins with police, he had been named 1988 "Australian Northern Territory Man of the Year" for inspiring the movie and putting "the Australian Outback on the map."[2]

In the end, after a two-day shooting spree, Crocodile Dundee shot dead a police officer and was killed by return fire during the confrontation. What motivated this shooting spree? In 1996, Australia adopted draconian gun control laws, banning certain guns (estimated at 60 percent of all guns), and requiring registration of all firearms and licensing of all gun owners. Apparently "Crocodile Dundee" believed the police were coming to confiscate the unregistered firearms he had refused to turn in and perhaps arrest him for falling outside the law. Distraught as he might have been for failed business ventures as some have claimed, Rod Ansell was a "wild man of the bush" and not likely to give up his guns without a fight.[2]

It's a fact that since the passage of the Australian gun control measures in 1996, the police can enter a person's home and search for guns, copy computer hard drives, seize records, and do it all without a search warrant! It's the law that police can go door to door searching for weapons that have not been surrendered in the highly publicized gun buyback programs. They use previous registration and firearm license lists to check for lapses and confiscate non-surrendered firearms.

The problem began with the Port Arthur (a Tasmanian resort) tragedy on April 28, 1996, when a crazed assailant opened fire and shot 35 people. Australians were shocked and the government reacted with knee jerk promptness. The Australian government adopted the National Firearms Agreement (NFA), an innocuous sounding, but, in fact, a far reaching gun control measure. The agreement was a draconian gun ban that seriously curtailed gun rights and led to major changes in the way of life for the people Down Under.

At the time, there were three major political parties in Australia: the center right Liberal Party, the socialist Labor Party, and the ultra-left Australian Democratic Party. The latter tilted the balance of power leftward toward stringent gun control at the expense of freedom.

As a result of the ban, all semi-automatic firearms (rifles and handguns) were and remain proscribed, including .22 caliber rabbit guns and duck-hunting Remington shotguns. Former California State Senator H.L. Richardson, Chairman of Gun Owners of America (GOA) wrote: "They outlawed every semi-auto, even those pretty duck guns, the Browning A5 and the Remington 1100s. They even struck down pump shotguns: the Winchester model 12 and the Remington 870...Do you own a Browning BAR rifle? Banned. How about a Winchester Model 100? Out of luck, all semi-auto hunting rifles were outlawed as well. They didn't miss a one."[2]

Be that as it may and at a cost of $500 million, out of an estimated seven million firearms (of which 2.8 million were prohibited), only 640,000 guns were surrendered to police. What were the consequences of Australia's gun ban? The same consequences England suffered. Like Great Britain, crime Down Under escalated immediately after the ban. Twelve months after the law was implemented in 1997, there was a 44 percent increase in armed robberies, an 8.6 percent increase in aggravated assaults, and a 3.2 percent increase in homicides. That same year in the state of Victoria, there was a 300 percent increase in homicides committed with firearms. The following year, robberies increased almost 60 percent in South Australia. By 1999, assaults had increased in New South Wales by almost 20 percent. And prior to the ban, crime in Australia had been on a downward trend.[2]

Waves of Crime in the Australian Countryside

Two years after the Australian gun ban, there were still increases in crime: armed robberies up by 73 percent; unarmed robberies up by 28 percent; kidnappings up by 38 percent; assaults up by 17 percent; manslaughter up by 29 percent, according to figures posted by the Australian Bureau of Statistics. These figures were subsequently removed, and were no longer available after several months, veritably erased from the statistical record.

Apparently denying and falsifying the record is what the Australian government chose to do, embarrassed to tell the truth about what really happened after the gun ban. The Australian government claimed that reducing the number of guns in Australia reduced homicides and suicides during this period. But how can Australian government statistics be trusted when the numbers are suddenly changed in mid-course and figures cannot be verified by outside observers?

There is no question crime increased for three years after the Australian gun ban went into effect. The question now is whether there have been reductions in crime rates since that time, despite the curtailment of freedom and the increase in government intrusion. Also we must consider the fact that over the previous 25-year period before the ban, Australia had shown a steady decrease both in homicide with firearms and armed robbery—that is until the ban. The most recent statistics show a mixed bag of data, but definitely demonstrate that despite the claim by the Australian government that the ban has resulted in a decrease in violent crime, no such conclusion can be drawn, and plotted graphs illustrate that crime rates have decreased in some areas and increased in others (see graphs). My figures were corroborated by data collected not only by the NRA and GOA but also by other investigators, as we will demonstrate shortly. Incidentally, the NRA has also had an ongoing feud with the Australian government over the statistics.

Finally, after being lambasted for years for claiming that Australia's draconian gun laws had not resulted in a significant improvement in the crime rate, a 2005 article written by Robert Wainwright, a journalist for

The Sydney Morning Herald, substantiated much of what the NRA had been saying. Because Australian anti-gun activists claimed that the statistics were misquoted and statements taken out of context by the NRA, and also because I fear the Wainwright article may also vanish into thin air, I quote in full the first five paragraphs of that report:

> *Gun ownership is rising and there is no definitive evidence that a decade of restrictive firearms laws has done anything to reduce weapon-related crime, according to New South Wales's top criminal statistician.*
>
> *The latest figures show a renaissance in firearm ownership in the state—a 25 percent increase in three years. And the head of the Bureau of Crime Statistics and Research, Don Weatherburn, said falls in armed robberies and abductions in NSW in the past few years had more to do with the heroin drought and good policing than firearms legislation.*
>
> *Even falls in the homicide rate, which have been steady, began long before the gun law debate provoked by the Port Arthur massacre in 1996.*
>
> *Nationwide, the proportion of robberies involving weapons is the same as it was in 1996, while the proportion of abductions involving weapons is higher, the latest Australian Bureau of Statistics figures reveal. They show a mixed result in fire-arms-related offences since the mid-1990s. There has been a fall in firearms murders (from 32 to 13 percent) but a rise (19 to 23 percent) in attempted murders involving guns.*
>
> *'I would need to see more convincing evidence than there is to be able to say that gun laws have had any effect,' Dr Weatherburn said. 'The best that could be said for the tougher laws is there has been no other mass killing using firearms [since Port Arthur].'*[3]

We have had to wait nearly a decade to obtain independent confirmation of what we feared was really happening in Australia, at least in New South Wales, and it is ironic that, as we shall see, we had to wait even longer for the next reliable independent report to come out from Down Under. Nevertheless, this article gives us a glimpse at what was actually happening in Australia behind the government smoke screen and corroborates the facts we mentioned earlier that if there was a drop in homicide with firearms "it began long before the new laws and has continued on afterwards." Weatherburn also confirmed our earlier claim to a rise in crime following the ban. He was quoted as saying, "There has been a more specific…problem with handguns, which rose up quite rapidly and then declined. The decline appears to have more to do with the arrest of those responsible than the new laws. As soon as the heroin shortage hit, the armed robbery rate came down. I don't think it was anything to do with the tougher firearm laws." That is perhaps as much of an admission as we can expect to get from the head of the Bureau of Crime Statistics and Research.

Some Australian politicians quit in frustration over the gun ban and the further useless restrictions extinguishing individualism and liberty. The Shooters Party MP John Tingle retired in 2006 frustrated in his attempts to prevent further gun control measures. Tingle declared, "If the laws had worked there would be much less illegal gun crime…we are continuing this perception that if you tighten firearm laws you are going to control firearm crime, even though the opposite is true. Restrictive laws against legitimate ownership and use do nothing to stop gun-related crime because only law-abiding citizens will adhere to laws."[3]

Unfortunately, the NSW police commissioner continued to support the ban despite the statistics and admitting to the genuine grievances of gun owners by praising the work of MP Tingle in advocating fairly for the right of Australia's once lawful "shooters." Ten years later, the NRA published an Investigative Report by Ginny Simone that confirmed the grievances and disclosed that billions of dollars spent on mass confiscation and disarmament of Australians had resulted in loss of freedom but no reduction in crime.[4]

Australia is a semi-arid, isolated continent, a vast nation-state whose history in many ways parallels that of the United States. In the 1850s and 1860s, it had gold rushes and pioneering settlers, reminiscent of American westward migration. In World War I and World War II, Aussies fought with the allies.

Although Australia gained its legislative independence from Britain in 1986, it remains a commonwealth with close ties to the British crown. With only 24 million people, Australia has an impressive flora and fauna, but also plenty of varmints, including dingoes that wreak havoc on livestock, large rats and other rodents, and deadly poisonous snakes. Yet, hunting has become prohibitively difficult for all but a handful of Australians with private lands and the usual political connections.

No Right to Self, Family, or Home Protection

The ban on firearms and the disarmament of ordinary Australians has left criminals free to roam the countryside. Bandits, of course, kept their guns. As in America, only the law-abiding, by definition, obey the law. Yet, the successive leftist or left-of-center politicians in the Australian government responded by passing more laws; for example, in 1998 Bowie knives and other knives and items including handcuffs were banned. Apparently the large urban cities of Australia dictate to the rest of the continent what can be done and restrict the liberty of the people in the hinterland at will. Australians need an Electoral College for better and fairer representation of the entire population. It seems the people in the rural countryside, admittedly less populated but which nevertheless include vast areas of the continent, are not fairly represented in the government as to be capable of asserting their political rights to self and family protection.

As in Great Britain and Canada, armed self-protection and the legal right to self-defense are not recognized in Australia. No one should then be surprised that licensing for firearms remains difficult, even for victims of crime and those who show a need for personal protection. Self and family protection are not considered valid reasons to own firearms. Like Americans, at one time, Australians loved and possessed rifles and handguns—but they were not vigilant enough, the ban was passed, and it changed their way of life for the worse.

Two decades later, the Australian gun ban still stands and crime persists. Policies such as firearm confiscation and disarming Australian citizens have not made them safer. In 2013, the New South Wales Police Commissioner Andrew Scipione admitted that gun violence was still a huge problem, stating,

"There is no single source of gun violence. Guns have fallen into the hands of organized crime, outlaw motorcycle gangs, mid-level crime groups and petty thieves, and the lines are often blurred."[4]

And yet, America's progressive (authoritarian socialist) politicians continue to praise the draconian gun laws of Australia and point to them as if they offer a panacea for mass shootings and criminal gun usage. Using the occasion of the tragic 2015 mass shooting in an American black church in Charleston, South Carolina, comparing it to the aftermath of the Port Arthur massacre in Australia in 1996, President Barack Obama chimed, "It was just so shocking—the entire country said, 'Well, we're going to completely change our gun laws,' and they did. And it hasn't happened since."[4]

Down Under (Australia) does have an advantage over the U.S. in her criminal justice system, an important issue that has been neglected, perhaps deliberately, by gun prohibitionists. This is the fact Australia does not have an indulgent criminal justice system, unlike that of the United States which coddles criminals. Australia may catch killers and robbers at similar rates as the U.S., but once arrested, criminals are likely to go to jail and stay locked up. Australia has a high conviction rate for both homicides and robberies. In New South Wales, persons arrested for robbery have a 90 percent conviction rate and 60 percent of them go to jail for longer than five years.[5] Violent crimes in association with guns are severely penalized and the maximum sentence is life in prison. Compare these facts, with U.S. statistics. In New York City, only one percent of felony arrests lead to a state prison term and only nine percent of felony convictions lead to more than one year in jail. In the U.S. as a whole only 13 percent of felony convictions leads to incarceration for one year or more![5]

Australia, then, does not have a penal system with revolving prison doors, and violent criminals, especially those convicted of guns crimes or in possession of firearms, are locked up, reducing the overall crime rate. This is not the case in the United States, where the judicial system, in general, and the Democrat Party, in particular, at both the national and state levels, routinely stands for the "rights" of criminals at the expense of victims. The politicians of the Democrat Party militate for early release, plea bargaining, shorter sentences, as if indirectly encouraging the rise in the crime rate, so that then they can pass more gun laws penalizing law-abiding citizens who unfairly are disproportionately affected by such legislation.[4]

In Australia the criminals on the loose do remain armed and continue to circumvent the law, and the government's tactics continue to be confiscatory gun policies and more rounds of federal amnesty programs in an attempt to get criminals to give up their guns. They never do. Only law-abiding citizens comply and submit, which is the usual story we have been relating in this book.

An NRA-ILA report in 2017 reviewed the issue and found:

> In 2013, the U.S. Department of Justice's National Institute of Justice reviewed the available research on Australia's NFA firearm confiscation program and issued a memorandum that concluded that the effort had no effect on crime generally. In coming to this determination, the memorandum cited work from University of Maryland Professor Peter Reuter and Jenny Mouzos, aptly titled, 'Australia: A Massive Buyback of Low-Risk Guns.' The NIJ memo made clear that the researchers 'found no effect on crime.'[4]

In fact, repeated federal amnesties and recent confiscations have resulted more in the sequential removal of remaining family heirlooms and disarming the law-abiding citizens of Australia than "in getting rid of guns off our streets." The registering, banning, confiscation, amnesty programs, and destruction of firearms have not made an impact on the persistent increases in crime, and not just burglaries, but assaults and home invasions. To make matters worse, the Australian government is so committed to the gun ban laws that the government's published crime figures cannot be trusted unless verified by outside sources.

In short, gun control has eroded the rugged individualism of Australians, and now, within a vast continent, they must depend on faraway government protection. Freedom and personal independence have been extinguished. A way of life has ended.[6]

Great Britain and Gun Control

Let's now cross the Indian and Atlantic Oceans to the nation of Great Britain to examine the crime and gun control measures in that country. I must confess that I have gone down this path before and—even though I am an admirer of Great Britain, her history and her former empire—when it comes to crime and gun rights, it has not been a pretty path for the past half century. Thus, when I wrote an article for *World Net Daily* back in 2003 about gun control in Great Britain, I felt compelled to write an apologist introduction that is still pertinent today. For this chapter I must cite an additional reason for the caveat. Great Britain has been a staunch ally "in the war on terror" and a proven friend to the United States. And almost alone, the U.S. and Great Britain seem to be the only western powers restraining the tide of globalization suffocating freedom and the national movements toward self-determination.

I regret the British persistence in using strict gun control, restricting freedom and individual liberty, instead of instituting crime control. In addition, the British deny citizens self-protection, even the right of the people to protect their homes and families. All of this, despite the wave of illegal immigration, crime, and Islamic terrorism assailing Europe—a destructive wave enveloping European civilization and way of life. Great Britain should realize by now that she has not been immune to these developments. In 2003, I wrote:

> *Difficult as it is to be critical of a friend and ally in the war on terror, Great Britain has instituted a cruel and unjust gun-control policy, a worsening evil, upon her law-abiding citizens that needs correcting. The title of this essay comes from the seemingly paradoxical unrelenting tide of thievery and burglaries that has swept Great Britain, and was so dubbed by the London Sunday Times in 1998—A Nation of Thieves.[7]*

I proceed now to tell the story of a miscarriage of British justice. I refer to the shameful case of Mr. Tony Martin, who was introduced to American readers in the October 2003 issue of *America's 1st Freedom* by Wayne LaPierre, NRA executive vice president.[8] LaPierre revealed with perfect clarity how Great Britain's stringent gun control laws and the abolishment of the right to self-defense have brought the birthplace of classical liberalism beyond absurdity to the footsteps of authoritarian socialism.

Who Are the Bad Guys in Good Old England?

Briefly, 57-year-old British farmer, Tony Martin, who lived in a remote farmhouse in England and had been terrorized several times by burglars, shot and killed an intruder in his home. Another thief-accomplice escaped. For this act of self-defense in his own home—and ironically in the same country where the great statesman Sir Edward Coke (1552—1634) declared boldly that a man's home is his castle—Tony Martin, a free citizen, was sentenced to life imprisonment as "a danger to burglars!"[8]

While Martin languished in an English prison, the other thief was freed after serving only 18 months in jail. The British government granted the felon, who had previously been convicted of 34 crimes, £5,000 of taxpayer money as legal aid to file a lawsuit against Martin for emotional distress. This is incredible, but true! The nation that for centuries had established the basis for the most equitable system of Anglo-American jurisprudence that men have ever devised and extended the horizons of liberty to the entire world, had now come down to this—coddling thieves while punishing citizens for protecting themselves and their property.

It is not surprising, then, that in London, a person's chance of being mugged is six times greater than in the Big Apple! Nor should it surprise anyone that in England, day burglary is commonplace and dangerous because burglars know that even if the homeowners are present in the domicile, they are defenseless and literally at the "mercy" of the criminal.[7,8]

Tony Martin was finally released after serving four years in prison. Subsequently, he was forced to live in safe houses in fear for his life. Pardon the vulgar conversational style that follows as I quote the threats made against Martin's life by other thieves and relatives of the dead burglar: "He will get it. Something will happen to him, it's got to...To those who say it's just talk, I'd say wait and see. The detectives can't be with him all the time, can they?"

And as reported in *America's 1st Freedom*, another conspirator boasted, "He is a dead man...It will be a proper hit man, a professional job."[8]

The police cannot protect Martin from the thieves; nor as a convicted felon, can he leave Britain. Least of all, he cannot use a gun for self-protection. For nearly two decades, he has been in an unsustainable catch-22 situation because the gun-prohibitionist system of British justice has failed him miserably. In 2014, it was reported that Martin had abandoned his house, and had to live with acquaintances or in his car, a flighty existence and untenable situation for any citizen. Before his mishap, Martin had been a lawful citizen who owned a prime 300-acre farm worth an estimated £3 million. But he lost everything and now subsists in a deplorable condition. He was arrested again in 2015 for allegedly possessing a firearm for personal safety.[9]

Imagine the irony of this shameful story, of all places, taking place in the country that gave the world the legal minds of the great jurists of liberty, Sir Edward Coke and Sir William Blackstone!

Under these conditions, we can ask ourselves, who really fared better: Crocodile Dundee being shot dead in Australia in 1999 or Tony Martin, in 2015, living in such deplorable circumstances and in constant fear for his life in what should have been Merry Old England? Patrick Henry answered that question at the outset of the American Revolution in his unforgettable speech that ended with, "Give me liberty, or give me death."[10]

In Great Britain today, draconian gun control laws remain firmly in place and there is no right to armed self-defense. All handguns are banned in places of business and even in the home. Just as the NRA and GOA had warned, firearm registration in Great Britain facilitated disarmament and confiscation in 1998. Simple possession of a firearm carries a 10-year prison sentence; and yet, England's permissive criminal justice system emphasizes rehabilitation of hardened criminals with revolving prison doors for all habitual thieves and burglars.[11]

The Rise in Crime and Violence in Britain

In America in the 1990s, violent crime steadily decreased and remained low in most cities (with the notable exceptions of Washington, D.C., Chicago, and Baltimore) up to the present time, despite the fact there are more guns in

America than ever before and record numbers of citizens are carrying legally concealed firearms. However, the same cannot be said for Great Britain.

Notwithstanding draconian gun control laws and the erosion of the civil liberties, crime steadily increased in Britain during the 1990s and has remained relatively high to the present time. Consider the lamentation:

> *Britons are chagrined by the findings of a U.S. Department of Justice study that says a person is nearly twice as likely to be robbed, assaulted or have a vehicle stolen in Britain as in the United States. The Trans-Atlantic cousins can take comfort in the fact that the United States remains far ahead of Britain in violent crimes, including murder and rape, although the gap is narrowing there as well.*[12]

Additionally, criminologist David Kopel revealed "In 1995…there were 20 assaults per 1,000 people or households in England and Wales but only 8.8 in the United States."[13] While the U.S. still leads in the most violent crimes, rates for serious crimes, such as murder, are coming down relative to Great Britain. In fact, the *Associated Press* reported that U.S. murder rates reached a 30-year low and "serious crimes reported by police declined for the sixth straight year in 1997."[14]

A study conducted by a Cambridge University professor and a statistician from the U.S. Department of Justice reported in *The Washington Times* that several types of crimes rose steadily in Britain while declining in America. For example, "Robberies rose 81 percent in England and Wales but fell to 28 percent in the United States. Assault increased 53 percent in England and Wales but declined 27 percent in the United States. Burglaries doubled in England but fell by half in the United States and motor vehicle theft rose 51 percent in England but remained the same in the United States."[12] It should be noted these comparable trends in serious crimes that began in the 1990s have held largely to the present time. In fact major crimes in the U.S. continued to decline until the small spike in firearm deaths for the short period of 2014–2016, which we mentioned earlier in Chapter 12.

To make matters worse for England (and this is also true for Canada), in those countries where citizens are disarmed in their homes, day burglary is commonplace and dangerous because criminals know they will not be shot at, even if caught in *flagrante delicto*. In the U.S., burglars try to make sure homeowners are not at home to avoid being shot at by intended victims; this is not so in Great Britain where they do not fear citizens. The *London Sunday Times* reporting on this dangerous and rising tide of thievery and burglaries in England dubbed Britain "a nation of thieves." The *Times* noted, "More than one in three British men has a criminal record by the age of 40. While America has cut its crime rate dramatically Britain remains the crime capital of the West." "Where," asked the British author, "have we gone wrong?"[15]

Ironically, the most drastic ascendancy of crimes in Britain was found in those types of felonies where recent studies in the U.S. have shown that guns in the hands of law-abiding citizens not only save lives and protect private property but also reduce injuries to good people and crime is generally deterred.[16]

The British are as proud of their gun control efforts, fruitless as these efforts might be, as they are of their socialistic National Health Services, despite the long queues and waiting lists. They are so proud of these national policies that they have been shown to lie about their statistics. In this book, of course, we will only consider crime statistics, deceptive statistics that gun prohibitionists tout in the United States in defending the UK civilian disarmament policies.

Consider the fact that while the FBI's reported number of U.S. homicides is inflated because the numbers are compiled from preliminary data at the time of death and therefore misleadingly include justified self-defense shootings among the criminal homicides, the United Kingdom's Home Office does the complete opposite and uses methodologically different criteria that deliberately create low numbers. Instead of compiling crime figures by counting dead bodies with evidence of foul play, as the FBI does, the Home Office's tallied numbers depend on conviction. And these delays in adding numbers, not only deflates the true figures but, further obfuscates the true picture:

> *Since murder cases often take years to be resolved, statistics for a given year tend to reflect events actually occurring in previous years. For example, Home Office figures appear to indicate a massive spike in murders culminating in 2003; in actuality, this is the year in which the victims of prolific serial*

killer Harold Shipman—who murdered throughout his long
career—were reported.[14]

Obviously by using different criteria, U.S. murder rates will be a lot higher
than those in the UK. The other method used in the UK, the Crime Survey,
conducted by the Office for National Statistics, is likewise problematic. It
relies incredibly on "interviews of individuals, not law enforcement data."[14]
Therefore comparing U.S. homicide data with the British statistic thrown out
nonchalantly by gun control activists is misleading, if not outright fraudulent.
Doing so would be tantamount to comparing apples to oranges at best and
using artful disingenuousness at worse.

Careful examination of the British data over decades revealed an
increase in the number of homicides in the UK in the mid-1990s, which only
worsened after the 1997 British gun ban; the climbing murder rate only sub-
sided after a massive expansion of the police forces in Britain. Nevertheless,
crime remains too high for comfort, especially when citizens cannot protect
their lives or property. It goes without saying that in the UK a burglar can
sue a homeowner for damages sustained after breaking into a home.

Yet, the legerdemain with the UK crime statistics gets worse than just
different methodology. As early as 1996, the *London Daily Telegraph* admitted
that British crime figures were a "sham," noting that "pressure to convince
the public that police were winning the fight against crime had resulted in a
long list of ruses to 'massage' statistics," and "the recorded crime level bore
no resemblance to the actual amount of crime being committed." Dave Kopel
and associates at the Independence Institute concluded that comparing crime
rates between America and Britain is fundamentally flawed. In America, a gun
crime is recorded as a gun crime. In Britain, a crime is only recorded when
there is a final disposition (a conviction). All unsolved gun crimes in Britain
are not reported as gun crimes, grossly undercounting the amount of gun
crime in the UK. To make matters worse, British law enforcement has been
exposed for falsifying criminal reports to create falsely lower crime figures.[14]

Despite playing fast and loose with statistics to tout the supposed
achievement of their drastic gun control measures, the truth is getting out. In
October 2017 Breitbart's headlines spotlighted the shocking reality: "London
is Falling: UK Capital Now More Dangerous Than NYC…More Rape, More

Robbery, More Violence." It cited the latest crime figures for England and Wales that revealed an overall increase in violence and crime that astounded the authorities—a 22 percent rise in rape, 26 percent rise in knife crimes, and a dramatic and even steeper rise in gun offenses, compounding the ascent that was noted in 2016.[15]

If Great Britain was dubbed "a nation of thieves" and the "crime capital of the West," London could very well now be dubbed "the murder and rape metropolis of the industrialized world." And this has happened under the administration of Labor leader and London's Muslim mayor, Sadiq Khan, who had previously boasted that "London is the safest global city in the world," while encouraging the police to reach out to criminal elements rather than increasing arrests and cracking down on crime.[15]

Crime in London has only steadily gotten worse. Further statistics compiled in the fall of 2017, disclosed that London officially surpassed New York City in the number of homicides for the first time since 1800. The increase in London homicides has occurred with guns and knives, both of which are already prohibited. The article also attributed the increase in murders in part as "a consequence of Mayor Khan's campaign against using stop and search on ethnic minorities, with London police chief Cressida Dick admitting that constables have become 'fearful' of confronting suspects as they 'might get into trouble or might not be supported if they had a complaint.'" In short, compared to New Yorkers, Londoners are now six times more likely to be burgled, three times more likely to be raped, and one and a half times more likely to be robbed. Guns and knives are not the only weapons used; throwing acid and other corrosive substances, criminal practices that may have originated in India and other southeast Asian countries, are also very common at more than 800 offenses per year.[15]

The Thieves of the Gulag Archipelago

In my frequent re-examinations of the epic volumes of Aleksandr Solzhenitsyn's *The Gulag Archipelago*, I came across some psychosocial observations noted by the illustrious Nobel Prize-winning author and political philosopher. In Volumes III and IV, I found something about the nature of common thieves in the former USSR, those supposedly "in freedom" (e.g., in the USSR at large), as well as in the gulag's corrective (destructive) labor camps. We learn for example that in the Soviet Union, even at the height of Joseph Stalin's reign of terror and bloody purges (at a cost of 20 to 40 million lives), the thieves were considered "socially friendly" elements, and were useful and used extensively by the Soviet government.

The thieves not only terrorized the population, as haters and defilers of private property, but also were used as informants by the police; and in the gulag, served as "instructors" in the cultural and educational sections, or as actual officers by the internal security police (the MVD). Needless to say, they were also useful to the repressive apparatus as the proverbial stool pigeons and enforcers of hard labor and terror against ideological (political) prisoners. When needed, they even worked hand in glove with the security forces in carrying out mass murder in the extermination camps of the gulags.

While citizens were arrested, hauled off to the gulags for slave labor and saddled with long prison sentences (10- and 25-year sentences were typical), Solzhenitsyn wrote:

> Sentences [for the thieves] were bound to be reduced and of course for habitual criminals especially. Watch out there now, witness in the courtroom! They will all be back soon, and it will be a knife in the back of anyone who gives testimony! Therefore, if you see someone crawling through a window, or slitting a pocket, or your neighbor's suitcase being ripped open—shut your eyes! Walk by! You didn't see anything! That's how the thieves have trained us—the thieves and our laws![17]

In the destructive-labor camps of the Soviet Union (1918–1956), the thieves robbed, tortured and murdered political prisoners with impunity. Indeed, they were rewarded with higher food rations, better living space and other privileges for collaborating with the guards and fomenting terror.

It makes hair stand on end when we see that parallels can be drawn between today's coddled thieves of the social democracy of Great Britain and the erstwhile, hard-left communist dystopia of the former USSR.

And If You Cannot Flee or Be Heard—Shout!

Solzhenitsyn wrote that fear of exceeding the limits of self-defense for individual Soviet citizens "led to total spinelessness as a national characteristic" on the part of the individual and total omnipotence on that of the criminal state. When a military officer, mind you a Red Army officer, defended himself from an assailant and killed the hoodlum with a penknife, the officer got 10 years for murder. "And what was I supposed to do?" the officer asked. The Soviet prosecutor replied, "You should have fled!"[17]

"Flee!" That distant Soviet echo reverberates in modern British society—"Scream, run, shout!"—and not only in the United Kingdom but also in other territories of the British Commonwealth, such as Canada and Australia. In those nations, there is no recognized right to self-defense, and citizens are also told to run and flee from assailants. Human dignity—self-defense, private property—out the window! But what if the victims cannot run and their shouts are not heard? Are women supposed to allow sexual predators to rape them? The British constable told Tony Martin, who lived on an isolated 300-acre ranch, that he should have shouted! The lamentable absurdity is palpable, or laughable, were it not for the indignity suffered by the honest British subjects at the expense of pandering to the base criminal elements.

The incidents in this chapter will help the reader understand why many, in fact the majority, of the state legislators in America have supported the Castle Doctrine and passed "stand your ground" legislation, so that Americans have the legal right, as well as moral prerogative, to protect themselves, their families, and their homes with dignity and without having to abandon them. We also have concealed carry weapons (CCW) and "Constitutional Carry" (CC) rights, which will be discussed in Chapter 25.

Like the Soviets, British Subjects Have No Right to Self-Defense

Let's return to the instructive Soviet parallels, *The Gulag Archipelago*, and to life in the Soviet labor camps, which for some citizens in the social democracies is looking more and more reflective of what is happening in their soft-left, socialist "free countries."

Astonished we learn (or relearn) from Solzhenitsyn that in the heavily militarized Soviet Union, "The State, in its Criminal Code, forbids citizens to have firearms or other weapons, but does not itself undertake to defend them!"[18] The communist State defended itself ferociously with its famous KGB, the Sword and the Shield of the Soviet State, but the State would not commit itself to defend its citizens from non-political criminals, particularly, the "socially friendly" thieves. Solzhenitsyn wrote:

> *The State turns its citizens over to the power of the bandits—*
> *and then through the press dares to summon them to 'social*
> *resistance' against these bandits. Resistance with what? With*
> *umbrellas? With rolling pins? First they multiplied the bandits*
> *and then, in order to resist them, began to assemble people's*
> *vigilantes (druzhina), which by acting outside the legislation*
> *sometimes turned into the very same thing.[18]*

It is of historic interest that similar scenarios took place in Cuba in 1959 when Fidel Castro, in ascending and consolidating power, called forth his political "vigilantes," either the Committees for the Defense of the Revolution (CDR) that envious riffraff flocked to join, or the peoples' *milicianos*, "the militia," used to intimidate and disarm the opposition and eventually the people at large. The Cuban *milicianos*, like their Russian counterpart, the *druzhina*, were used to fight farmers resisting collectivization. The farmers were then demonized as "bandits" and "enemies of the people" by the State.[19]

In the U.S., some people may be afraid to go out at night in the big cities, but Americans have a right to defend themselves, and most states now allow law-abiding citizens to carry concealed firearms for self-protection. American women, especially, have an extended right to defend themselves with firearms to prevent being raped or murdered by sexual predators.

Yet, in England, people live in fear in their homes, afraid of muggers and burglars—not even possessing the right to self-defense with any weapon, much less a firearm!

But wait! If this is any consolation, English women do have one "viable" option according to the Police National Legal Database, a website operated by local police constabularies to help disseminate information to the public. In response to a woman's question, "Are there any legal self-defense products I can buy?" The police responded, "The only fully legal self-defense product at the moment is a rape alarm." Another woman was instructed not to display a knife in order to ward off an intruder and potential assailant. If those examples don't express the absurd state of natural rights in England, I would be hard pressed to say what does.[20]

One cannot avoid seeing a resemblance between the permissiveness and obsequiousness extended to the thieves in Great Britain and in the Soviet gulags as "socially friendly" elements, as opposed to the abuse and indignities made to suffer by the honest, law-abiding citizens in the British Empire and the political prisoners in *The Gulag Archipelago*. Are law-abiding British citizens today playing the hapless role that the ideological political prisoners played in the former Soviet Union? If so, who does the British government consider the real domestic enemies—thieves, terrorists, or honest citizens?

We are still hopeful that eventually freed from the European Union, the British come to their senses and begin punishing the real criminals instead of coddling them and allowing lawful, honest citizens to keep firearms for self and family protection, and cease their unjust policy of citizen disarmament. In other words, punish the thieves and real criminals and allow the lawful citizens to exercise their natural right of self-defense at home and in the street.

CHAPTER 21

GUN CONTROL AND THE HALLMARKS OF TYRANNY

*The people of the various provinces are strictly forbid-
den to have in their possession any swords, short swords,
bows, spears, firearms, or other types of arms. The possession of unnecessary implements makes difficult the collection of taxes and dues and tends to foment uprisings.*

—Toyotomi Hideyoshi (1537—1598),
shogun (dictator) of Japan, August 1588

*One of the hallmarks of dictatorship is that its laws are deliber-
ately vague. A dictator wants vague laws in order to make obe-
dience difficult so that he may call you guilty whenever he likes.*

—Alan Stang,
journalist, quoted in *The New American*, May 4, 1992

Georg Hegel (1770—1831), the father of dialectical idealism, which Karl
Marx transmogrified into Marxist dialectical materialism, lamented that
what we do learn from history is that man does not learn its lessons. Despite
what we have learned about the deleterious effects of draconian gun control,
as always preceding tyranny and even the mass killing of the people by their
own government (democide) in the last bloody century, Barack Obama and
the usual suspects in the Democratic Party used every shooting tragedy to
resume the beating of the drums to call for new authoritarian gun control

measures. But Americans knew that those freedom-curtailing measures only punished the vast majority of lawful gun owners and did nothing to stop the criminal elements. Those measures were defeated. So the gun grabbers fell back to an old refrain: gun violence as a public health menace and the need for more gun research, more gun studies! So Obama called for more gun research, by executive order.

We are now learning that research and more gun studies dealing with gun violence need to be directed elsewhere, such as the realm of sociology and criminology, not public health. We are learning that many shooting rampages are committed by mentally ill, deranged individuals who fell through the cracks of the mental health system, or by homicidal individuals full of hatred, or by criminal copycat killers, who have flouted our lenient criminal justice system. Seeking notoriety, America's new pathological craving, many of the mentally deranged were enticed to mass shootings by the sirens of the popular culture and Hollywood, hypocritical cultures glorifying violence for profit, while at the same time frequently calling for gun control. Such pathological shooters are often bent on achieving notoriety and morbid celebrity status even if it ends with their own death![1-2] We will revisit this issue in the next chapter, but for now let's return to the State and the inception of tyranny.

Five Essential Ingredients for Creating and Sustaining Tyranny

As any student of history knows, loss of individual freedom concomitant with government repression features prominently in the inception and development of totalitarian States. These features recur: First is the centralization and empowerment of a national police force with a vast network of surveillance and informants to spy on the suspected population. Second is the issuing of national identification cards to keep tabs on the whereabouts of all citizens. Third is control of education, which is necessary for the indoctrination of the youth and the neutralization of moral instruction normally inculcated by the family and churches. Fourth is control of the mass media by outright control of the press or at least making it pliable to the dissemination of State propaganda, while silencing the opposition. Fifth is civilian disarmament via gun registration and restrictive licensing, followed by banning and confiscation of firearms.[3]

Thus gun control, along with loss of liberty and increasing repression, necessarily and prominently feature in the unfolding, authoritarian designs of a burgeoning police state. For the total empowerment of national police forces—which our Founders called "standing armies" operating with vast surveillance capabilities and networks of informants to spy on the population (not foreign enemies)—draconian gun control measures become a necessity.

In Cuba and the Soviet Union, as we have seen, the informants upon which these agencies rely are usually the dregs of society. These stool pigeons are often unreliable ruffians or underworld elements willing to be snitches, so they can remain at liberty to commit their own common, non-political crimes. In the Soviet police State and the gulag, these valuable criminal informants were referred to as "socially friendly" elements by the guards of the labor camps and the secret police (KGB).

In America, we already have myriad agencies of law enforcement from the Drug Enforcement Administration (DEA) to the Bureau of Alcohol, Tobacco, Firearms, and Explosives (ATF). We should pause and be reminded of the misadventures of the ATF, always a standing army, frequently an army of rogue agents. When serving friendly Democrat and RINO ("Republican in name only") administrations, the ATF launched open war against certain elements of American society considered politically incorrect and vulnerable and thus liable and subject to intimidation. Once targeted by the ATF, the nonconformist and politically incorrect elements become subject to harassment and to the violation of the law that a man's home is his castle. It was this type of open season entrapment and harassment that was responsible to a significant degree for both the tragedies at Ruby Ridge, Idaho (1992) during the George H.W. Bush administration, and Waco, Texas (1993) during the Clinton administration. The ATF, empowered to control illegal firearms in the U.S., has been found on more than one occasion to be deeply steeped in crime and corruption. During the Obama administration, the ATF was responsible for the infamous Fast and Furious Operation, selling illegal "assault weapons" to Mexican drug lords as well as attempting to register legal guns and compiling lists of lawful gun owners in illegal databases.[4] In fact, had there been a Republican in the White House, this scandal would have brought him down. Larry Pratt, Executive Director Emeritus of Gun Owners of America summarized the Fast and Furious episode as follows:

The government's reckless pursuit of a political agenda cost the lives of almost 200 people—mostly Mexicans, so maybe they don't matter to the administration? Over 1,000 guns were lost by the Bureau of Alcohol, Tobacco, Firearms, and Explosives. And we learned only recently that one of those Fast & Furious guns was a .50 caliber sniper rifle that found its way into the hands of El Chapo [Mexican drug overlord now in prison]. All of this happened on Attorney General Eric Holder's watch. Yet there have been no prosecutions of any high-ranking official involved in Fast & Furious.[4]

Education and the Media Controlled by the State

The first two points were only briefly enumerated because an in-depth analysis is beyond the scope of this book. The next three points are discussed at more length because of their relevance to what is happening in today's educational environment and the propaganda power of the media; the fifth point, gun control, is discussed throughout the book.

So as it regards control of the media, we have also seen that even in free countries the press, of its own volition purely and by sharing political ideology with a political faction, can become a willing tool, a propaganda organ of the opposition to the legal government in power or vice versa. In fact, this is happening in the U.S. as I write these words. No president in American history has had to suffer the sustained open media attack that the American print and electronic media has launched against President Donald Trump, the legally elected president of the United States. Some media personalities have even called openly for his assassination.[5]

New revelations have just come to pass with disgraced and roguish ex-Acting Director of the FBI, Andrew McCabe, reluctantly admitting that with devious U.S. Deputy Attorney General Rod Rosenstein—fifth columnists within those agencies of intelligence and law enforcement, no less—an attempt to overthrow the duly elected President of the United States was made. This veritably attempted coup d'état by the entrenched political and bureaucratic establishment, the "Deep State," could not have taken place without the assistance of a continuous barrage of negative propaganda and hostility displayed toward President Trump. Compare this belligerence against Republican President Trump with the obsequiousness that the establishment's media observed for Democrat President Obama.[6,7]

The fourth point is that the media and their power of disseminating propaganda and exerting mass indoctrination of the population can conversely help prop up a dictatorship or help establish one that shares their ideology.[8,9] These events took place in Cuba as witnessed by the author: The invaluable assistance rendered to Fidel Castro by the media both in Cuba and in the United States in the overthrow of Cuban President Fulgencio Batista, and then the assistance rendered by the government-run media in the sustenance of the communist dictatorship of the Castro Brothers, which continues to this day. To ensure control of the press, one of the first things Fidel Castro did after his takeover was to silence the potential media opposition and then take over all media organs, press, radio, and television.[10]

Not surprisingly, private education in reference to the third point of a dictatorship also ended in Cuba immediately after the communist takeover. The government-controlled public education system that followed became a vast and necessary organ for the mass indoctrination of the Cuban youth, emphasizing the importance of the third major point of tyranny or dictatorship, as previously outlined.[11]

How education and the press were taken over by the communist State in Cuba, I've described in my book, *Cuba in Revolution: Escape From a Lost Paradise*. In fact, I described how all five major points of tyranny were implemented on the island, suffocating a way of life and ending freedom. And while what happened in Cuba took place by revolution, similar steps are taking place in the United States by evolution. Sadly, it is becoming obvious that what happened in Cuba, can also happen here. It can take place in this country despite interludes of elected Republican administrations because the media, academia, and the established elites have joined forces against the working and middle class of this country.[12] Their armies are the idle, disaffected envious elements and the eternal malcontents who live at the expense of the other half, and no matter how much they receive in handouts referred to as benefits, it is never enough.

Lump Them Together So They All Smell

Since 2016, the mainstream liberal media has openly joined the progressive leftist camp and even use old Soviet tactics to defame their conservative opponents. Take for instance, Lenin's (1870—1924) advice to his communist party followers, later the Soviet government: "We must be ready to employ trickery, deceit, law-breaking, withholding and concealing truth. We can and must write in the language which sows among the masses hate, revulsion, scorn, and the like, toward those who disagree with us." The directive was further elaborated in 1943 by the Communist Party of the USSR: "When certain obstructionists become too irritating, label them, after suitable build ups, as Fascist or Nazi or anti-Semitic…In the public mind constantly associate those who oppose us with those whose name already have a bad smell. The association will, after enough repetition, become 'fact' in the public mind."[13]

So that is exactly what the mainstream liberal media has been trying to do with Trump's presidency and the Republican Party—lump mainstream conservatism with smelly racists and anti-Semites, then charge mainstream conservatism with racism and anti-Semitism and refer to it as the far right. They did so with the 2017 confrontation in Charlottesville, Virginia, categorizing Unite the Right marchers as conservatives and lumping them with the "smell" of the Ku Klux Klan and Neo-Nazis, neither of whom are conservative groups but more akin to the left in the political spectrum.[14] The media used the event not only to attempt to discredit all conservatives, following the old advice of Lenin and the Communist Party Directive of the Soviet Union, but also to help incite the disturbance in the first place.

The comparison between media coverage of events in Charlottesville to those that followed on August 14, 2017, when radical protesters in Durham, North Carolina tore down a Confederate monument, is informative.[15] In Durham, the protesters were led by members of the Workers World Party (WWP), an extremist communist group and outshoot of the Socialist Workers Party (SWP), but that incident and the nature of the participants were downplayed. The WWP is a far-left group that has sponsored violent demonstrations in the United States and stands by such violent actions as were carried out by the Black Panthers and the Weather Underground, and openly still supports the communist government of North Korea, a rogue nation that until recently was threatening nuclear war against the United States. You can be certain the members of WWP were not lumped with the respectable left and the progressive movements to which both the mainstream media and academicians belong.

Respectable Socialism and Critical Thinking

Yet, socialism has become respectable thanks to the failed but popular candidacy of Senator Bernie Sanders (I-VT), an openly socialist politician who ran as a Democrat in the 2016 U.S. presidential election. Millennials flocked to him when he falsely claimed the moral high ground of socialism and promised them free higher education. It is no wonder the students flocked to him in droves. In addition to the promise of free college education, the way had been well prepared by the government teachers, well-primed in lower education with political correctness; and subsequently indoctrinated in the college campuses and universities with the nuances of socialism, the "fairness" of wealth redistribution, and the evil inequalities of capitalism.[16]

The fact is that young impressionable minds are being indoctrinated, as in Cuba, only more subtly so and using more high-tech methodology, and they don't even know they are being brainwashed with "fairness" sophistry and the modish intellectual expression of learning to use critical thinking. The only problem is that the thinking being promoted is only in one direction—e.g., critical of conservative ideals and institutions, but the liberal contradictions, moral shortcomings, and outright failures of socialism and progressivism are evaded and swept under the rug. Our youngest daughter, who is now attending college, recently questioned us on this subject that I referred to as unidirectional critical thinking, and asked us for an example. My wife mentioned the difference in the reception and course of events with Eldridge Cleaver's two books, *Soul on Ice* (1968) and *Soul on Fire* (1978). The first book, written by a militant Cleaver, a bitter rival to Huey Newton and at one time the leader of the most belligerent wing of the Black Panthers, is still read and considered a literary masterpiece, a political science classic on college campuses today. Yes, she knew that book. On the other hand, *Soul on Fire*—which Cleaver wrote after travelling the world as an American fugitive, coming full circle to repudiate Marxism, returning to the U.S. to face American justice, and regaining his Christian faith—is ignored and remains unknown, virtually unmentioned in academia. No, she did not know that one. The same can be said for the acclamation at one time for the work of David Horowitz as a radical, and subsequently the criticisms heaped on his life and works by the left after his conservative conversion.[17] Political ideology certainly continues to prevail over critical thinking in the academic circles of the left!

Once these mechanisms of oppression are firmly in place, persecution and elimination of suspects and political opponents follows, and then every social, political and economic policy the State desires can then be implemented. This happened with the National Socialists in Nazi Germany, fascist states such as Italy under Mussolini, and communist powers, such as the former Soviet Union (and its satellites behind the Iron Curtain) and Red China.[14,18,19] It was therefore astonishing and quite disturbing that Americans were being assailed by President Obama with an avalanche of dangerous presidential decrees leading to the construction of the type of freedom-eroding scaffold which is anathema to individual liberty and the legacy of freedom our Founding Fathers bequeathed to us as responsible citizens capable of self-governance. Take for instance Obama's Social Security gun ban. This executive action, decreed after the San Bernardino shooting, allowed Social Security bureaucrats to search the records of federal disability recipients, and if anyone other than the recipient had processed their checks for any reason (and without any fraud involved), the recipient would lose their guns. Repeal of the Social Security gun ban was a priority for GOA, and it was a significant triumph for the organization when the obnoxious decree was repealed by President Trump in February 2017.[20] Under the Obama administration everything possible was attempted to take the guns away from citizens. Many of these edicts are still in place, such as Obama's executive decree ordering the resumption of biased gun (control) research.

Construction of an authoritarian scaffold for gun control has been attempted with a number of anti-gun bills that have been introduced and re-introduced in Congress banning "assault weapons," requiring that all "qualifying firearms" in the hands of citizens be registered. The usual suspect politicians have been involved: Senators Dianne Feinstein (D-CA), Elizabeth Warren (D-MA), and Charles Schumer (D-NY), and their counterparts in the House, such as Rep. David Cicilline (D-RI) and John Conyers (D-MI). A more recent entry into this anti-gun club is Senator Chris Murphy (D-CT).

Hegel was right: What we do learn from history is that man does not learn its lessons. This is regrettable for we are condemned to live in ignorance, repeating errors. As we shall see, progressive (socialist) politicians have proven very adept in their arrogance at confirming this truism.

Gun Registration and Confiscation

Retaining lists of gun owners leads to registration, which in turn results in confiscation. In this regard, the New York City experience is instructive. In the 1960s, municipal authorities required registering long guns. They assured citizens they would never use such lists to confiscate firearms. Laws have no verbal memories and keep no oral promises, and on August 16, 1991, New York City Mayor David Dinkins signed Local Law 78, which banned the possession and sale of certain rifles and shotguns. Confiscation soon followed. Those who refused to comply with the ban suffered police raids. In 1992, the police raided a resident of Staten Island and seized his guns. Soon more knocks on the doors of other citizens followed, and confiscation in the city began in earnest.[21]

Citizens of Detroit and Washington, D.C. also suffered confiscation of their firearms, following a similar government formula. In 1989 California passed a law that banned certain semi-automatic firearms. Californians were also assured that proscribed guns could be legally kept, if they were registered prior to the ban.

In the spring of 1995, a gun owner planning to move to California inquired from the state Attorney General's office whether his SKS Sporter rifle would be legal in that state. The gun owner was assured the rifle was legal, and based on that assurance (from the Attorney General's office no less), he relocated to the Golden State. It did not take long for California to reverse course and in 1998 the state began seizing firearms from lawful citizens. Confiscation remains the threat, or rather, it's now the law in California. The legislation was passed by the state assembly and signed by the governor, although its constitutionality is being fought in the courts.[22]

In other countries, such as Greece, Ireland, Jamaica, and Bermuda, gun registration has also been followed by banning and confiscation.[23] Disarming the civilian population via government confiscation can then be followed by more drastic measures because the people are unable to defend themselves from persecution and tyranny. This is what happened in the Soviet Union, Nazi Germany, China, Cambodia, and Cuba. We will be saying more about the issue of gun control, tyranny and genocide briefly later in this chapter and more thoroughly in Chapters 23 and 24.

Legislating Gun Control Boondoggle

Certain gun control proposals, so far defeated in Congress, would have required that all gun owners be fingerprinted, licensed with passport-size photographs, and forced to reveal certain personal information as conditions for licensure. Registration lists, as we have seen, would make it easy for municipal, state, or even the federal government to seize the registered firearms under orchestrated excuses or using a tragedy as pretext.

The re-introduced Assault Weapons Ban of 2012, for example, was eerily reminiscent of the Australian experience, an expanding list of proscribed firearms as to include over 50 percent of all guns already lawfully possessed by Americans. Moreover, as we now know, Barack Obama bypassed the authority of Congress ordering the CDC to repudiate the congressional gun research restrictions issued in 1996. Obama ignored the fact that accumulated data from numerous anti-gun public health investigators had been shown to be faulty, politicized, and based on result-oriented research—that is, that the research was preordained to prove that gun availability to citizens result in crime and that guns are a serious menace to the public health and therefore should be banned. Such biased "research" could only be characterized as junk science.[24,25] Obama even seized the opportunity to encourage physicians to use their positions of authority to spy on their patients and ask them about gun ownership—in effect, using physicians as snitches for the government![26]

Legislation proposed by Senator Dianne Feinstein and rejected by Congress mandated that gun owners register their firearms[27], in essence establishing a national gun registry through the back door, as was the case in Canada. The Canadian experience itself should be instructive. Lorne Gunter, writing in the *Edmonton Journal* as early as October 13, 2000, revealed that the Canadian Outreach program to register all gun owners was failing. The result and cost of this Outreach campaign not only failed to bring in the expected 1.4 million gun owners (to only one-third of that, 486,000) but also exceeded the projected price tag many times over. By December 2002, the Canadian registry boondoggle was already costing nearly $1 billion. The cost has escalated well beyond the $1 billion mark and has proven to be a complete failure.[28] One trait of progressive politicians is hubris; lessons are ignored and errors repeated because they arrogantly believe that what fails in the hands of others will work magically in theirs. Gun control, like socialism, is another evil and spectral idea that, despite repeated failures, refuses to die and continues to be conjured up and resuscitated by leftist politicians—or rather, political demagogues.

The Canadian experience has shown the excessive cost and ineffectiveness of a gun registry as well as the fact that rather than helping track criminals and their guns as claimed, registration of firearms is dangerous to the liberty of law-abiding citizens, and as we shall see, counterproductive in dealing with criminals.

Civilian Disarmament Leads to Tyranny and Genocide

Unbeknownst to many Americans who have seen and experienced mostly the goodness of America, gun registration is the gateway to civilian disarmament, which often precedes genocide. In the monumental compilation *Lethal Laws*, published by Jews for the Preservation of Firearm Ownership, we learn that totalitarian governments that conducted mass killings of their own population (genocide) first disarmed the citizens. The recipe for accomplishing this goal went as follows: demonization of guns, registration, then banning and confiscation with total civilian disarmament.[29]

Following disarmament, enslavement of the people follows with limited resistance, as was the case in Nazi Germany, Poland, Hungary, the Soviet Union, Red China, Cuba, and other totalitarian regimes of the 20th century. Frequently, when presented with these deadly chronicles and the perilous historic sequence—namely, that gun registration is followed by banning, confiscation, civilian disarmament, and ultimately by totalitarianism—naive Americans opine that it cannot happen here. The Germans of the Weimar Republic thought the same until Hitler came along only a few years later!

Governments have a penchant to accrue power at the expense of the liberties of individual citizens.[30] Civilian disarmament is not only dangerous to one's personal liberty but also counterproductive in achieving collective safety.

Two great books have further attested the dangers to a disarmed population. One book by University of Hawaii professor R.J. Rummel is *Death by Government*. The second book is *The Black Book of Communism*, edited by Stéphane Courtois and written by a coterie of notable scholars. These books make it clear totalitarianism frequently sprouts from authoritarianism, and both are dangerous to the health of humanity. During the 20th century, more than 100 million people were killed by their own governments bent on destroying liberty and building socialism and collectivism, hells on earth.[29,31]

The Absurdity of American Gun Registration

Another fact Americans need to understand is that registration is directed at law-abiding citizens, not criminals. Not only do convicted criminals by definition fail to obey the law but also they are, astonishingly enough, constitutionally protected against any registration requirement. In *Haynes v. United States*, the U.S. Supreme Court in 1968 ruled seven to one that compelling registration by those who may not lawfully possess firearms amounts to a violation of the Fifth Amendment's proscription against forced self-incrimination. In other words, the court said that if someone "realistically can expect that registration [of a firearm] will substantially increase the likelihood of his prosecution," the registration requirement is unconstitutional. Incredible, but it's true.[32]

The ruling has, in fact, been expanded and some courts have more clearly stated that registration of firearms only applies to lawful citizens, not to felons. This has been underscored by legal scholar Don B. Kates mentioning, for example, the *Kastigar v. United States, 406 U.S. 441* (1972) decision. Do court arguments leading to the exemption of felons from gun registration sound irrational? They certainly sound like *argumentum ad absurdum*!

If gun registration were to be implemented in the United States, criminals and felons could very well not be expected to register their weapons, since they are already felons proscribed from legally owning firearms. Requiring them to register their guns, some courts may opine, would necessarily incriminate them, and this would violate their Fifth Amendment rights.[32]

In Conclusion

As Edmund Burke, founder of modern conservatism and champion of British liberty, now forgotten in his own country, once orated, "The people never give up their liberties but under some delusion." Americans must therefore remain informed and vigilant to preserve their traditional and constitutionally protected liberties, and prevent enactment of gun control legislation rooted at best in passion and emotionalism, and at worst in the authoritarian inception of tyranny. Oppressive laws that impact the law-abiding and not the criminals are unjust and tyrannical. Government efforts should be directed against criminals and felons, and should therefore best be directed towards crime control rather than gun control.

Governments that trust their citizens with guns are governments that sustain and affirm individual freedom because as Thomas Jefferson affirmed, "The natural progress of things is for liberty to yield and for government to gain ground."[33] Indeed, governments that do not trust their citizens with firearms tend to be despotic and tyrannical. And, as our history of Prohibition in the 1920s has shown, Americans obey just and moral laws but disobey or flout capricious and tyrannical laws.

Finally, let's heed again the admonition of the English philosopher John Locke (1632—1704), who was greatly admired by the American Founding Fathers and who opined, "I have no reason to suppose, that he, who would take away my Liberty would not when he had me in his Power take away everything else."[34]

PART 7

MASS SHOOTINGS AND THE MEDIA

CHAPTER 22:
SHOOTING RAMPAGES, MENTAL HEALTH, AND THE SENSATIONALIZATION OF VIOLENCE

Legitimate defense can be not only a right but a grave duty for someone responsible for another's life, the common good of the family or of the State. Unfortunately, it happens that the need to render the aggressor incapable of causing harm sometimes involves taking his life. In this case, the fatal outcome is attributable to the aggressor whose actions brought it about, even though he may not be morally responsible because of a lack of the use of reason.

—Pope John Paul II (1978—2005),
From his Encyclical Letter from 1995, EVANGELIUM VITAE

Gun violence and the much sensationalized and senseless shooting rampages arouse emotional points of debate in the American and international media with repercussions in politics in the U.S. and globally. Following the Newtown, Connecticut tragedy on December 14, 2012, Democrats capitalized on the tragedy as usual and worked frantically to try to pass stringent gun control laws in Congress. In the United Nations (UN), the Small Arms Treaty was discussed and approved in March 2013.

The American media and proponents of gun control assert that the problem lies in the "easy availability of guns" in America. Second Amendment and gun rights advocates, on the other hand, believe the problem lies elsewhere, including a permissive criminal justice system that panders to criminals; the failure of public education; the fostering of a culture of dependence, violence, and alienation engendered by the welfare state; and the increased secularization of society with children and adolescents growing up devoid of moral guidance. I agree with the latter view, but believe there are additional contributing, and in the case of rampage shootings, more proximate causes—e.g., failures of the mental health system and the role of the media and popular culture in sensationalizing violence. These issues have not been but need to be specifically pointed out and discussed. I will do so in this chapter.

Sensationalizing Violence, Celebrating Shooting Madmen

The debate over the role of firearms in society returned with a fury in the United States after the shooting rampage at Sandy Hook Elementary School in Newtown, Connecticut, on December 14, 2012. Politicians were once again calling for gun control without examining other psychosocial factors that play a tremendous role in gun violence. The Connecticut shooting, which took the lives of six adults and 20 children, was indeed a lamentable tragedy, and like all previous mass shootings, it was difficult to find the words to convey the tragic horror and express the magnitude of the loss of innocent human life. This mass-shooting incident was carried out by 20-year-old Adam Lanza, a loner with a personality disorder, who it was obvious was in critical need of mental health evaluation and psychiatric treatment. Once again, evidence mounted that deadly rampages are the result of the failure of the mental health system in association, as we will suggest later in this chapter, with the systematic sensationalizing of violence by the mass media and popular culture.

In a previous rampage-shooting incident on January 8, 2011, another disturbed individual, 22-year-old Jared Loughner, shot U.S. Representative Gabrielle Giffords in Arizona. Six people, including a nine-year-old student, a judge and one of Giffords' staffers, were killed in the incident and 13 others were wounded. Again, prior to the shooting, there had been signs of psychiatric illness and social psychopathology that should have alerted those around him that Loughner should have been referred for psychological evaluation and psychiatric treatment. But Loughner, like Lanza, fell through the obvious cracks of the mental health system.

The case in Arizona is particularly revealing because a consensus was reached that Loughner should have been mentally evaluated and psychiatric treatment administered.[1] The same conclusion was reached with Adam Lanza in Connecticut. Once severe instability and the potential for violence and criminal acts have been ascertained, firearms should be kept away from such deranged individuals. "Convicted felons and mentally unstable people," as I stated in a previous article, "forfeit the right to possess arms by virtue of the fact they are a potential danger to their fellow citizens. This has been demonstrated further by the tragedies that took place in Arizona and in Aurora, Colorado; and not only in the United States but also in Oslo, Norway."[2]

The case of the senseless massacre in Norway on July 22, 2011 is also instructive. After bombing a government building in Oslo and then taking over an island, Anders Behring Breivik, a homicidal killer, massacred 77 of his fellow citizens, systematically hunting down unarmed youths at a camp, methodically killing the defenseless teenagers. Imagine the alternative scenario that could have taken place, if just one person had carried a gun and had used it to defend his or her life and the lives of others. Breivik was heavily armed but one citizen armed and familiar with firearms could have stopped the killer. One bullet is all that it takes. Although Norway has one of the least stringent gun control systems in Western Europe and Scandinavia, it is still restrictive enough so that no civilian would have been allowed armed in the camp. Thus a deranged individual was able to enter and kill with impunity.

Investigation and further legal developments in these three aforementioned incidents represent cases of criminal derangement, and in at least the first two cases and probably the third as well, associated with regrettable failures in mental health systems, rather than the assignation of blame with the clichés of "easy gun availability" or "too many guns in the hands of the people."

Later in the chapter, I cite two contrasting cases that occurred in Aurora, Colorado, in the spring and summer of 2012. One incident was widely reported; the other, where a citizen stopped a rampage and saved the lives of others, was not.[3] In the U.S., the vast majority of citizens—those who hunt, participate in shooting sports, and most importantly, those who possess firearms in their homes for family protection or legally carry concealed weapons for self-protection—use firearms responsibly.[2,4,5,6,7]

Rampage Shootings and Armed Citizens

In 2000, a *New York Times* study revealed that in 100 cases of rampage-shooting incidents, 63 cases involved people who "made threats of violence before the event, including 54 who threatened specific violence to specific people." Nothing was done about the threats. Moreover, more than half of the shooters had overt signs of mental illness that had gone untreated. For these troubled individuals, a precipitating event in association with failures in life and long-term mental illness finally triggers the shooting rampage, giving "the appearance of being at the same time deliberate and impulsive."[8]

In 2012, a study by *Mother Jones* magazine also suggested the majority of mass shooters in the past 30 years evinced signs of mental health problems prior to the killings. This conclusion is supported in the medical and legal literature. While the figures in the *Mother Jones* article are for the most part correct, unfortunately the analysis and conclusions are not, because, like many other studies on gun violence, they are tainted by passion and ideology, resulting in overt biased and result-oriented, preordained conclusions.[9] For example, while it is true that the number of rampage shootings has increased in recent years, the rate of violent crimes and homicides for both blacks and whites (including those committed with firearms) has decreased significantly over the same period, despite the tremendous increase in the number of firearms in the U.S., according to both the FBI Uniform Crime Reports and the U.S. Bureau of Justice Statistics.[10,11,12] In fact, the number of firearms increased from approximately 200 million in 1995 to 300 million in 2012, in association with a significant decrease not only in violent crimes but also in all property crimes since 1990 to the present.[11,12]

I would also be remiss if I did not point out the *Mother Jones* article was incorrect when it further claimed, "In not a single case was the killing stopped by a civilian using a gun."[9] And yet *Mother Jones,* along with the mainstream liberal media, is not alone in ignoring the beneficial aspects of firearms by armed citizens. Public health researchers deny and most often ignore defensive uses of firearms. We must suppose these researchers exist in their own hermetically sealed, liberal environments that prevent any information, contrary to their own views, to enter their set-in-concrete bastions of liberalism and trouble their minds.

Take for instance, Daniel Webster of the Johns Hopkins Bloomberg

School of Public Health, a center that along with the Harvard School of Public Health, make up perhaps two of the most strident academic institutions militating for draconian gun control, masquerading as objective gun research. Webster, the Center's director for Gun Policy and Research, erroneously wrote in a recent article:

> To listen to open-carry advocates, mass shootings would be far less common if only we had enough armed citizens at the ready to take down active shooters. In the context of mass shootings, though, it's incredibly rare that someone successfully interrupts and stops an event. In fact, out of the 111 mass shootings analyzed by researcher Louis Klarevas in his 2016 book, Rampage Nation: Securing America from Mass Shootings, an armed civilian never—not once—intervened to end it.[13]

Both Webster and Klarevas then are part of the problem—that is, they are perpetuating erroneous information and outright lies. Are these errors related to ignorance? Or are they deliberate lies, overt mendacity, and academic dishonesty? If the latter (mendacity), do they think they can get away with it? If the former (ignorance) is the case, how can they be ignorant of the facts, when they are supposed to be the experts? How can they not be aware of the many instances in which armed citizens have ended mass shootings in progress and even prevented further killings by holding the assailants under the gun until the police arrived? In many other instances, the citizens have caused the killers to take their own life, and as a last resort, have even shot dead the madman on the scene. How can they deny that these documented cases took place or do they think they can spin them off out of existence? Consider the following cases:

In November 1990, Brian Rigsby and his friend Tom Styer left their home in Atlanta, Georgia, and went camping near Oconee National Forest, not far from where I live in rural Georgia. Suddenly, they were assaulted by two madmen, who had been taking cocaine and who fired at them using shotguns killing Styer. Rigsby returned fire with a Ruger Mini-14, a semi-automatic weapon frequently characterized as an "assault weapon." It saved his life.[14]

In January 1994, Travis Dean Neel was cited as "citizen of the year" in Houston, Texas. He had saved a police officer and helped the police arrest three dangerous criminals in a gunfight, street-shooting incident. Neel had helped stop the potential mass shooters using once again semi-automatic, so-called "assault weapons" with high capacity magazines. He provided cover for the police who otherwise were outgunned and would have been killed.[7]

The January 16, 2002 case of three law students at the Appalachian School of Law in Grundy, Virginia, who prevented a mass shooting is also very revealing. The media reported the incident but left out one inconvenient detail. According to the *Washington Post*, they "pounced on the gunman and held him until help arrived." What the media left out was the fact that one of the students was armed, and thus they felt safer in carrying out the courageous act they performed. In his book, scholar John Lott recounts the incident:

> *Mikael and Tracy were prepared to do something quite different: Both immediately ran to their cars and got their guns. Mikael had to run about one hundred yards to get to his car. Along with Ted Besen [who was unarmed], they approached Peter [Odighizuwa, the gunman] from different sides. As Tracy explains it, 'I stopped at my vehicle and got a handgun, a revolver. Ted went toward Peter, and I aimed my gun at [Peter], and Peter tossed his gun down. Ted approached Peter, and Peter hit Ted in the jaw. Ted pushed him back and we all jumped on.'[15]*

In 2007, a brave woman, Jeanne Assam, a former police officer, who had volunteered to work security at the New Life Church in Colorado Springs, Colorado, prevented a shooting rampage when she shot and killed a man storming the building who intended to kill as many people as possible at the church.[16]

Just days after the 2012 Sandy Hook Elementary School shooting, an off-duty police officer prevented a shooting rampage at the Mayan Palace Theater in San Antonio, Texas, by shooting the gunman before he had a chance to kill anyone.[16] This incident "sparks memories" of the mass slaying at "the gun-free zone" Cinemark movie theater in Aurora, Colorado, in the summer of 2012, widely reported by the media, where citizens had been virtual sitting ducks.[2] In contrast, as I alluded earlier, the media did not widely report the shooting incident that took place three months earlier (April 2012) in the same town, Aurora, Colorado, where a law-abiding citizen, an armed churchgoer, shot another human predator and stopped a shooting rampage, saving his life and the lives of others in the process.[3]

In another shooting rampage on November 5, 2017, a young white man dressed in black and armed with a Ruger AR-556 rifle entered the First Baptist Church in Sutherland Springs, Texas, and opened fire killing 26 people and wounding 20 other parishioners. The gunman then exchanged fire with an armed citizen, Stephen Willeford, a former NRA instructor, and fled the church but was pursued by Willeford, who recruited another citizen on the scene, Johnnie Langendorff. After a high speed but short 11-mile chase, the gunman suddenly lost control of his car and ran into a ditch. Apparently, Willeford had wounded him, and then, as many of these killers are prone to do once resistance is encountered, he turned the gun on himself. The killer was found dead with three wounds, including his self-inflicted gunshot head wound.[17] Willeford and Langendorff, two Texas heroes, were the responsive citizens and their quick actions stopped what could have been a series of rampage shootings. The killer had more arms and ammunition in his Ford Explorer.

The deranged assailant was identified as 26-year-old Devin Patrick Kelley, who had served in the Air Force, had been court-martialed for battering his wife and child, had been imprisoned for one year, and then dismissed from the Air Force with a bad conduct discharge. Since that time, Kelley had also used physical violence against his second wife, and the church he attacked was the one where his mother-in-law (with whom he also had domestic problems) worshipped. Luckily, she was not there that Sunday.

Why was this man in possession of a firearm after a military conviction of a serious domestic violence charge and dismissed from the Air Force with a bad conduct discharge? In fact, Kelley tried to get a gun license, but was denied by the Texas Department of Public Safety. Simply, the Air Force failed to report the verdict so the FBI could place Kelley in the NICS. The system failed, once again, despite the $1 billion per year cost, compliments of the American taxpayers.

But as the story unfolded, yet more details came to light. There had been other opportunities to stop the madman before he struck and perpetrated the massacre on the small Texas congregation gathered for that fateful Sunday service. Kelley had escaped from a mental health hospital in New Mexico in 2012 and brought guns into a military base and there threatened his superiors. He was also a suspect in a 2013 sexual assault in his hometown in Texas, barely 35 miles from the scene of the horrific church attack.[17]

It has become clear that the mental health system failed. Why wasn't there mental health follow up after all these incidents, and why wasn't Kelley back in for treatment? Authorities fumbled at least three opportunities where he could have been stopped and his access to guns impeded, thus possibly avoiding the massacre. Thankfully, an armed Texas citizen ended the massacre and probably prevented other killings.

Additional Cases, Armed Citizens Stopping Mass Shooters

The following additional cases bring to light the inconvenient fact that armed citizens save lives. These cases were ignored not only by the investigative journalists of the mainstream media but also missed by the *Mother Jones* study claiming, "in not a single case was the killing stopped by a civilian using a gun."[9] Let's look at these additional cases:

In 1997, in Pearl, Mississippi, 16-year-old Luke Woodham used a hunting rifle to kill his ex-girlfriend and her close friend and wound seven other students. Assistant Principal Joel Myrick retrieved his handgun from his automobile and halted Woodham's shooting spree. Myrick held the young delinquent at bay until the police arrived. Later it was discovered that Woodham had also used a knife to stab his mother to death earlier that morning. Even though this shooting incident was widely reported, the media ignored the fact that Mr. Myrick, an armed citizen, had prevented a larger massacre by retrieving and using his handgun.

Then in 1998, in Edinboro, Pennsylvania, a deadly scenario took place when 14-year-old Andrew Wurst killed one teacher and wounded another, as well as two fellow classmates. A local merchant, James Strand, who used his shotgun to force the young criminal to halt his firing, drop his gun, and surrender to the police, halted the Edinboro shooting rampage.

In another unreported incident in Santa Clara, California, Richard Gable Stevens rented a rifle for target practice at the National Shooting Club on July 5, 1999, and then began a shooting rampage, herding three store employees into a nearby alley, and stating he intended to kill them. When Stevens became momentarily distracted, a shooting club employee, who had a .45 caliber handgun concealed under his shirt, drew his weapon and fired. Stevens was hit in the chest and critically wounded. He was held at bay until the police arrived. A massacre in the making was prevented. The press ignored the valiant deed performed by the armed employee, another unsung hero. Why are these and other similar incidents, where the tables are turned, and citizens use guns to protect themselves and others, only seldom reported by the mainstream media?[2,5,7]

The fact, as we have recounted here, is that many crimes and rampage shootings have been prevented or stopped by armed citizens. Consider the case at the Clackamas Town Center in Oregon in December 2012, where another shooter murdered two people, then turned the gun on himself. In that case there was a concealed carry permit holder that took aim at the deranged gunman but did not shoot because of a bystander. It is suspected that the deranged killer killed himself when he saw the citizen taking aim at him.[16] As with all types of crimes, the police cannot be everywhere at all times to protect us. By the time the police arrive at a crime scene, most dramatically at a shooting rampage, it's usually too late for the victims. An armed citizen could already be there, identify the shooter, and at least stop the carnage. Only if one of the intended victims already at the scene is armed, can he or she prevent or stop the shooting, as in some of the aforementioned described cases.[3,6,7,14,15,16,17,18]

Instructive Cases, Lessons to Be Learned

Because guns have been demonized and because "gun-free zones" have been allocated in so many places, neither armed citizens nor the police are able to stop, much less prevent, many rampage shootings.

The Charleston church shooting took place in a historic Emanuel African Methodist Episcopal Church on June 17, 2015 during a prayer service. Nine people were killed and three other wounded by 21-year-old white supremacist

Dylann Roof. The mass shooter reportedly wanted to start a race war, instead he was convicted in federal court of murder in 2016 and sentenced to death in 2017.[19] An armed citizen at the Charleston church would have prevented or ended the massacre sooner, just as Jeanne Assam had done at the New Life Church in Colorado Springs, Colorado.[16]

But we soon heard more news from historic Charleston, South Carolina. On August 24, 2017, "a disgruntled, fired dishwasher" shot a chef at a downtown restaurant. This shooting represents yet another occasion where the criminal justice system failed, as well as another example of a copycat shooting. In this incident, a wild-eyed but composed dishwasher, who recently had been fired from Virginia's restaurant, walked in, declared "There is a new boss in town," and fatally shot the head chef. After holding another person hostage for three hours, the shooter was critically wounded by police. The dramatic incident took place in a tourist stretch of shops and fine restaurants along historic King Street in downtown Charleston, only a few blocks from the Emanuel AME church where the June 2015 shooting had occurred. The assailant turned out to be not only "a disgruntled former employee," but also a violent felon with a lengthy criminal record spanning more than three decades that included "prior convictions for assault and battery with intent to kill in 1983, receiving stolen goods in 2009, possession of LSD and cocaine in 2010, strong arm robbery in 2012 and larceny in 2015"—in short, a repeat violent offender. Why was this felon in possession of a firearm? Why was he even out of jail? All we can say is that the permissive criminal justice system with its revolving prison doors was responsible for this shooting; and that quick police action prevented further casualties.[19]

The Columbine High School Massacre took place on April 20, 1999 near Littleton, Colorado. The perpetrators, Eric Harris and Dylan Klebold, a pair of deranged senior students, had meticulously planned the massacre with numerous explosives and bombs to supplement the shooting rampage. They murdered twelve students and one teacher, and injured 21 other people, then committed suicide.

The shooting ignited another confrontational debate on gun control that invoked the same old public health paradigm calling for the eradication of "the epidemic of gun violence," as well as conjuring new themes—school bullying, the gothic culture and social outcasts, video game violence, avid teenage internet use, and the use of antidepressants in teenagers—some of which may have played roles. In reality, plenty of signs had been available as to the psychopathic tendencies of the pair: internet death threats to fellow students (reported to the Jefferson County Sheriff's office); felonious thefts of equipment; threats to other students and teachers; illegal drug use; juvenile "diversionary" and juvenile probationary system failures; anger management classes and substance abuse classes that the pair failed to attend. Although one of the perpetrators continued to see a psychiatrist, no further mental health intervention was made, and the pair went on to carry out their planned high school massacre. This was a clear failure of two separate juvenile systems—e.g., the juvenile mental health system and the probationary criminal justice system—failing to take the necessary preventive measures to stop these psychopathic young delinquents from going on further and committing mass murder.[20]

This deadliest high school mass shootings in U.S. history could have been prevented by more aggressive mental health and juvenile delinquency intervention. If only an armed teacher had been available to assist the security guard assigned to the school (who actually exchanged gunfire with the shooters), the young criminals perhaps could have been stopped sooner, as in Pearl, Mississippi, in 1997, when Assistant Principal Joel Myrick retrieved his handgun from his automobile and halted 16-year-old Luke Woodham's shooting rampage. Myrick held the young delinquent at bay until the police arrived.

The incidence of mass shootings with the usual intensive media coverage, and concomitant sensationalization, give the impression that we are about to be swamped by mass shooters. The truth is that the incidence of mass shootings is very low by any standard. John Fund, a former columnist for *The Wall Street Journal* and distinguished *National Review Online* (NRO) columnist, correctly noted, "The chances of being killed in a mass shooting are about what they are for being struck by lightning." And despite the draconian gun control laws in Europe, "until the Newtown horror, the three worst K-12 school shootings ever had taken place in Britain and Germany."[18] Moreover, the Norway massacre of July 22, 2011, described previously, claimed a total of 77 lives, mostly teenagers. These statements are not repeated here to trivialize shooting tragedies nor intended to detract from the need to be concerned about them, but to place the matter in a more precise sense of statistical proportion and recognize that other countries, including those with draconian gun control laws, are not immune.

In the wake of the Sandy Hook Elementary School shooting in Connecticut, the National Rifle Association (NRA) called for armed guards to protect all schools in the United States. In the short term, this may sound like a good idea but, as we have seen, a single security guard in the Columbine shooting did not prevent the massacre. Moreover, is this major proposal feasible? We could begin by hiring security guards and police officers, but the police are stretched to the limit as it is, and budgets are tight with the American middle class already squeezed dry, sustaining as it is a myriad of entitlement and social welfare programs. Thus, I suggest the employment of volunteer citizens, who must be psychologically evaluated, pass a background check, and then undergo training in the use of firearms and gun safety, to serve as "school sentinels," or better yet, allowing concealed carry weapons (CCW) licensed teachers to carry guns to school for student protection.

According to a study conducted between 2005 and 2007 by research-ers at the University of Wisconsin and Bowling Green State University, the police across the country were convicted of firearm violations at an 0.002 percent annual rate, which is about the same rate as concealed-carry gun (CCW) permit holders in the states with "shall issue" CCW laws.[18] As we have previously demonstrated, research conducted by criminology professor Gary Kleck and constitutional lawyer Don B. Kates has shown that firearms are used more frequently by law-abiding citizens to repel crime than used by criminals to perpetrate crime. Moreover, Professor Kleck has noted that citizens acting in self-defense kill at least twice and up to three times more criminals than do the police.[6]

Jim Kouri, the public information officer of the National Association of Chiefs of Police, told Fund at the time of the theater shooting in Aurora, Colorado: "Preventing any adult at a school from having access to a firearm eliminates any chance the killer can be stopped in time to prevent a rampage."[18] In fact police, occasionally outgunned by criminals, have also been assisted by armed citizens, although again these incidents have been downplayed by the mainstream media.[4,7] On February 22, 2018, in the after-math of the Stoneman Douglas High School shooting in Parkland, Florida (February 14), President Trump endorsed arming teachers in schools to protect students.

Unfortunately, the American media does not give the defensive uses of firearms the attention they deserve, and they go unreported. By and large, to read about the cases where law-abiding citizens use firearms for self and family protection, one has to read independently published books such as Robert A. Waters' excellent tome, *The Best Defense,*[7] or read news accounts published by the NRA, GOA, and other gun rights organizations. Rarely do these cases get publicized in the mass media; and even less frequently are they published and disseminated in the medical journals, as public health investigators do with one-sided reporting of the criminal aspects of guns and violence.

Three Cases of Terrorism Inspired by Jihad or Political Hatred

We could say that all mass shootings are inspired by hatred, but as we have seen, some are carried out by deranged individuals, susceptible to violence but possessing no clear and distinct political or religious motives. These disturbed, mentally unstable people are unhinged by the strain of the postmodern age and what they see and experience, receptive to the influences of the perverse degeneration of the popular culture, media sensationalism, and the pursuit of celebrity status, even if they pay with their own lives to achieve the dubious notoriety.

The following three rampage shootings are clearly of a different variety from those previously described. They were triggered by fanaticism, entwined with a specified hatred. The first was motivated clearly by Jihad and "home grown" Islamic radicalism. The second was similarly motivated by the ongoing war that Islamic terrorism has been waging against America and the West. The third, perhaps the most odious, was the result of perverted political ideology and the increasing hatred boiling over from the frustrated political left in the United States.

The San Bernardino terrorist attack took place on December 2, 2015, when 14 people were massacred and 22 others were injured in the mass shooting and attempted bombing of the Inland Regional Center in San Bernardino, California. The perpetrators were a married couple, both of Pakistani descent, who had been radicalized by Islamic fundamentalism in the United States. Their target was a Department of Public Health Christmas party at a rented banquet room with about 80 employees in attendance, including the husband who was a public health inspector. After the shooting the couple escaped but were pursued and later killed in a shootout with police. The motive was Islamic terrorism, incited by jihad and apparently seeking martyrdom. Several friends and family members were subsequently arrested under a variety of charges ranging from conspiracy to provide material support to terrorists, perjury, sham marriages, and immigration fraud. An armed citizen could have stopped the shooting rampage, but in a restricted public health setting, we must admit that armed self-defense would have been highly unlikely. Besides the fact that a group of public health workers are unlikely to have among them CCW holders, the Inland Regional Center is also most likely designated a gun-free zone (GFZ) that consigns those present to be hapless and defenseless victims in a mass shooting incident.[21]

The Orlando nightclub shooting took place on June 12, 2016, when Omar Mateen, a 29-year-old security guard opened fire and killed 49 people and wounded 58 others inside Pulse, a gay nightclub in Orlando, Florida. The mass shooting was a terrorist attack aimed at homosexual members of the LGBT community. Since the nightclub was hosting "Latin night," most of the victims were Latinos. Mateen had sworn allegiance to the Islamic State (ISIS) and in a 911 call made during the rampage openly declared that the shooting was in retaliation for U.S. forces killing a terrorist in Iraq, American intervention in the Middle East, and the alleged U.S. bombings in Iraq and Syria.

This mass-shooting incident was the deadliest terrorist attack on U.S. soil since September 11, 2001. Initially both the media and the Obama administration sought to politicize the event and blame the tragedy on guns, then a hate crime against LGBT people—ignoring the fact Mateen had ties to ISIS, as revealed by the 911 call he made in the midst of the rampage.[22,23]

Another point that was lost in the attempt at politicization was that the terrorist, knowing about the event, lack of security, and probably the presence of unarmed individuals at the gathering, chose the time and place for maximum damage. But the fact remains had only one patron or bouncer there been armed, the shooting rampage could have been stopped sooner. Instead, the shooting turned into a horrible massacre followed by a tense standoff for three uncertain hours—until Mateen was shot and killed by Orlando police. A state of emergency was even proclaimed by the governor of Florida for the city of Orlando.

Before closing on the issue of Islamic terrorism, a word should be said about the most recent incident in New York City, which underscores not only the increasing new terroristic threat to American cities but also the use of cars and trucks to plow into unsuspecting crowds with mass casualties of innocent civilians. A vehicle driven into a crowd is becoming the terrorists' weapon of choice in Europe and the sanguinary practice seems to be taking hold in the U.S. as well. The Halloween truck attack on October 31, 2017 in Manhattan a few blocks from the site of the Twin Towers is an egregious example. The atrocity also emphasizes a switch from mass shootings caused by deranged citizens to deliberate jihad by foreign and domestic Islamic terrorists. The courts' initial disapproval of President Trump's ban on immigration from seven countries with strong ties to terrorism permitted dangerous individuals to enter the country. Our faulty immigration laws and virtually open borders facilitate Islamic terrorism in this country, whether by mass shootings or the use of vehicles to plow into crowds.

It is because of this political inaction largely on the part of obstructionist Democrats, who block efforts, and their media allies, who continually criticize Trump and the GOP, that terroristic mass killings are happening with more frequency—and not because of easy gun availability. That is why truck driver Sayfullo Saipov, an Uzbekistan national, plowed into a group of people, killing eight in a Halloween incident. Saipov was shot and wounded by hero NYPD Officer Ryan Nash, who stopped Saipov from escaping and prevented the attack from becoming more deadly. It could have been even less deadly, if an armed citizen had been present and had shot the terrorist before he could have harmed anyone. Incidentally, the terrorist left behind notes written in Arabic pledging loyalty to ISIS and a picture of the ISIS flag. What (or who) was at fault here? Virtually open borders to Islamic nations with ties to jihad and terrorism, or easy availability of trucks? We are left to wonder, but not for long. Gun prohibitionists are relentless. One *New York Times* journalist was unfazed and called for gun control after the truck terror attack! And, incredibly, he was not alone. New York City Mayor Bill de Blasio and New York Governor Andrew Cuomo also talked about firearms, assault weapons and gun control, but not terrorism, after the truck attack.[23]

We also have politically-motivated rampages, such as the shooting at the Republican congressional baseball practice on June 14, 2017 in Alexandria, Virginia, which was the direct result of the increasing hatred that the left has been openly expressing and actually generating since the election of Donald Trump as President of the United States.[24,25] In this rampage, left-wing hatred-spewing activist, James Hodgkinson, shot three people—including the third highest ranking Republican in the House of Representatives, Congressman Steve Scalise, at a GOP congressional baseball practice prior to a charity event. Scalise was critically wounded in the hip with profuse internal bleeding from torn bone, blood vessels, and damage to internal organs.

This mass shooting was stopped only because Congressman Steve Scalise, as House Majority Whip, had police protection. After a 10-minute shootout, police officers finally mortally wounded Hodgkinson, who later died at a local hospital. Congressman Scalise "received multiple blood transfusions and underwent several surgeries to repair internal damage and stop the bleeding."[26] He was in and out of intensive care for the next two weeks. As of August 2017, he was still recuperating from his wounds. Several witnesses reported their lives were saved only because of the presence of the armed Capitol Police, and had Scalise not had police protection, there would have been another massacre. Congressman Scalise returned to work at the Capitol in September 2017, and in early October gave an interview that we will refer to later in the chapter.

Everything we have said about the benefits of armed self-defense applies to these political and terrorist shootings. An armed citizen in place could have stopped them. In fact, after the congressional shooting, the U.S. Congress began debating the adoption of security measures, including issuing concealed carrying weapons (CCW) permits to members of Congress, and allowing those who have a CCW license in their home states to be able to carry their guns to work in Washington, D.C.[26]

The De-institutionalization of the Mentally Ill

The United States is a federal republic, and the 50 states of the Union have some leeway in passing and enforcing gun laws. In America, we already have more than 20,000 gun laws on the books. We do not need more statutes. The societal failure for violence, with guns or otherwise, lies elsewhere.

Killers operate with impunity in states that do not allow people to carry guns for self protection, and most states in the U.S. already have a "zero tolerance" for guns in schools, which amount to "gun-free zones" where firearms are strictly prohibited. This is another reason to consider allowing teachers to have CCW licenses to protect students. It would be a sensible and easy strategy to protect the children in this mad, dystopic world that liberals have been creating, with a society too permissive to criminals and protective of the rights of repeat criminal offenders, while easily blaming guns and proposing more laws to limit the rights of lawful citizens in society at large.

Guns are inanimate objects. The responsibility for crime rests on the criminal elements and those who facilitate their crimes! Failures in the criminal justice system pandering to criminals with too much leniency for repeat offenders, and the revolving prison door system in place, allow many of the same criminals to commit the vast majority of serious crimes.[4] I would now elaborate on the failures of the mental health system that began with de-institutionalization of the seriously mentally ill.

De-institutionalization of mental patients began in the 1960s, and it rapidly placed thousands of mental patients including some dangerously ill back on the streets. It has only worsened in recent years due to the drive for containment of health care costs coupled with the decades-long, misguided mental health strategy of administering mental health care via community outreach and outpatient treatments. In many cases, these strategies have failed because of inadequate follow-up and poor compliance by patients, as well as legal restraints placed on families.

Another problem is the current privacy laws in association with the forced legal emancipation of children from their parents in educational and health care laws, which has made it difficult for parents to obtain confidential mental health records on their children, even if the adult child is still dependent upon the parents for health insurance coverage.

With the passage of the ObamaCare law requirements, children up to age 26 can be covered under the parent's health insurance. This coverage should allow the emendation of privacy laws to allow parents access to the mental health information on their dependent children. ObamaCare or not, these problems need to be corrected by reforming privacy laws, allowing parents to exert more control of their children in the psycho-socially challenging, difficult years of adolescence and young adulthood, when many cases of schizophrenia and other psychopathology first become apparent.

Unfortunately, instead of emphasizing family support and quick preventive action, ObamaCare and myriad executive rulings issued during President Obama's tenure, underscored government reporting and general data collection

on the mentally ill. Admittedly, a good balance between mental health reporting and privacy rights needs to be reached before gun rights are severely
restricted. Yet, family members and neighbors should not fear reporting—in
good faith—individuals with a history of violence and possible serious mental
illness to the appropriate mental health agencies and law enforcement. For
this to happen, the removal of potential legal repercussions is salutary policy.
A step further is to take legal action: Potentially dangerous individuals known
to possess firearms should be constrained from possessing guns by seeking
a "gun-violence restraining order" (GVRO), a process that will be discussed
shortly. Beyond these measures, institutionalization of the violence-prone,
mentally ill patient may be necessary for those who do not respond to counseling, psychotherapy or drug treatment in the outpatient setting.

But for this to be feasible, legal impediments to medical commitment
for those severely ill and potentially dangerous individuals in need of long-
term psychiatric hospitalization should be removed. Steven P. Segal of the
University of California at Berkeley has shown that "a third of the state-to-
state variation in homicide rates was attributable to the strength or weakness
of involuntary civil commitment laws."[16] David Kopel, coauthor of the law
school textbook, *Firearms Law and the Second Amendment* (Aspen, 2012),
has correctly noted the detrimental drastic drop in long-term institutionalization of the mentally ill:

"In the mid-1960s, many of the killings would have been prevented
because the severely mentally ill would have been confined and cared for in a
state institution. But today, while government at most every level has bloated
over the past half-century, mental health treatment has been decimated."
Kopel then cites the dramatic statistics released by the Treatment Advocacy
Center in July 2012: "The number of state hospital beds in America per capita
has plummeted to 1850 levels, or 14.1 beds per 100,000 people."[16]

Another view is advanced by practicing psychiatrist and Distinguished
Life Fellow of the American Psychiatric Association, Robert B. Young, M.D.
A strong advocate for both the mentally ill as well as gun rights, Dr. Young,
who is also DRGO editor, pointed out towards the end of Obama's second
term in 2016:

> *One of the outcomes of the President's announcement is great*
> *concern that physicians and mental health care providers*

will now be reporting everyone's mental illness to the FBI,
which runs the NICS [National Instant Criminal Background
System]. We all want to identify people who are prohibited
from buying guns for good reason, but the prospect that
anyone in emotional distress could be prohibited from legal
gun ownership for life is reasonable cause for panic. It would
devastate the privacy necessary to the trusting relationships
that treatment requires.[28]

In agreement with my view that those who could be identified as a serious risk for gun violence should be prohibited from buying firearms, he has reiterated, nevertheless, his view that the vast majority of the mentally ill are peaceful and "far more likely to become victims than attackers."[28]

While it is true that only a small fraction of the mentally ill are dangerous, it is also true that among mass shooters, the majority of the perpetrators have been found to be mentally deranged individuals who—prior to the shooting—should have been under psychiatric treatment and perhaps institutionalized. There are two main types of mass shooters, and in the United States, so far, the majority of shooters—unlike other parts of the world where political or religious fanatics predominate—have been seriously deranged individuals, not hard-core terrorists. Yet, in view of the two recent cases of Islamic fanaticism we presented under the previous heading, the situation may be changing, so we must remain vigilant.

I also agree with Dr. Young that emotional distress and transient "mental illness" are not sufficient of themselves to bar anyone from possessing firearms. As Dr. Young further explained: "Half of all Americans experience at least one episode of diagnosable psychiatric illness during their lifetimes. Prohibiting all of those would vastly restrict the number of Americans who could retain their constitutional right to keep and bear arms over time." Fear of losing one's Second Amendment rights could be counterproductive. He adds, "The fear of their guns being confiscated could also increase the chances that many in need of psychiatric treatment, and perhaps those at highest risk of violence, would avoid it."[28]

In short, the mental health field is ripe for getting more aggressive in researching, identifying, diagnosing, and treating the individuals who are prone to violence. In fact, a 2004 study conducted by the U.S. Secret Service and the U.S. Department of Education found that in 81 percent of school shootings the deranged individuals gave indications of their intent to harm at least one and in 59 percent more than one person. That should be a start. In the meantime, there is a legal process by which family members, relatives, and others can be empowered to impede a troubled individual access to firearms. Several versions of this law have been enacted, including one in California that took effect in 2016. This legal process intended to prevent deranged individuals from carrying out gun crimes, including mass shootings, is referred to as a gun-violence restraining order (GVRO).[28]

The GVRO permits a spouse, parent, sibling, or person living with a disturbed and potentially violent individual to petition a court for an order enabling law enforcement to suspend that individual's Second Amendment right temporarily. Conservatives and gun rights proponents should consider supporting GVROs in their states, as long as several conditions are met: Petitioners should be limited to family members or people who live with or intimately know the individual; clear and convincing evidence of the danger that the individual poses to others should be provided; due process and the opportunity for a hearing within 72 hours should be provided for the respondent (e.g., the potential offender) to contest the claim; and the GVRO should automatically lapse after a period of time, unless evidence is provided that the respondent continues to pose a public threat. While we await the effect of the law in California, we should consider enacting such laws in other states as we balance the rights and privacy of the individual vis-à-vis public safety.

Sensationalizing Violence in the Media and the Popular Culture

Finally, there is another even more sinister and perhaps more insoluble contributing factor—namely, the problem of how the media report and how popular culture sensationalize violence, which in association with the fruitless pursuit of celebrity status in vogue today has become all pervasive. What more evidence is needed for the "15 minutes worth of fame" phenomenon[29] than the immense popularity of absurd and very frequently vulgar "reality" television shows?

It is not a big step to link extensive coverage of rampage shootings in both the press and the flashy electronic media as a major contributing factor to the pathologic wish and morbid pursuit for the attainment of celebrity status even in death. In his review of Sharyl Attkinson's book, *The Smear*, Dr. Michael S. Brown, an active DRGO member, who considers himself a pragmatic libertarian, discusses how far the media will go not only to sensationalize the news but also actually to lie for political or financial reasons. Lies may misinform and deceive, but sensationalization of mass shootings is causing mayhem and death; they need to stop both.[30]

I have previously reported on the excellent work of Dr. Brandon Centerwall of the University of Washington School of Public Health. Centerwall's studies found that homicide rates in Canada were not related to easy gun availability in the population as he had expected, but to the incitement of aggressive behavior from watching violence on television. He found that homicide rates not only in Canada but also in the U.S. and South Africa soared 10–15 years after the introduction of television in those countries.

In the U.S., there was an actual doubling of homicide rates after the introduction of television. Moreover, Centerwall noted that up to half of all homicides, rapes, and violent assaults in the U.S. were directly attributed to violence on television. That was when the violence was nothing compared to the rampant and graphic violence depicted today on television, in the cinema, and now in videos on the internet.[31]

In 2004 Loren Coleman also reminded us of the copycat effect, as a social phenomenon, incited by the way the media report the news and the velocity with which it travels throughout society in the modern information age. Serial killers and shooting rampages have also been subject to the copycat phenomenon because of the sensationalization of violence. Coleman relates that copycat incidents are not new to the 21st century. In 1774, Johann Wolfgang von Goethe's publication of the romantic tragedy, "The Sorrows of Young Werther," triggered a number of copycat suicides in Europe in the late 18th century.[16]

Responsible journalists should be able to collect, write, and disseminate information to the public, while remaining unbiased, objective professionals who report the objective "news." Excepting of course, op-ed pieces, they should not use emotionally charged, atrocious crimes purely to incite even more passion or make heroes out of criminals to sell newspapers or television time, or to promote their gun control agenda. The media moguls, frankly, need to convene a meeting of the minds to systematically de-sensationalize crime and cease making morbid celebrities out of criminals.

Banning "Assault" Weapons and Confiscating Guns During Natural Disasters

In medicine, surgeons cannot guarantee results. Serious complications and even sometimes death may occur. The same can happen with misuse of guns. Firearms in the hands of terrorists, criminals, or the mentally deranged are very dangerous. Senator Dianne Feinstein (D-CA) and other politicians have attempted to capitalize on firearm tragedies whenever they occur. She used the Newtown, Connecticut tragedy to reintroduce the Assault Weapons Ban and other gun control measures on the first day Congress reconvened in 2013.[32] It did not faze her that when this Assault Weapons Ban was in full force, it failed to prevent the infamous 1999 Columbine High School shooting in Littleton, Colorado, nor did the Assault Weapons Ban reduce crime. This is because gun control laws affect only law-abiding citizens and not criminals, psychopaths, or deranged individuals who are in need of committal to prisons or to mental health care facilities.[1,17,18,29,33]

The ban expired in 2004 in accordance with its sunset provision, and despite repeated efforts by Senators Dianne Feinstein, Charles Schumer (D-NY), and other gun prohibitionists in Congress, the Assault Weapons Ban wisely was voted down when it was re-introduced in the Senate in 2013. In fact, despite the senators' passionate appeal, the Feinstein ban failed by the wide margin of 40 to 60.[34]

In fact, history has repeatedly shown that firearms, including so-called "assault weapons," can be very useful and life-saving tools following natural disasters, such as Hurricane Hugo in 1989 and Hurricane Andrew in 1992, and during times of civil unrest, as during the Rodney King L.A. riots of 1992.

In 2005 with Hurricane Katrina approaching, the New Orleans police used the excuse of enforcing compliance with the mandatory evacuation order to confiscate firearms. They went door-to-door seizing guns from the people who stayed behind hoping to ride out the storm. These were the same firearms that the citizens might need to protect their lives and property in the aftermath of the disaster.

New Orleans Mayor Ray Nagin's police chief superintendent said that the only guns allowed would be "in the hands of law enforcement." Stacy Washington, a decorated Air Force veteran, writing for the NRA *America's 1st Freedom*, pointed out:

> *Guns were confiscated with disastrous results: Utter lawlessness ensued, and the police were spread too thin to respond to all the mayhem. Before total gun removal was completed, the NRA stepped in, first gaining a preliminary injunction and then an order putting a stop to the ill-conceived plan. The sheriff had to return more than 1,000 firearms to their respective owners.*[35]

Gun-grabbing Mayor Nagin should have known that confiscation of firearms from persons, who have not committed a crime, is a violation of the Second Amendment—and under the dire circumstances of a natural catastrophe, an inexcusable and unforgivable misjudgment, as well as an affront to the people of New Orleans.

Gun confiscation at the time of the Hurricane Katrina disaster—when they are most needed by citizens to protect their families and property—was such an outrage that several states and the federal government passed laws to prevent that egregious constitutional illegality from ever taking place again.

In 2006 Congress passed the Disaster Recovery Personal Protection Act that became incorporated as an amendment to the Department of Homeland Security Appropriations Act of 2007. It was signed into law on October 4, 2006. This federal legislation prevents the government from confiscating legally owned firearms during times of major disasters or states of emergency. Following the example of the federal government, most state legislatures adopted similar versions of this law.

Notwithstanding U.S. law, on September 5, 2017, in preparation for contending with Hurricane Irma, the Governor of the U.S. Virgin Islands, Kenneth Mapp ordered the National Guard to confiscate firearms and ammunition from the people of the islands. Confiscation was supposedly necessary so the authorities "could carry out their mission." Whatever that may have been, we were left to wonder! Point of reference: The Islands are ruled by federal law approved by Congress in 1954 in the "Revised Organic Act of the Virgin Islands." The NRA threatened to file a lawsuit against the Islands government and confiscation plans were supposedly stalled, but not before they left many citizens defenseless, causing considerable mayhem in the territory, including looting and lawlessness.[36]

Ms. Washington further wrote:

> *Time after time during natural disasters, reports of looting*
> *and increased armed criminal action have been reported. The*
> *primary reason for firearms purchases is to protect self and*
> *loved ones, and this is especially important at times when the*
> *police are overtaxed and crimes of opportunity are more likely*
> *to occur. Natural disasters offer criminals an opening too*
> *sweet to resist—and once an individual or group of marauders*
> *is at your door, it's too late to ask the National Guard for your*
> *guns back.[35]*

Exactly!

Florida has led the way in how to handle some of these natural disasters. In 2015, in addition to the well-known concealed carry weapons (CCW) licensing, the state passed a separate law that permits all adults (but not felons), to carry concealed firearms during emergencies "for up to 48 hours after issuance of an evacuation order."[36]

Some states like Maine and Vermont have "Constitutional Carry" laws, which allow all law-abiding citizens to carry firearms without a permit—emergency or not. In such states, as well as in Florida with its expansive CCW license laws, citizens act as deterrent to crime during natural disasters and emergencies because criminals and the marauding thugs do not know who is armed—a potential victim could very well be an armed citizen and deadly to rob or victimize.

Revising American History and the "Gun Culture"

Better said and repeated than not said at all. There are already an estimated 300 million firearms in civilian possession in the U.S., a number equivalent to the population of the nation. Like it or not, firearms and civilian gun ownership have been part of American history from its inception, and have become part of the culture—as American as mom and apple pie. And it should remain so for lawful citizens. Not that my assertion based on historical reality would be accepted by some undaunted public health researchers, as will be briefly recounted.

One researcher, an Emory University professor and Bancroft Prize winner, Michael A. Bellesiles, faked data to "prove" in his now discredited book *Arming America: The Origins of a Natural Gun Culture* (2000) that gun ownership in early America was fiction. Bellesiles contended that guns were uncommon in the civilian population during the colonial and early periods of the Republic and that guns were rare during those early periods. Consequently, most Americans were not proficient with guns. Bellesiles argued, citing non-existent probate court records, that widespread firearm use came for the civilian population only after the U.S. Civil War, and that became possible only because of the mass production of cheap guns with greater accuracy.[37]

Only one of those contentions was correct; that mass production decreased the cost of firearms while increasing quality and accuracy. The rest was fabricated mendacity. His conclusions were wishful thinking, tailor-made for the liberal intelligentsia, who received his book with great élan, and enthusiastically supported and acclaimed his "historic" work. Yet, his conclusions, going against well-known facts of American history, were preposterous for anyone with even a modicum of historical knowledge. How could early Americans survive the wilderness without possessing firearms and not be proficient in their use? How could colonists in the frontier, subject to Indian raids all the time, protect their families? How could the colonial militia be ready at a moment's notice not only to fight Indian raids but also to join the British army in fighting in the French and Indian War (1756–1763), as Colonel George Washington and his militia did to fulfill their duty? And most astounding of all, how could the celebrated event in American history we now refer to as Patriot's Day (April 19, 1775) have taken place without availability and familiarity with firearms? How could the minutemen (summoned by Paul Revere in his famous ride, warning the country side, "The British are coming!") assemble so quickly and with their muskets fire "the shot heard around the world" on that day? Why would the American patriots prevent the British army's attempt to disarm them and seize the arm depots at Concord, while passing by Lexington in the Colony of Massachusetts? How could they harass the Redcoats all the way back to Boston?

This preposterous attempt at historical revisionism was truly audacious; only an anti-gun "scholar" with a supremely exceeding capacity for arrogance and hubris would have attempted such mendacity, but such dishonesty was only an illogical extension of the politicized, dishonest gun research that we have been exposing all along.

So it didn't take long for true scholars to prove Bellesiles' "scholarship" was fraudulent and his conclusions fabricated, his book a bag of lies conceived to reach the preordained conclusions that the American gun culture was a relatively new phenomenon, the result of a tragic civil war and an overabundance of cheap mass-produced weapons. His mendacity cost him his reputation, his coveted Bancroft Prize, and his professorial position at Emory University—sadly also the alma mater for my post–doctoral neurosurgical training.

There is actually a real misconception of the Old West that truly needs correcting. That is the notion of an uncivilized Wild West, where antisocial and violent behavior was the norm, and where citizens were afraid to leave their homes, afraid of rampant crime and in fear for their lives. This savage perspective turns out to be incorrect—false assumptions of the Old West based on sensationalist press, the Buffalo Bill Wild West Show of the 1880s and '90s, and subsequently cowboy shows and Hollywood movies. Bands of working cowboys and good citizens did not go about town in their leisure time challenging, outdrawing, and shooting each other in a systematized orgy of violence and gunfights as portrayed in the movies.

Bad men and violent outlaws did kill each other, but almost always left the good people of the towns alone. The famous gunfight at the O.K. Corral in 1881 in Tombstone, Arizona, in which Wyatt Earp and his brothers, Virgil and Morgan, with Doc Holliday, killed three of the outlaw "Cowboys," became a celebrated incident not only because of the unique circumstances but also because brother lawmen killed brother outlaws in a historic shootout. Even then it was newsworthy and certainly not a daily occurrence.

In his book, *Gunfighters, Highwaymen, and Vigilantes: Violence on the Frontier*, historian Roger D. McGrath has corrected the historic record with substantive scholarship. After studying the Sierra Nevada frontier towns of Aurora and Bodie, he found that those mining towns, where audacious young men and gunmen roamed freely packing either Colt Navy .36 six shot pistols in Aurora or Colt double action "lightning" or "peacekeeper" revolvers in Bodie, were peaceful towns, except for the quarrels in the carousing and gambling saloons. Otherwise, both towns carried on well, and everyone not interested in whoring, drinking, and gun fighting were left alone.

True, the homicide rate was high among those carousing and looking for fights in the saloons, but in the rest of the populace, the old, the ladies, and those not willing to pick fights, homicides were rare. Likewise, robberies, burglaries, and rape were rare. Murder was confined to the "drunkards upholding their honor." The homicide rate for Aurora and Bodie were 64 and 116 per 100,000, respectively, compared to Washington, D.C., at 72 per year in the 1990s. Likewise, the burglary and robbery rates were 6 and 84 per 100,000, respectively, for Bodie; compared to 2,661 and 1,140, respectively, for New York City in 1980.[38] The townspeople, although they might have carried guns, respected each other, and townspeople did not even bother to lock their doors at night. Similar observations have been made by other researchers studying the supposedly violence and crime-ridden Lincoln County, New Mexico; the Kansas towns of Dodge City and Wichita in the 1870s; and the Texas frontier towns from 1875 to 1890.[38]

Returning to the issue of the possible confiscation of American firearms in the current era, consider the practical obstacles, not to mention the constitutional protection. Trying to blame, register, ban, and confiscate (one step usually follows the other) over 300 million firearms owned by Americans would bring about a tinder box situation, at least an order of magnitude worse than Prohibition, for Americans obey just and moral laws, but not capricious or tyrannical laws, and a veritable police state would be required to enforce the draconian gun laws that would be necessary to carry that out.

Thus, those politicians who sadly continue to use the latest tragedy (and the emotionalism and the passions elicited in its wake) to push for the usual round of gun control while ignoring the accumulated objective research published in the social sciences and the criminological literature[4,6,15], are not sincerely lamenting the deaths of the innocents or sympathizing with their families, but attempting to score political points, political points at the expense of the victims or good citizens. They are also further polarizing America and tearing apart the fabric of this great nation by using emotionalism rather than common sense to bolster their unwise, political actions.

Let's stop demonizing guns and end the shootings by incarcerating the criminals and identifying and healing the mentally ill, for much work needs to be done in the psychiatric and mental health arenas and in the task of reducing violence. Media sensationalization of violence, heaped day after day by the press, the electronic media and the internet—upon impressionable individuals subject to our increasingly dumbed down, popular culture and public education—is having a malevolent effect that needs to stop.[33,39,40]

Las Vegas Massacre and the Mass Shooting Derangement (MSD) Syndrome

As I was working on the manuscript for this book on Sunday, October 1, 2017, I was astounded and horrified to learn about the terrible carnage of the Las Vegas shooting. This massacre left America in a state of shock.

How can anyone be driven by personal demons to massacre innocent people to such a horrific extent? In the context of this heinous carnage, many of us experienced in astonishingly rapid succession the five stages of grief for the victims, as described by the late Dr. Elisabeth Kübler-Ross—e.g., denial, anger, depression, bargaining, and acceptance. Except some of us, instinctively and categorically, reject four of the stages as unacceptable. So that now only anger remains towards the killer, deranged or not. Needless to say, as usual, the Democrats used this tragic occasion not to mourn but to push for drastic gun control measures, banning more guns, even though only 4 percent of guns used in crimes are legally obtained. Universal background checks were also called for, even though background checks did not stop this shooter.

One voice opposing this chorus calling for gun control was that of U.S. Representative Steve Scalise (R-LA), the congressman who was the subject of the serious mass-shooting incident described earlier. He told Fox News anchor Martha MacCallum that the shooting "fortified" his view on gun rights. He further stated, "Because first of all you've got to recognize that when there's a tragedy like this, the first thing we should be thinking about is praying for the people who were injured and doing whatever we can to help them, to help law enforcement. We shouldn't first be thinking of promoting our political agenda."[41] Incidentally, on November 9, 2017, the U.S. Congress honored the officers who responded to Scalise's attack, presenting them with the U.S. Capitol Police Medal of Honor, awarded "to those who exhibit great courage and voluntarily risk their life to help others." Scalise attended the ceremony and praised the officers, but he still required two walking canes for assistance.

We know that 64-year-old mass shooter Stephen Craig Paddock, who opened fire on innocent victims attending the outdoor music festival, killed 58 people, injured another 538, and then turned the gun on himself. His body was found on the 32nd floor of the Mandalay Bay Resort with an arsenal of weapons. Reportedly, he used a bump fire or "trigger activator" device to convert his semi-automatic weapons to full automatic action, simulating machine gun fire.[42] Fully automatic weapons have been tightly regulated since the Firearm Act of 1934 and are not legally obtainable without a full background check and written permission from local law enforcement authorities. Fully automatic weapons are in fact the true assault rifles used in combat and not generally found in the American civilian population.

This shooting rampage was reminiscent of the University of Texas Tower shooting in 1966, when Charles Whitman, a former marine sharpshooter, shot sixteen people and injured thirty-one others from atop the 28th floor observation deck of the Main Building tower at the University of Texas at Austin. Whitman was killed by police and at autopsy was found to have a brain tumor that may have contributed to his derangement.[43]

The shooting rampage in Las Vegas surpassed the 2016 jihadist terrorist shooting at the Pulse nightclub in Orlando, Florida, as the deadliest mass shooting by a single gunman in American history. We need to find ways to identify these deranged individuals before they strike and the simple parroted solution of the gun prohibitionist movement—e.g., more gun control—is not the answer. We have had plenty of guns in American society, and yet, this type of mass murder at one time was very uncommon. I have coined the term Mass Shooting Derangement (MSD) syndrome for a violent disorder that needs to be studied in a hurry, as we did with AIDS, utilizing sound medical, mental health, and criminal research—not public health—so that effective solutions can be found. The public health model for the study of gun violence must be rejected. It was misapplied for over three decades and, as we have shown in this book, was found wanting, riddled with faulty, preordained, politicized gun research masquerading as science.

Mass shooting deaths, enormous in human pain and suffering and tragic as they are, represent approximately one percent of all homicides in the United States. Shooting rampages, as we have previously stated, come in three distinct types. The first type is the politically motivated shooting, as with the 2017 infamous Republican congressional baseball practice shooting in which House Majority Whip Steve Scalise was shot and wounded along with three other people. The second type are those motivated by terrorism, which in our day is almost always Islamic terrorism inspired by jihad, whether home grown or foreign. The third type and the most common in the U.S. is what I like to call the MSD syndrome, which I have come to categorize as a sociopathic disorder, and the narrative that follows concerns only this last type.

Paddock's motives are yet to be ascertained but we now know he was "a high stakes gambler," which I take to be a gambling disorder as categorized in psychiatry in the Diagnostic and Statistical Manual of Mental Disorders (DSM-5). Details were slow to come in but according to police, "his casino transactions were in the tens of thousands of dollars prior to the shooting."

Equally puzzling and requiring further investigation is that Paddock's father was a bank robber who escaped from a federal prison and made it onto the FBI's most-wanted list in 1969, and was described by the FBI as "psychopathic" with "suicidal tendencies."[44] Suffice to say we are only beginning to study psychopathy and unprovoked human aggression with biochemical and genetic markers, radioisotopes, and neuroimaging techniques. Much work still needs to be done to add to what we know from neuropsychiatry and clinical psychology.[45,46]

In my investigations of mass shootings and their media reporting, I believe these shooters are either deeply deranged, psychopathic, and sociopathic individuals, prone to unprovoked aggression, violence, and crime, who seek celebrity status, even if achieving it ends with their death; or they are disturbed or malcontented persons who have a bone to pick with society and blame others for their personal failures and shortcomings in life. They take it upon themselves to hunt down and kill innocent victims to find deadly outlets for their pent up resentment, satisfy their own sense of dissatisfaction, and even fulfill their morbid fantasies in the process.

Informed consent should be obtained from those shooters who have been apprehended and convicted of mass murder (or from their families when appropriate) so they can be studied. Federal grants should be awarded to private psychiatric facilities that agree to diagnose, treat and study those deranged inmates who survive the attacks. These facilities should be secure for that purpose. These are dangerous individuals. The fact that these psychopaths-sociopaths might be diagnosed with the MSD syndrome should not in anyway be construed as proof of mental incompetence or insanity, which are legal terms, and not medical terms. The MSD syndrome should be considered within the context of a severe Antisocial Personality Disorder (APD; DSM-5). Rather than overtly displaying some of the characteristics of APD, some of these individuals are able to hide their pent-up resentment until they finally explode. But, they have carried with them their inherent psychopathic tendencies, such as secretiveness, mendacity, unconcern for others, and violent tendencies, as well as sociopathic motivations and blaming others for their personal failures and mishaps in life. When they finally act, these sociopaths meticulously plan their violent acts, in this case mass shootings, with complete lack of empathy or consideration of the lives of others; and if they survive, display a dispassionate lack of remorse for the people they hurt and the innocent lives they have taken. They should therefore be considered competent and legally sane despite the underlying diagnosis of psychopathy—MSD syndrome. Those who succeed in carrying out such heinous acts should know they would be stigmatized as sociopathic freaks of nature and not gain the desired fame and notoriety they so crave.

The incitement of the politics of envy and class warfare hatred by political demagogues, constantly hammered in by the academic establishment and the popular culture, is a major contributor to this alienation and derangement disorder by contrasting the shortcomings of these psychopathic-sociopathic individuals. Their maladjustment breeds resentment and engenders hostility, until these individuals come to believe that they have not received their "fair share" of the economic benefits and the social contentment that others enjoy.

Mental health research needs to be intensified with a multidisciplinary approach in the study of the MSD syndrome, including not only psychologists but also sociologists and criminologists. Just the fact that we categorize the MSD syndrome as a mental disorder, subject to medical investigation and studies, may serve enough of a deterrent for some of those seeking notoriety and inflicting punishment on society for their personal failures. We must find effective citizen empowerment and law enforcement solutions to the MSD syndrome without extinguishing liberty from the rest of society.

Causes of MSD and Constructive Solutions

I would be remiss if I did not admit to and express openly some feelings of apprehension regarding the fact that after all the figures are analyzed, there might actually be an increased incidence of mass killings for the year 2017, not just in the United States, but throughout the world, whether arising from deranged mass killers, jihad-inspired terror, or the political hatred of the left or right. They are all ramifications of the socialistic, egalitarian ethos.

We have discussed in detail the October 1, 2017 Las Vegas shooting, because of a man suffering from MSD syndrome with the aspiration of a "successful high stakes gambler," turned out to be a loser who had lost "quite a bit of money on his gambling." We had the October 31, 2017, Halloween truck massacre in New York City, where an Islamic terrorist plowed into a crowd in the name of jihad and ISIS. Why are we allowing all of these potential and actual terrorists into this country? It is utter madness. We must implement drastic security measures against the enemy so that we can preserve our way of life and freedom. Yet our borders are porous if not wide open, and obstacles have been placed in the way of President Trump in his attempt to exercise his prerogative as commander in chief with his order to ban immigration from countries with strong ties to terrorism or build the wall across our southern border in order to safeguard our national security.

Che Guevara, an icon of the left, thought that socialism and egalitarianism would create a new socialist man dedicated to the common good without the need of material incentives to work and live. Che lived long enough to see it did not, although he persisted. Socialistic policies have instead created deranged individuals who resent the gains of others, blame society for their failures, and at some point become killers.

It does not bode well for us as a society that we have a broken criminal justice system with revolving prison doors that panders to criminals and forgets the victims. We have the popular culture of Hollywood, which led by producers like Harvey Weinstein and actors like Kevin Spacey, glorify antiheroes. We have a mainstream liberal press that sensationalizes crime and grants celebrity status to mass killers, while it has moved so far to the left that it has become a propaganda organ of the Democrat Party. It glorifies sex, vulgarity, and violence, and then clamors for gun control and not crime control.

It does not bode well that the socialistic egalitarian ethos promulgated by the liberal press, the progressive academic establishment, and the popular culture, has so permeated our society that when borderline individuals and outright malcontents, are not able to reach for the stars and succeed to the grandiose dreams of equality of outcomes promised by the intelligentsia, they blame society and seek deadly revenge on others.

Men have been told they are equal, and because of the limits of public education, the meaning of the phrase has not been explained to them that they are equal in front of the law and in their freedom to pursuit happiness, but not in looks, IQ, motivation, intellect, industry, or what they ultimately attain in life. When their great expectations are not fulfilled and their delusions come crashing down, they seek victims because they believe they have been cheated.

There is no doubt in my mind the progressive zeitgeist of the last several decades has contributed immensely to the MSD syndrome: the institutionalization of government dependency; the nauseating and depraved popular culture on TV and cinema, especially the garbage coming from Hollywood; the incitement of the politics of envy and class warfare hatred by political demagogues (constantly underscored and hammered in by the academic establishment and the mass media). All of these have been major contributors to this alienation and derangement disorder we see so clearly in America.

All the politically correct nonsense such as gun free zones, zero tolerance for guns (including, ludicrously water guns and even pictures of firearms, all banned in schools and which have resulted in young children being suspended from schools) must cease. Demonizing guns, inanimate objects, at the same time that criminals are pandered to in the criminal justice system—must stop! More armed good citizens are needed in crowded places, including teachers in schools and ministers in churches.

PART 8

AMERICA, GUNS, AND FREEDOM

CHAPTER 23

AMERICA, GUNS, AND FREEDOM— A RECAPITULATION OF LIBERTY

Before a standing army can rule, the people must be disarmed; as they are in almost every kingdom of Europe. The supreme power in America cannot enforce unjust laws by the sword; because the whole body of the people are armed, and constitute a force superior to any band of regular troops that can be, on any pretence, raised in the United States.

—Noah Webster (1758—1843),
Examination of the Leading Principles of the Federal Constitution, 1787

The role of gun violence, and more importantly how to unobtrusively as possible restrict civilian gun ownership, remains a subject of great discussion among national and international organizations, including the United Nations (UN) and the European Union (EU). Because the Second Amendment to the U.S. Constitution protects the individual right of American citizens to own private firearms, the right of free people to keep and bear arms remains an insurmountable problem for the global elite, who seek to disarm Americans so they can rule as they please worldwide.

Freedom along with the number of firearms is greater in the U.S. than the rest of the world. Although the American people continue to purchase and possess firearms in record numbers, homicides and violent crimes have, at the same time, diminished for several decades because guns in the hands of the law-abiding citizens do not translate into more crime.

In addition, unlike the rest of the world, America has not been invaded by any nation since the War of 1812 at which time Great Britain, the greatest power in the world, finally gave up any ideas of trying to subjugate the United States and bring it back into her empire. Indeed, the British Red Coats, who had defeated Napoleon's Grande Armée at Waterloo, were picked off like in a dove shoot by American irregulars—e.g., citizens, pirates, soldiers, farmers, and adventurers that constituted the army of General Andrew Jackson at the Battle of New Orleans in 1815.

Abraham Lincoln was correct half a century later in his famous observation:

> *From whence shall we expect the approach of danger? Shall some trans-Atlantic military giant step the earth and crush us at a blow? Never. All the armies of Europe and Asia...could not by force take a drink from the Ohio River or make a track on the Blue Ridge in the trial of a thousand years. No, if destruction be our lot we must ourselves be its author and finisher. As a nation of free men we will live forever or die by suicide.*[1]

Other nations were not so fortunate as we have witnessed in some of the terrible events of the 20th century.

Dateline: Warsaw, Poland, 1943

In the spring of 1943, the inhabitants of the Warsaw Ghetto, having become aware the Nazis were deporting the remaining Jews to the gas chambers of Treblinka, took up arms, whatever they could find, and rebelled against the German occupiers. These determined insurgents had only homemade Molotov cocktails and a handful of small arms, revolvers, pistols, and a few military or hunting rifles. Yet, it took time and resources as well as vastly superior Nazi forces to subdue the rebels, and the Germans suffered up to 300 casualties in pacifying the city.[2]

There were several other armed struggles and Ghetto uprisings, and Warsaw and the Poles remained a serious problem for the Germans during the remainder of the war. The Polish Jews continued to procure whatever arms they could find to defend themselves in their struggle, repeatedly disrupting the timetable of the Nazi high command and the German war effort.

The last major Polish uprising in August 1944 was to be launched in concert with the liberating Soviet Red Army. But, the advancing Red jugger-naut suddenly and inexplicably halted. Advised by General Georgi Zhukov, Stalin rejected the appeals of the Western allies to assist the insurgents. For two months, the courageous Poles fought the Nazis in heroic, urban warfare without any assistance. Stalin had deliberately halted the advance of the giant Red Army to allow the Germans to destroy the noncommunist freedom fighters: 200,000 Poles perished and 800,000 were deported to the death camps.[3] Warsaw was erased by orders of Adolf Hitler, and the Soviets at the outskirts of the city did nothing.[4]

Dateline: Budapest, Hungary, 1944

During the summer of 1944 in the ongoing carnage of World War II, German troops were retreating on multiple fronts. Hungarian troops, allied to Germany, were defending their country from the onslaught of the Soviet Red Army; yet in the midst of the chaos, nearly 500,000 Hungarian Jews were rounded up and deported to the Nazi death camp Auschwitz-Birkenau, where 90 percent of them were summarily exterminated in the gas chambers. A reign of terror ensued for those who remained in Hungary; thousands of them were tortured, robbed, or murdered; Jewish women were raped; property was looted or confiscated.[5] These atrocities were carried out with a minimum of Nazi troops. While seated in a restored synagogue in Budapest a few years ago, a friend of mine listened in utter disbelief as this story was recounted. How could this have happened? How could these atrocities have been carried out with only a minimum of Nazi troops? The Hungarian state had outlawed the possession of firearms for its citizens. Simply put, this happened without resistance because the Hungarian people had been disarmed.

Dateline: Havana, Cuba, 1959

Here is a story with which I am intimately familiar. After the triumph of the revolution in 1959, Fidel Castro reneged on his promise to establish democracy in Cuba. In response, the Revolutionary Directorate (RD), the opposing, noncommunist group that had also fought President Fulgencio Batista, threatened to renew the insurrection this time against the revolutionary government of the Castro brothers. To back their demands with substance or perhaps even expecting a showdown, the RD seized arms from the San Antonio de los Baños Air Force Base in the western part of the island.

Fidel Castro reacted characteristically in a speech at the Maestre Barracks of San Ambrosio, artfully commanding the situation by accusing the RD of seizing the arms and then, in a masterpiece of rhetoric, asking, *¿Armas para que? ¿Para luchar contra quién? ¿Contra el gobierno revolucionario, que tiene el apoyo del pueblo?* ("Guns, for what? To fight against whom? Against the revolutionary government that has the support of the people?") With public jubilation, Fidel Castro defused the situation and neutralized the defiance of the RD. Shortly thereafter, Castro commenced his longterm campaign to disarm not only his purported confreres in the Revolutionary Directorate, who had at last joined him, but also in due time all opponents of his regime. A 100,000-member "militia" (*milicia*) was organized to seek out the political opposition and disarm it.

Unfortunately, they had a welldrawn blueprint to follow—the local firearm registration lists that the former dictator, Fulgencio Batista, had established. All the *milicianos* had to do was to seize the registration (licensing) lists and then go door to door searching for and confiscating firearms. The militia tried to disarm my father, a physician, and the episode is recounted in my book *Cuba in Revolution: Escape from a Lost Paradise.*[6]

During the Batista dictatorship (1952–1958), Cubans were free to leave the country with family, personal possessions, and their wealth, anytime they wished, but not so in communist Cuba.

Since the triumph of the revolution in 1959, the best figures we can glean are that between 30,000 and 40,000 Cubans were either executed *en los paredones de fusilamiento* (on the firing squad wall) or died at the hands of their communist jailers. Between 1960 and 1965, hundreds of anticommunist rebels, many of them former RD members, went back to the hills of the Escambray Mountains in my native Las Villas province to fight the new communist dictatorship of the Castro brothers. The mostly peasant insurgents, who were defending their lands, lacked sufficient weapons to overcome the well-armed, communist Cuban military forces. Thus, most of these peasant insurgencies were annihilated by 1966. The Escambray rebellion against Castro's communist government, which actually took a larger human toll than the struggle against Batista, was referred to by the communists derisively as the War Against the Bandits.[6-8]

Moreover, between 1960 and 1993, 36,000 Cubans perished at sea trying to escape Fidel Castro's communist inferno. If we include all of those who died escaping the regime, those who were shot or died in custody, the figure well exceeds 100,000 casualties. In fact, the late scholar Armando M. Lago, PhD (1939—2008) arrived at a death toll of 105,000 victims directly attributed to the regime of Fidel Castro.[6,7]

Countless thousands of other Cubans have died indirectly as a result of Fidel and Raúl Castro's collectivist policies, unspeakable privations, malnutrition, and the general desolation of a once prosperous island—the island Christopher Columbus called the "Pearl of the Antilles."

One day, as happened in the Soviet Union, we will learn the truth and more accurate numbers will be available, recording the full extent of the brutality and destruction wrought by communism in Cuba. One reason this happened and Cuba today remains a totalitarian state, despite the collapse of Soviet communism, is because the Cuban people were disarmed.[6-8]

Firearms and the U.S. Constitution

[Those] who are trying to read the Second Amendment out of the Constitution by claiming it's not an individual right (are) courting disaster by encouraging others to use the same means to eliminate portions of the Constitution they don't like.

—*Alan Dershowitz, Harvard Law School*

In the wake of President Barack Obama's re-election on November 6, 2012, and the virtual demoralization of Republicans, GOP partisans should have recognized that the political mastery of the left does not last forever, despite the liberal media rejoicing and claiming that the end of the GOP was near. Even with that defeat, three new conservative, pro-Second Amendment senators and several freshmen representatives were elected. A solid Republican majority was preserved in the House of Representatives. So, the election did not mean complete defeat for the GOP.

Better tidings awaited with the election of 2016 when Donald Trump was elected president with a sweeping victory in the electoral map. Republicans retained the House of Representatives and the Senate. Republicans also garnered a large majority of state legislatures, and most importantly, Trump was able to fill in the seat of the great jurist Antonin Scalia with another superb jurist, Neil M. Gorsuch, who has already participated in Supreme Court proceedings and whose talent promises to follow the legal path blazed by Scalia. But we cannot leave everything in the hands of the courts.

Education of children and remaining informed and vigilant citizens are important because freedom comes with responsibilities. Children should be taught not only the basic academic subjects but also instructed in civics, the constitutional principles of government, and the meaning of liberty. Simply restated, education is important and should also serve the purpose of supporting constitutional governance that teaches the price of freedom and the benefits of attaining and preserving individual liberty. Yet, it comes with concomitant duties, responsibilities, and sometimes, personal sacrifices. Liberty requires that the empowered population remain informed and vigilant—the people themselves, the ultimate guardians of their rights and freedoms.[9-12]

Political battles will continue as every generation must safeguard the freedoms bequeathed by their forefathers. Thus, conservatives and gun rights advocates must keep their eye on the ball, particularly in regard to the constitutional right that ultimately preserves all others—the Second Amendment.

After the re-election of Barack Obama, not a friend of the Second Amendment, many of us were disheartened. In an attempt to preserve morale within the conservative ranks, I wrote in my local newspaper, "Yes, the political pendulum has swung to the left, but it will not remain there. After the 'reign' of FDR and the presidency of Harry Truman came Dwight

D. Eisenhower (for two terms), and after Jimmy Carter came the great Ronald Reagan."

Our present GOP champion, President Donald Trump, has already become another "great communicator," bypassing the liberal media and reaching the people. Trump has already transcended political correctness, given a salutary blow for freedom of speech, and in this alone, not to mention the Supreme Court appointment, he has provided a great service. It will not be easy draining the swamp of Washington, breaking the stranglehold of the entrenched bureaucracy and the Deep State, and ending the political correctness and intolerance of progressive academia.

The important thing is that conservatives and gun owners must regroup to preserve the gains already achieved on gun rights. In President Donald Trump, conservatives have a champion of the Second Amendment. They also have a revitalized Supreme Court, which had already ruled that the right to keep and bear arms was an individual right not a collective privilege arbitrarily granted by government.

The Bill of Rights

The first 10 amendments to the U.S. Constitution (the Bill of Rights) were added to the document to specifically limit the power of government and enumerate certain fundamental individual rights, so that their enumeration provides specific protection from the monopolistic tendency of government to wrest power away from the people and usurp the rights of citizens. James Madison, the master builder of the U.S. Constitution, framed the Second Amendment as an essential part of the American Bill of Rights and an inalienable natural right of citizenship guaranteed by the Constitution.

According to Joseph Story (1779—1845), foremost American jurist and intellectual alter ego of Chief Justice John Marshall, the solution to the dilemma of government as a necessary evil was found in the Second Amendment.

Supreme Court Justice Story wrote (1833):

> *The right of the citizens to keep and bear arms has justly been considered the palladium of the liberties of a republic; since it*

> *offers a strong moral check against usurpation and arbitrary*
> *power of rulers; and will generally, even if these are successful*
> *in the first instance, enable the people to resist and triumph*
> *over them.*[13]

These are strong words better said by an American founder in explaining the reason for the Second Amendment than to be left unsaid to a posterity that could have forgotten why the natural right of gun ownership was even written into the U.S. Constitution, and especially for those brainwashed by the liberal media and progressive academia who have no inkling why the amendment was written. It certainly was not written to protect duck hunting or skeet shooting and it most certainly is not outmoded and obsolete.

As we have already pointed out in Chapter 16, for the last several decades, most American legal scholars have concluded that the Second Amendment protects an individual right to keep and bear arms. Nevertheless, gun prohibitionists, in justifying their crusade for gun control in place of crime control, erroneously maintained that the Second Amendment only permitted the National Guard or the police to possess firearms for collective police functions. This was a ludicrously ignorant assertion given the hostility the founders held against standing armies!

Recent U.S. Supreme Court Decisions on the Second Amendment

The U.S. Supreme Court finally confirmed what many of us had known for years. On June 26, 2008 in the *District of Columbia v. Heller* decision, the Supreme Court of the United States struck down a Washington, D.C. handgun ban, which had forbidden American citizens from owning and possessing firearms in the District of Columbia. The Court ruled that U.S. citizens have an inalienable, personal right to keep and bear arms in the federal district of the nation, a preexisting natural right guaranteed in the Second Amendment to the U.S. Constitution.

Then on June 28, 2010 in the *McDonald v. Chicago* case, the Supreme Court of the United States struck down a similar Chicago handgun ban, reconfirming that the Second Amendment protects an individual right of all citizens to possess firearms in their homes for self-defense. In the *McDonald* decision, the U.S. Supreme Court incorporated the Second Amendment as a fundamental right of citizenship applicable to all the states and municipalities of the nation via the Due Process Clause of the Fourteenth Amendment.

Under legal tradition, a constitutional right is protected and inalienable under the Fourteenth Amendment's Due Process and Equal Protection Clauses, if it is considered a fundamental natural right rooted in American history and jurisprudence.[14]

And yet, as I have said previously, citizens must remain alert to the circuitous ways of American jurisprudence. Even now that President Trump has appointed to the Supreme Court Justices Neil Gorsuch and Brett Kavanaugh, pro-Second Amendment jurists, the people must preserve their vigilance as to other appointments to the Supreme Court and to the lower courts. In fact, even as I write this, the Democrats are blocking presidential appointments to important vacant lower judicial courts. Keeping in touch with and from time to time calling and writing your Senators and Representatives are essential duties to help keep politicians' feet to the fire.

And don't forget, the pro-Second Amendment majority in the Supreme Court is still razor-thin at five to four. Moreover, the highest court has confounded many of us by refusing to rule on whether the Second Amendment protects the right to keep and bear arms outside the home. As a result, several states and municipalities still ban or restrict the right to conceal carry in public.

On July 25, 2017, by a two-to-one decision, the DC Circuit Court of Appeals struck down a District of Columbia law burdening applicants with the requirement that they must "demonstrate a need for self-protection distinguishable from the general community." This was not the first time anti-Second Amendment municipal officials tried to circumvent the law by placing additional impediments and restrictions on the right to keep and bear arms. The District of Columbia had ignored previous landmark Supreme Court rulings—e.g., *District of Columbia v. Heller* (2008) and *McDonald v. Chicago* (2010)—that the Second Amendment was an individual right that predated the Constitution. The highest court had previously struck down the District of Columbia ban on citizen possession of handguns in the *District of Columbia v. Heller*, and a district court had also nullified the D.C. ban on carrying handguns in *Palmer v. District of Columbia* (2014).[14]

Be that as it may, the Supreme Court has turned down several attempts to challenge the various Circuit Court decisions upholding restrictive concealed carry legislations in Maryland, New Jersey, and most recently California. In California, the Ninth Circuit Court denied that the Second Amendment protects the right to carry concealed weapons in public. Justices Clarence Thomas and Neil M. Gorsuch expressed regrets that the Supreme Court did not take the challenge of the case in California and believe it is high time the Supreme Court rules on the issue of concealed carry legislation and also affirms the Second Amendment right outside the home. In the words of Justice Thomas, "The Court's decision to deny certiorari in this case reflects a distressing trend: the treatment of the Second Amendment as a disfavored right." Thomas further wrote in his dissent, "For those of us who work in marbled halls, guarded constantly by a vigilant and dedicated police force, the guarantees of the Second Amendment might seem antiquated and super-fluous. But the Framers made a clear choice: They reserved to all Americans the right to bear arms for self-defense."[14]

Open carry is another issue that has not been settled to the satisfaction of gun owners, and the topic came to the forefront in Florida, the state that interestingly enough in 1987 passed the landmark concealed carry legisla-tion. The case was that of Dale Norman, a Floridian with a concealed carry permit who in 2012 was arrested in Fort Pierce openly carrying a gun in a holster. He was fined and convicted of a misdemeanor. He appealed on con-stitutional grounds. The U.S. Supreme Court declined to hear the case and effectively let stand a Florida Supreme Court ruling in March 2017 stating that the open-carry ban of the state did not violate the constitutional right of citizens to bear arms. Attorneys for the state successfully argued that lawful citizens may already carry concealed weapons legally by obtaining permits without undue burden. They also cited the fact that the U.S. Supreme Court has yet to rule that the Second Amendment protects open carry in public.[15]

The issue of the constitutionality of "assault weapons" has also not been settled. These beneficial semi-automatic firearms with paramilitary looks have been under attack at both the federal and state levels. Despite their usefulness for sports shooting as well as life-saving tools during natural catastrophes, urban unrest, and self-defense against multiple criminal assailants (as we have seen, particularly in Chapters 16 and 22), these firearms have been so maligned that some courts are yet to rule favorably on their constitutionality. On November 27, 2017, the U.S. Supreme Court refused to take up Maryland's assault weapons ban. The Fourth Circuit Court of Appeals upheld Maryland's Firearm Safety Act of 2013, banning the AR-15 "and other military-style rifles and shotguns." Again, semi-automatic "assault weapons" were confused with fully automatic "assault rifles" and characterized as military weapons, and thus excluded from Second Amendment protection. Interestingly, the judge who wrote the majority decision stated, "Put simply, we have no power to extend Second Amendment protection to the weapons of war that the *Heller* decision explicitly excluded from such coverage." Curiously, it was precisely in *Miller v. U.S.* (1938), the last federal ruling on the Second Amendment until the *Heller* decision in 2008, that ownership of military-style weapons were specifically protected as a pre-existent individual right by the Second Amendment.[15] Let's hope the U.S. Supreme Court does not delay too long, as it did between the *Miller* (1938) and *Heller* (2008) decisions, before it decides these important constitutional questions.[15]

The Eternal Threat of the UN Small Arms Treaty

Even before these landmark rulings, Americans had refused to give up their natural and constitutional right to keep and bear arms. Nevertheless, many politicians bent on prohibiting gun ownership have tried ingenious ways to curtail gun rights and institute gun control through the back door. One legal approach has been to attempt to apply the treaty power of the U.S. Constitution, using the UN deceptively as the vehicle to circumvent and contravene the document and disarm Americans.

I refer to the Supremacy Clause, Article VI, paragraph two of the U.S. Constitution:

> *This Constitution, and the Laws of the United States which shall be made in pursuance thereof; and all treaties made, or which shall be made, under the authority of the United States, shall be the supreme law of the land; and the judges in every state shall be bound thereby, anything in the constitution or laws of any state to the contrary notwithstanding.*

While in the landmark case *Reid v. Covert* (1957), the Supreme Court ruled that the U.S. Constitution supersedes the power of treaties, many left leaning, liberal scholars have tried to circumvent that ruling with creative arguments, claiming the treaty power vested in the Constitution supersedes other internal U.S. laws, even if these are duly enacted laws, and even if the treaty itself contravenes the U.S. Constitution. Other conservative legal minds disagree. For them, it is axiomatic that a creature is never greater than its creator.

For years, so encouraged, several influential politicians and members of the Democratic Party have worked hand in glove with their political counterparts in the United Nations to pass several versions of the UN Small Arms Treaty. The most recent attempt, the Arms Trade Treaty (ATT), was tabled in July 2012. According to Gun Owners of America (GOA), the United Nation's Secretary General Ban Kimoon called "the unraveling" of the ATT merely a "setback." Experts at the UN expect further discussions and the taking of votes at future General Assembly sessions.[16]

The Obama administration supported the treaty and tried to get the U.S. to join it. This stance to implement gun control through the back door is as disingenuous as "Operation Fast and Furious," in which American officials of the Bureau of Alcohol, Tobacco, Firearms, and Explosives (ATF) in the Obama administration, under the supervision of the Department of Justice, were running illegal guns to Mexican drug lords creating mayhem, so they could push for gun control in America while simultaneously pushing for the UN treaty.[17]

Former U.S. Representative Paul Broun (R-GA) in an open letter published back in June 2010 described what this UN treaty would entail:

> *If passed by the UN and ratified by the U.S. Senate, the UN Small Arms Treaty would almost certainly force national governments to: enact tougher licensing requirements, making law-abiding citizens cut through even more bureaucratic red tape just to own a firearm legally; confiscate and destroy all 'unauthorized' civilian firearms; ban the trade, sale and private ownership of all semi-automatic weapons; create an international gun registry, setting the stage for full-scale gun confiscation.[16]*

The truth is the UN Small Arms Treaty has failed to materialize because of the inability of negotiators to reach a consensus, but according to GOA, "It would be a mistake to believe that it spells the end of the effort to regulate small arms worldwide." Indeed, for years the UN has been trying to formalize a global, civilian disarmament treaty with the intention of circumventing the Second Amendment rights of American gun owners. After all, the UN has dictated national policy to other sovereign nations, as it regards environmental, criminal, and even global tax issues, so why not enforce gun control? Thus, the struggle to preserve the right to gun ownership is an ongoing effort, even for Americans who already possess it.

It is not only the United Nations that citizens of the civilized world have to worry about in the globalists' drive for gun control. In August 2017, the Czech Republic, that had promised to preserve their citizens' right to gun ownership in entering the European Union (EU), filed a legal challenge to the EU's onerous gun control European Firearms Directive. The central European nation, "filed suit in the European Court of Justice, demanding that the new gun controls be scrapped, postponed, or that certain countries be given exemptions from the measure."[18]

In 1938, Czechoslovakia, mother country of the Czech Republic, was sacrificed, betrayed by its Western allies, Great Britain and France. Czechoslovakia was invaded and annexed to the Nazi empire, soon after British Prime Minister Neville Chamberlain, deceived by Hitler, returned to England with a piece of paper claiming that he had brought "peace in our time."

Czechoslovakia and some of the other central and eastern European nations, like Poland and Hungary, which we introduced at the beginning of the chapter, knew better. The EU seeks to impose severe restriction on the civilian ownership of firearms, reduce gun owner privacy, and make it very difficult for State-issued firearms licenses. The new gun control laws of the European Firearms Directive went into effect on June 13, 2017.

Citizenship and the Beneficial Aspects of Gun Ownership

> *Laws that forbid the carrying of arms disarm only those who*
> *are neither inclined nor determined to commit crimes. Such*
> *laws make things worse for the assaulted and better for the*
> *assailants; they serve rather to encourage than to prevent*
> *homicides, for an unarmed man may be attacked with greater*
> *confidence than an armed man.*
>
> —*Cesare Beccaria,*
> *"On Crimes and Punishment," Italian criminologist quoted in*
> *Thomas Jefferson's Literary Commonplace Book*

Scholarship published in the criminological, sociological, and legal literature in the last 30 years show that *the defensive uses of firearms by citizens amount to up to 2 million to 2.5 million uses per year and dwarf the offensive gun uses by criminals. In the United States, between 25 and 75 lives are saved by a gun in self and family protection for every life lost to a gun in crime.*[19] *Medical costs saved by guns in the hands of law-abiding citizens are 15 times greater than costs incurred by criminal uses of firearms. Guns also prevent injuries to good people and protect billions of dollars of property every year.*[19-22]

Moreover, the actual U.S. health care costs of treating gunshot wounds was calculated to be approximately $1.5 billion, which was less than 0.2 percent of the U.S. annual health care expenditures calculated in the 1990s. The $20-40 billion figure cited in the medical literature in those same years has been found to be a deliberately exaggerated estimate of lifetime productivity lost. Reality points otherwise: Many "victims" are criminal elements who have been killed in the act of perpetrating serious crimes, either by the police or by law-abiding citizens acting in self-defense.[19,21] In fact, 61 percent of murder victims and the vast majority of murderers, 76 percent, have prior criminal records. The majority of murders occur among violent criminals.[23]

In 2015, *Mother Jones* published a study on the economic costs of "gun violence" and arrived at a figure of $229 billion for the year 2012. As one would expect, the *Mother Jones* researchers not surprisingly ignored justifiable homicides and failed to compare the financial benefits of defensive gun uses.[22]

Assuming that only 1.5 million defensive gun uses took place during 2012 and that in 16 percent of cases without defensive gun use "almost certainly someone would have been killed" (from Kleck's 1992 survey response), accepting *Mother Jones* assumptions and figures on economic costs, Dr. Robert Young calculated that "the economic savings to this country—just from thwarting criminal assaults—was over $415 billion in lives plus $95 billion in injuries, totaling more than $511 billion in that year alone."[22]

Thus we can confirm that not only the lives saved by a gun surpassed those lost, but also the economic savings outstrip those incurred by criminal misuses of firearms.

In the previously mentioned and still cited 1986 *New England Journal of Medicine* (*NEJM*) paper, Drs. Arthur Kellermann and Donald T. Reay claimed that defending oneself or one's family with a firearm in the home is dangerous and counterproductive, originating the mantra, "a gun owner is 43 times more likely to kill a family member than an intruder."[24] This conclusion, though, has been severely criticized by numerous investigators, who have pointed out methodological and conceptual errors in the study, and most significantly, that the authors had failed to consider and underestimated the protective benefits of guns.[19-22] These and other serious deficiencies stemming not only from methodological errors but also from ideological bias and partisanship have been repeatedly noted with the standard public health model of gun control, which also erroneously maintained that guns are a disease that must be eradicated in order to combat crime and promote what public health researchers deem desirable gun control laws.[19,22,25-33]

In another blow to the gun prohibitionists, John R. Lott, Jr., using the standard criminological approach, reviewed the FBI's massive yearly crime statistics for all 3,054 U.S. counties over 18 years (1977–1994), the largest national survey on gun ownership and state police documentation in illegal gun use. The data show that *while neither state waiting periods nor the federal Brady Law was associated with a reduction in crime rates, adopting concealed carry gun laws that allowed law-abiding citizens to carry concealed weapons for self-defense cut death rates from public, multiple shootings (e.g., as those which took place in 1996 in Dunblane, Scotland, and Tasmania, Australia, or the infamous 1999 Columbine High School shooting in Littleton, Colorado in the United States)—by an amazing 69 percent.*

Allowing law-abiding citizens to carry concealed weapons deters violent crime without any apparent increase in accidental death. In Lott's survey, children 14 to 15 years of age were found to be 14.5 times more likely to die from automobile injuries, five times more likely to die from drowning or fires and burns, and three times more likely to die from bicycle accidents than they are to die from gun accidents.[34] Incidentally, these figures on children's accidental deaths are consistent with the work of attorney David Kopel in the book *Guns: Who Should Have Them* as outlined in his chapter, "Children and Guns."[35]

In the United States, if states without concealed carry gun laws had adopted them in 1992, according to Lott's estimates about 1,570 murders, 4,177 rapes, and 60,000 aggravated assaults would have been avoided annually. Moreover, when concealed carry gun laws went into effect in a given county, murders fell by eight percent, rapes by five percent, and aggravated assaults by seven percent.[34]

For this important, groundbreaking research, John R. Lott has received the accolades he certainly deserves both from his peers in the social sciences and from the freedom-loving citizens of the United States. Nevertheless, his work and findings need wider dissemination among the people, and the elected representatives of the emerging democracies of the world are still unaware of his work and freedom-promoting message.

In the next chapter, we conclude with the experience of the United States in juxtaposition with the rest of the world in terms of the relationship of civilian disarmament to the development of tyrannical governments and genocide. In a better light, the next chapter ends with a discussion of how armed citizens can preserve their freedom by a form of government more commonly referred to as representative democracy, but more accurately described as a constitutional republic.

CHAPTER 24

AMERICA, GUNS, AND FREEDOM—AN INTERNATIONAL PERSPECTIVE

Besides the advantage of being armed, which the Americans
possess over the people of almost every other nation, the existence
of subordinate governments, to which the people are attached,
and by which the militia officers are appointed, forms a barrier
against the enterprises of ambition, more insurmountable than
any which a simple government of any form can admit.

—James Madison (1751—1836),
The Federalist Papers, No. 46

In this chapter the celebration of America's historic "gun culture" as a beacon of liberty continues, while the relationship of civilian disarmament to tyrannical governments and genocide in other countries is further explored. Incidents in which liberty has been extinguished because firearms have been banned and citizens disarmed by increasingly oppressive governments; and the converse, countries where armed citizens have preserved freedom are described in the pages of this chapter. We affirm from analyzing the historic record that guns in the hands of law-abiding citizens deter crime, and nations that trust their citizens with firearms have republican forms of governments, which sustain liberty and affirm the individual freedom of citizens. Governments that do not trust their citizens with firearms tend to be despotic and tyrannical, and are a potential danger to good, lawful citizens, and a peril to humanity.

The celebrated book, *The Samurai, The Mountie, and The Cowboy*, by gun rights attorney, David Kopel, makes the point that disparate countries such as Japan and Switzerland have low crime rates regardless of gun control laws because of close ties engendered in the traditional family. In those countries, parents spend time with children, who are then properly reared and imbued with a sense of patriotism as well as civic duty.[1] In this milieu, children can be brought up with firearms, instructed in their use and safety, and when they grow up, they should be allowed not only to own guns but also—given the endemic violence of the postmodern age and progressivism—to carry concealed weapons for self and family protection. In Switzerland citizens are allowed to keep guns in their homes and encouraged to participate in sport shooting. In this case, the country benefits and freedom roams. Japan does not have quite that freedom, and loses in the process with excessive regimentation and excessive constraints on personal liberty.

But with freedom comes responsibility, the duty of respecting the rights of others and the laws of the land. Criminals and mentally deranged people forfeit the right to keep and bear arms by virtue of the fact they are a potential danger to their fellow citizens or to themselves. This has been repeatedly demonstrated by FBI figures that show career criminals commit the vast majority of serious crimes; and that the mentally deranged are responsible for more than 50 percent of mass shooting tragedies as took place in Arizona[2] and in Aurora, Colorado[3]; not only in the United States but also in Oslo, Norway,[4] and other countries. These three specific cases represent overt failures in the criminal justice or the mental health system, rather than a problem with "too many guns" in the hands of law-abiding citizens.

Gun Violence, Street Crime, and Self-Defense

Dr. Mark Rosenberg, a former American public health official, once stated, "Most of the perpetrators of violence are not criminals by trade or profession. Indeed, in the area of domestic violence, most of the perpetrators are never accused of any crime. The victims and perpetrators are ourselves— ordinary citizens, students, professionals, and even public health workers."[5] That dramatic but erroneous statement is contradicted by available data, U.S. government data.

According to the United States Department of Justice, *the typical murderer has had a prior criminal history of at least six years, with four felony arrests in his record, before he finally commits murder.*[6,7] Federal Bureau of Investigation (FBI) statistics reveal that *75 percent of all violent crimes for any locality are committed by six percent of hardened criminals and repeat offenders.*[7,8] *Less than one to two percent of crimes committed with firearms are carried out by concealed carry weapons (CCW) permit holders.*[9-11]

Much has been said about "crimes of passion" that supposedly take place impulsively in the heat of the moment or in the furor of a domestic squabble. Criminologists have pointed out that homicides in this setting are the culmination of a long simmering cycle of violence. In one study of police records in Detroit and Kansas City, it was revealed that in *"90 percent of domestic homicides, the police had responded at least once before, during the prior two years, to a disturbance,"* and *in over 50 percent of the cases, the police had been called five or more times to that dysfunctional domicile.*[12]

These are not crimes of passion consummated impulsively in the heat of the moment by ordinary citizens, but the result of violence in highly dysfunctional families, in the setting of alcohol abuse, illicit drug use, or other criminal activities. Violent crimes continue to be a problem in the inner cities of the large metropolitan areas, with gangs involved in robberies, drug trade, juvenile delinquency, and even murder. Yet crimes in rural areas, despite the preponderance of guns in this setting, remain relatively low.[10,11,13,14]

Gun availability to law-abiding citizens does not cause but deters crime. It is a permissive criminal justice system with its revolving prison doors that exacerbates the problem of crime, which is further amplified in the context of gun prohibition in crime-infested cities, such as the District of Columbia, Chicago, Baltimore, and Los Angeles, where lawful citizens become sitting ducks, unable to defend themselves or protect their homes and families.

Prohibition tends to increase crime by criminalizing activities that should have been regulated rather than banned. Alcohol prohibition in the U.S. in the 1920s was a case in point. Following the passage of the XVIII Amendment, there was a significant increase in both homicide and suicide rates in the United States. Noncompliance and the mayhem generated by citizens in contempt of the law brought about a black market for illegal spirits and alcohol smuggling on a grand scale. It also brought violence and established organized crime in America. Crime came down only gradually after the repeal of Prohibition following the passage of the XXI Amendment in 1933. Homicide and suicide rates also increased for nearly a decade following the passage of the Gun Control Act of 1968 and very gradually decreased and stabilized with the passing of time.[15,16]

As to how citizens can protect themselves from criminal assailants when the police, more often than not, are not immediately there to protect them, we have discussed previously but it may be worth repeating at this point: The National Victims Data suggests that, *"while victims resisting with knives, clubs, or bare hands are about twice as likely to be injured as those who submit, victims who resist with a gun are only half as likely to be injured as those who put up no defense."* Of particular interest to women and self-defense, *"among those victims using handguns in self-defense, 66 percent were successful in warding off the attack and keeping their property. Among those victims using non-gun weapons, only 40 percent were successful."*[10] The gun is a great equalizer for law-abiding citizens in self and family protection, particularly women, when they are accosted in the street or when they are defending themselves and their children at home.[9,10,14,16-18]

Revisiting Multiple Shooting Massacres

Although not all citizens would want to carry a concealed firearm for self-protection, criminologists point out that criminals do make quick risk-benefit assessments about the looming, potential threat of a CCW citizen possibly being nearby. Thus, criminological studies consistently reveal that just the knowledge that one in five or six citizens in a public place could very well be armed can deter crimes and could very well avert massacres, as was the case in Israel, after the infamous Maalot Massacre,[19] Switzerland,[20] and the United States.[1,10,11,14,21] In Switzerland, for example, where gun laws are liberalized, there was not a single report of armed robbery in Geneva in 1993![20]) Except for isolated instances, Switzerland remains relatively crime free. Obviously, it is not all about guns; it is also about having a homogeneous population, and a civil and cultured society, as previously mentioned.

Now, let us re-consider the case in Norway. After bombing a government building in Oslo and then taking over Utoya, an island in a nearby lake, a homicidal killer perpetrated a horrible massacre.[4] He has declared himself an anti-Islamic fanatic, but instead of Muslims in a foreign land, Anders Behring Breivik massacred 77 of his fellow countrymen. Breivik systematically hunted down 69 unarmed people at a youth camp located on that island, methodically killing mostly teenagers who could not defend themselves (the other eight people died in the government building bombing in Oslo). Imagine if just one adult had carried a gun, knew how to use it, and was prepared to defend his or her life and the lives of others—the mass shooting could have ended with less loss of life.

Yes, there still may have been a massacre, but not 69 people shot haplessly in a virtual dove shoot. Just one individual armed and willing to protect his or her life and the lives of others was all that was needed to stop the carnage. Furthermore, even if the intended victim was prosecuted later for killing the madman in self-defense and for standing his or her ground, it would have limited the massacre and saved the lives of others. Probable prosecution of the hero or heroine not only in Norway but also in other European social democracies and Scandinavia is likely, given the anti-gun zeitgeist and the irrational degree of hoplophobia in those countries. Moreover, we have seen what has happened in Australia and Great Britain.

However, in most European countries guns have long been registered, or banned and confiscated. Citizens are disarmed in the course of "progress," and in those countries, no one even thinks about self-defense anymore. They depend on the government completely for protection, and where guns are banned only criminals have guns.[22,23]

In Macon, Georgia, we had the dramatic case of a businesswoman and grandmother, who was attacked by two thugs bent on robbing her and perhaps even raping and killing her. They followed the woman home at 1:30 a.m. as she left her convenience store business. The thugs pulled guns on her and demanded cash as she sat in her car. However, the grandmother was armed. Shots were exchanged. The woman wounded one assailant, who was later apprehended as he rushed to a local hospital. The other criminal also fired shots at her, but escaped. She was safe and sound. "I carry a gun all the time," she told a local newspaper reporter![24]

Of course in the southern United States this grandmother is a heroine and no one would consider prosecuting her.[25] That is not the usual course of events in some of our northern states or in other countries, particularly in Great Britain. In England, we discussed at length the case of Tony Martin, the British farmer who defended his home and possibly his life but who spent time in prison for shooting a burglar, who was a known dangerous criminal![23]

Another Look: Media Sensationalism or Propaganda?

The way the subject of "guns and violence" is broached by the popular media brings us to another problem. Most mainstream media reports are saturated with bias and sensationalism. One only needs to see the unprofessional manner Donald Trump has been treated in comparison with his "could do no wrong" predecessor. The mainstream liberal American press, just like their Western European counterparts, are overtly for gun control and look askance at citizens possessing firearms for self and family protection. With that in mind, let us recapitulate how the media reported some of the mass-shooting incidents in America that we have previously cited.

In 1997, in Pearl, Mississippi, 16-year-old Luke Woodham used a hunting rifle to kill his exgirlfriend and her close friend and wound seven other students. Assistant Principal Joel Myrick retrieved his handgun from his automobile and halted Woodham's shooting spree. Myrick held the young delinquent at bay until the police arrived. Later it was discovered that Woodham had also used a knife to stab his mother to death earlier that morning. Even though this shooting incident was widely reported, the fact that Mr. Myrick, an armed citizen, had prevented a larger massacre by retrieving and using his handgun was largely ignored by the media.

Then in 1998, in Edinboro, Pennsylvania, a deadly scenario took place when 14-year-old Andrew Wurst killed one teacher and wounded another teacher as well as two fellow classmates. The shooting rampage in Edinboro was halted by local merchant James Strand, who used his shotgun to force the young criminal to halt his firing, drop his gun, and surrender to the police.

In another unreported incident in Santa Clara, California, Richard Gable Stevens rented a rifle for target practice at the National Shooting Club on July 5, 1999, and then began a shooting rampage, herding three store employees into a nearby alley, and stating he intended to kill them. When Stevens became momentarily distracted, a shooting club employee, who had a .45 caliber handgun concealed under his shirt, drew his weapon and fired. Stevens was hit in the chest and critically wounded. He was held at bay until the police arrived. A potential mass shooting was prevented. The armed employee, an unsung hero, was ignored by the major media. Why are these and other similar incidents where the tables are turned and citizens use guns to protect themselves and others only seldom reported by the mainstream media?

Then we also have the shooting in Aurora, Colorado, on July 19, 2012, which resulted in the death of a dozen people because a deranged individual with criminal intent, James Holmes, was able to enter a theater with a posted "gun-free zone" sign, a designated public place where armed law-abiding citizens are not allowed to carry their concealed firearms. This theater had a "no guns policy," similar to the situation in Norway, which amounted to a dove shoot where only the predator, a hunter of humans, is armed.

The American media did not report another shooting incident that took place three months earlier in, of all places, Aurora, Colorado, where a law-abiding citizen, an armed churchgoer, shot another human predator and stopped a shooting rampage, saving her life and the lives of others in the process.[3] For a comprehensive review of the mass-shooting incidents, the reader may peruse the previous chapter and look up the reference sources there.

Recapitulating: Suicide, Accidental Shootings, Children, and Guns

Several gun researchers have written about suicides and have linked these fatalities to the availability of guns.[25] Medical critics, however, cite the overwhelming evidence compiled from the psychiatric literature that untreated or poorly managed depression is the real culprit behind the relatively high rates of suicide in the United States and other countries. In fact, the World Health Organization (WHO) considers suicide a major mental health problem worldwide. WHO points out that suicide is the second leading cause of death "among 15 to 29 year olds globally, and 78 percent of suicides occurred in low- and middle-income countries in 2015."[26]

Of the 36,861 total gun deaths for 2015, nearly two-thirds were suicides. This is a tremendous proportion, so gun control activists continue to insist that the possession of guns in the American civilian population is responsible for the high gun suicide rate. In other words, for the Democrats and their allies in the liberal press, the gun control propaganda arsenal must be replenished with suicide statistics because suicides outpace homicides every year by a two-to-one ratio.

A CNN article for example stated, "Gun-related suicides are eight times higher in the U.S. than in other high-income nations." But why select gun suicides? Why not compare the U.S. with other nations as to international suicide rates *by all means*? The data in the case of Japan is instructive. The latest figures (2016) show that Japan ranks 26th in international suicide rates; the Japanese commit suicide via hanging, suffocation, jumping in front of trains, and Harakiri at a rate of 19.7 per 100,000, much higher than the United States. In Japan, Seppuku (Harakiri) is, incidentally, still the fourth most common method of suicide. America ranks 48th and the rate is 14.3 per 100,000. Norway, Sweden, Belgium, Hungary, and many other European countries have higher rates of suicide than the U.S., and all of them have stricter gun laws. So obviously, worldwide, people use different cultural methods, or whatever means they have available, including guns, ropes, and herbicides, to commit suicide and they do so frequently at a higher rate than the U.S. But the mainstream liberal media choose to cherry pick and compare the U.S. homicide and suicide "gun" rates with other countries to make America deliberately look worse, a wasteland of homicides and suicides.

Why the caveat of "gun" suicides and "high-income" countries? With gun suicides, the progressive press eliminates the competition from other countries where suicides are committed by whatever means are available. "High income" countries means that most of the world doesn't count in the data compilation. As with homicides, I must suppose that only the lives of wealthy ("high-income") Europeans count and are worth comparing to the U.S., but such is the arrogance and condescending attitude of the gun prohibitionists.

Thus, the truth is that many countries, including Japan, Hungary, Lithuania, Belgium, and most of the Scandinavian nations—all of which have moderate to strict gun control laws and relatively low rates of firearm availability—have much higher rates of suicide than the United States. In those countries, citizens simply use other cultural or universally available methods, such as Seppuku (Harakiri) in Japan; drowning in the Danube as in Hungary; suffocation by poisonous gases from stoves or automobile exhausts; or hanging and strangulation, as in Belgium, Denmark, Poland, Lithuania, and Germany; or by drinking agricultural pesticides, as is commonly done by both sexes in Sri Lanka and most of the Asian third world. Moreover, in these countries, citizens commit suicide quite effectively by their own preferred methods and at higher rates than in the United States.[26]

A child's death from any cause is a tragedy. For 2015, the last year for which we have data, the CDC as usual mixing children with adolescents lumped apples with oranges and claimed 1,500 deaths for children and teens under the age of 18. Although the word "teens" was added, still mixing children with adolescents obfuscates the fact that children's deaths (age 14 or younger) are truly accidental shootings, while adolescent shooting are most often the result of criminal actions.

The truth is that accidental gun fatalities continue to fall because of the increase in gun safety and storage awareness by gun owners, including hunters, sports shooting enthusiasts and collectors, as well as education efforts by organizations such as the NRA and the Sports Shooting Association. As a result, according to the National Safety Council, there were only 59 children's deaths (ages 14 years or younger) from firearms in 2009.[27,28] On the other hand, in the last two years criminal activities and adolescent shootings have risen along with other serious crimes (as we discussed previously in Chapter 12).

Unfortunately, brainwashed pediatricians continue to obfuscate the statistics by using the term "children" to refer to adolescents who are young delinquents and gang bangers. Jacob Sullum observed in a recent article in *Reason* magazine, "This sort of misrepresentation is an old trick among gun controllers," as David B. Kopel noted in *Reason* 24 years ago. 'Gun-control advocates are hammering at the issue of children and guns as never before,' Kopel wrote, 'in the hope that it will be easier to enact gun controls aimed at adults in an atmosphere of panic about children.'"[27]

Gun Violence and Civil Liberties—Another Look Globally

Australians learned the lessons of indiscriminate, draconian gun control laws the hard way. In 1996, a criminally insane man shot to death 35 people at a Tasmanian resort. The government immediately responded by passing stringent gun control laws, banning most firearms, and ordering their confiscation. More than 640,000 guns were seized from ordinary Australian citizens.[22,29]

As a result of the government's action, there was a sharp and dramatic increase in violent crime against the disarmed law-abiding citizens, who in small communities and particularly in rural areas were unable to protect themselves from brigands and robbers. Two years following the gun ban/ confiscation, armed robberies had risen by 73 percent, unarmed robberies by

28 percent, kidnappings by 38 percent, assaults by 17 percent, and manslaughter by 29 percent.[29] All this mayhem took place in a nation where crimes of all types were decreasing before the ban. Crime rates did not stabilize until three years after the ban. No further reductions in crime rates have taken place despite repeated gun buyback programs as we described in Chapter 20.

Interestingly, the same phenomenon occurred in Great Britain. Following a 1996 massacre of school children by a madman in Dunblane, Scotland, the British government banned and ordered the confiscation of most firearms. Following the ban, a horrific crime wave took place in England and Scotland. In 1998, the United States Department of Justice declared that the rate of muggings in England had surpassed those in the United States by 40 percent, while assault and burglary rates were nearly 100 percent higher in England than in the United States. To make matters worse for England—and this was also true for Canada—in those countries where citizens were disarmed in their homes, day burglary was commonplace and dangerous because criminals knew they would not be shot at if caught in *flagrante delicto*. The criminals had nothing to fear from disarmed and helpless homeowners. Not so in the United States, where burglars try to make sure homeowners are not at home to avoid being shot at by the intended victim.[1,16,23]

The Sunday Times of London, on January 11, 1998, wrote about the rising tide of thievery and burglaries in England and dubbed Britain "a nation of thieves." The same article further noted, "More than one in three British men has a criminal record by the age of 40. While America has cut its crime rate dramatically Britain remains the crime capital of the West. Where have we gone wrong?"[23]

It does not have to be that way. A study performed by the United States Department of Justice, Office of Juvenile Justice and Delinquency Prevention tracked 4,000 juveniles aged six to 15 years, in Denver (CO), Pittsburgh (PA), and Rochester (NY) from 1993 to 1995. The investigators found that children who were taught to use firearms with parental supervision, as in hunting or target shooting, were 14 percent less likely to commit acts of violence and street crimes than children who had no guns in their homes (24 percent); whereas, children who obtained guns illegally, did so at the whopping rate of 74 percent.[30] This study also provided more evidence that in close nuclear families where children were close to their parents, youngsters could be taught to use guns responsibly. These youngsters, in fact, grow up to be more responsible in their conduct and more civil in their behavior.

This study confirms what many of us have argued since time immemorial that we must lay the blame for juvenile delinquency, street crime, and gun violence where it belongs: An increasingly permissive culture that for many years has been mired in political correctness and where public schools no longer teach traditional morality and the discernment between right and wrong, leading to situational ethics and moral relativism. To the detriment of children, building self-esteem has been placed ahead of the salutary and profitable teachings of both civics and morality. There is also a lack of discipline at home and in schools because parents and teachers are afraid of reprimanding the young for fear of being denounced by social workers, charged with child abuse, and prosecuted by the state.

Civilian Disarmament, Tyranny, and Genocide

Depending on the level of culture and social progress, violence can take different forms in different societies.[1,7] For example, in the midtwentieth century, the communist government of USSR dictator Joseph Stalin killed more Soviet citizens through privation, forced labor, and famine, than Russian soldiers died fighting the Germans in World War II on the battlefields of Russia.[31]

More recently, in 1994, the Hutuled Rwandan government massacred 800,000 to 1.1 million people, mostly Tutsis, in a genocide carried out largely with machete-wielding government forces. The massacre took place despite the presence of United Nations "peacekeeping" forces, armed with automatic weapons. The UN troops failed to intervene. The Tutsis were unarmed and helpless against the government assailants.[32]

Civilian disarmament has always preceded genocide in authoritarian and totalitarian states. In the gruesome, but monumental book, *Lethal Laws*, we learn that repressive governments that conducted genocide and mass killings of their own populations have first always disarmed the citizens.[33] The political formula for accomplishing this goal, hallmarks of tyrannical governments, is and remains: public propaganda against firearms, followed step-by-step by gun registration, banning, confiscation, and finally total civilian disarmament. Enslavement of the people then follows easily with limited resistance.[31-34] This is what happened in Nazi Germany, the Soviet Union, Red China, Cuba, and other totalitarian regimes of the twentieth century. In the previous chapter, we contrasted the American experience with short introductory vignettes about the ghastly incidents in Poland, Hungary, and Cuba as they relate to civilian disarmament in both war and peacetime.

When presented with these deadly chronicles and perilous historic sequences, the popular opinion is "it cannot happen here." We have also discussed the danger of such naïveté. As to the dangers of licensing of gun owners and registration of firearms, the same uninformed respondents frequently retort, "If you don't have anything to hide, then you don't have anything to fear!" This is followed by, "I see nothing wrong with gun registration and some restrictions on gun ownership, because we have to do something; there are just too many guns out there that fall into the wrong hands." These naïve attitudes ignore the penchant of governments to accrue power at the expense of the liberties of individuals.[1,17,31-35]

Civilian disarmament is not only harmful to one's freedom and potentially deadly to one's existence but also counterproductive in achieving safety. This has been further attested to by University of Hawaii Professor, Rudy J. Rummel, in his book, *Death by Government*,[31] and by the French scholar Stéphane Courtois and his associates in their monumental volume, *The Black Book of Communism*.[36] These books make it clear that authoritarian governments that limit their citizens' freedom and proscribe them from owning guns are always dangerous to liberty—and the health of humanity. During the 20th century, more than 100 million people were exterminated by their own repressive governments—police states bent on destroying liberty and building communism, socialism, fascism, collectivism, and other worker utopias that turned out to be hells on earth![31-34,36]

Armed People Victorious

In debunking the myth that "guns increase violent crime," Richard Poe, the former editor of *FrontPage Magazine*, rebutted the false assumption that America is more violent than other nations, again emphasizing that more people during the twentieth century were killed in other countries by their own governments than by war, while reaffirming that gun control laws have almost always preceded genocide or mass murder of the people (democide).[17,31]

While the United States and Switzerland have more guns per capita than any of the other developed countries, they also have been very effective historically in preserving their freedom and independence. Even Japan, a country that has embraced democracy and Western mores in many ways, still has the centuries-old tradition of subordination of individualism to the State, and the collective. Japanese citizens have less personal freedom than those of Switzerland where individualism is paramount, and all Swiss adult males are considered part of the militia and are permitted to keep their service rifles at home.

Japan may have a low crime rate, but citizens live in a virtual authoritarian state, where the police keep full dossiers on every citizen, and "twice a year, each Japanese homeowner gets a visit from the local police to update files" on every aspect of the citizen's home life.[1,17]

Switzerland, on the other hand, a small, landlocked country, stood up against the Nazi threat during World War II, because each and every male was an armed and free citizen. (The Swiss republic was the "SisterRepublick" that the American Founding Fathers admired.) Nazi Germany could have overwhelmed Switzerland during World War II, but the price was too steep for the German High Command. Instead, the Nazi juggernaut trampled over Belgium, Luxembourg, Holland, Norway, and other countries, and avoided the armed Swiss nation, the "porcupine," which was prepared for war and its military was ready to die rather than surrender.[17,37]

As to what an armed population, such as those of the original 13 American colonies that later became the United States, did to obtain their independence is a well-known story. Suffice to say, that the shot heard "around the world" on Patriot's Day (April 19, 1775) was precipitated when the British attempted to seize the arms depot at Concord and disarm the American militia at Lexington in the Colony of Massachusetts.[38,39] As to what an armed population can do to prevent the overthrow of their government by oppressive, communist movements, I recommend Larry Pratt's excellent little tome, *Armed People Victorious*. Larry Pratt is Executive Director Emeritus of Gun Owners of America (GOA). *Armed People Victorious* vividly recounts stories of how two countries, teetering on the brink of disaster and as dissimilar as Guatemala and the Philippines, turned defeat into victory when the governments recognized that allowing and encouraging the people to form armed militias to protect themselves, their families, and their villages from communist insurgents in the 1980s, helped to preserve their freedom.[40]

Civilian disarmament remains deadly in the 21st century. During 2018 Daniel Ortega in Nicaragua and Nicolás Maduro in Venezuela avoided popular overthrow and in 2019 continued to wage war against their respective populations because the opposition and the people were disarmed. Like Cuba, Venezuela was once a prosperous nation, but under a military regime bolstering authoritarian socialism, ten percent of the populace (3 million people) have fled, while the remaining citizens have suffered shootings, starvation, and unendurable privations. All of this happened in Venezuela because under Maduro's predecessor, socialist Hugo Chavez, the people were disarmed.[40]

Why is this so important to ordinary Americans? First, because we are all citizens with rights as well as civic duties, and we should understand the historical importance of attaining freedom and the constitutional necessity of preserving it.[32,35,38,40,41] Public health officials and researchers of gun violence have an obligation to reach their conclusions based on objective data, historical experience and scientific information, rather than ideology, emotionalism, expediency, or partisan politics. After all, the lessons of history sagaciously reveal that whenever and wherever science and medicine have been subordinated to the state—and individual freedom has been crushed by tyranny—the results for medical science, public health and society at large, have been as perverse as they have been disastrous, as the barbarity of Nazi doctors and Soviet and Cuban psychiatrists amply testified. Beyond the abolition of freedom and dignity, the perversion of science and medicine becomes the vehicle for the imposition of slavery and totalitarianism.[42-45]

Governments that trust their citizens with guns are governments that sustain and affirm individual freedom. Governments that do not trust their citizens with firearms tend to be despotic and tyrannical.

CHAPTER 25

OFFENSE IS THE BEST DEFENSE FOR ADVOCATING GUN RIGHTS

*I went to the store the other day to buy a bolt for my front
door, for, as I told the storekeeper, the Governor was coming
here. 'Aye,' said he, 'and the Legislature too.' 'Then I will need
two bolts,' said I. He said that there had been a steady demand
for bolts and locks of late, for our protectors were coming.*

—Henry David Thoreau (1817—1862),
Journal, September 8, 1859

Gun rights proponents must keep politicians' feet to the fire by ensuring they
do not propose and pass harmful legislation affecting gun owners and the
rest of the community. Given the level of violence and crime in our society,
gun rights and safety issues should be of importance to all citizens, and
effective methods of self and family protection should be paramount. In
this chapter we summarize some of the new issues and legislation coming
up in the gun rights versus gun prohibitionist debate and point out where
battle lines have been drawn. This includes the latest developments in
the expansion of concealed carry weapons (CCW) legislation; states and
national concealed carry (CCW) reciprocity; CCW on college campuses;
the status of self-defense and stand-your-ground legislation; and armed
home protection with the application of the Castle Doctrine.

Specific legislation of importance to gun owners, such as hearing
protection bills and lifting the prohibition against firearm suppressors, are
also discussed. Anti-gun aspects of the ObamaCare law still in place—and

that most citizens are unaware of—are cited and effective proposed remedies propounded.

Before we discuss proposed legislation, we should discuss some of the problems facing lawful citizens both in the street and in their own homes. With crime endemic and terrorism rising, it becomes obvious that extending gun rights proposals are of paramount importance, and that it is essential that citizens assume some responsibilities for their own protection and safety.

Burglaries, Home Invasions, and Forced Entries

Despite the fact that overall crime statistics remain down, the incidence of burglaries and forced entries (home invasions) remain high, too high for those who have been or will become victims. But there is hope on the horizon; recently we have seen more news reports of men and women defending themselves and their homes and families. Reports in NRA and GOA publications and local newspapers are describing citizens fighting back and defending themselves against assailants attempting to break in or in the act of burglarizing their homes.

The 2012 statistics for Macon-Bibb County, Georgia, where I resided until a few years ago, show that while aggravated assaults declined, residential burglaries were up six percent over the previous year. Frequently, repeat offenders and drug addicts perpetrating crime to feed their addictions commit the burglaries. As in many other communities, drug dependence and the associated violence and crime present major problems for law enforcement. And as we have stated repeatedly, the police cannot be everywhere at all times to protect homes and businesses. Visible police presence and patrolling neighborhoods may deter crime temporarily, but unless we turn society into a police state, a remedy worse than the disease itself, law enforcement measures alone will not suffice, and citizens must take some responsibility for their own protection. Firearm training and gun safety courses, and most importantly general awareness that responsible citizens should shoulder some responsibility for personal protection and be willing to defend their homes and families, would go a long way to alleviate the problem.

In 1966 to 1967, the Orlando, Florida local media publicized a gun training and safety course for women taught by the police department. The course was successful beyond expectations, and Orlando's rape rate dropped 88 percent in 1967, while remaining unchanged in the rest of Florida and U.S.[1]

In 1982 in my state of Georgia, the town of Kennesaw (near Atlanta) passed legislation requiring the head of the household to keep at least one firearm in the home for family protection. As you can imagine, an initial furor was raised about the law and its implications. Nevertheless, when all the dust had settled, the residential burglary rate had dropped 89 percent in the town, compared to the modest 10.4 percent drop in the state of Georgia as a whole. Ten years later, the residential burglary rate in Kennesaw was still 72 percent lower than it had been in 1981, before the law was passed.[2]

Statistical comparisons with other countries, as we have previously commented, demonstrate that burglars in the United States "are far less apt to enter an occupied home than their foreign counterparts who live in countries where fewer civilians own firearms." Burglaries occur in the United States with only a 12.7 percent occupancy rate; while in the social democracies of Great Britain, Canada, and Netherlands, the occupancy rate average for those three nations was 45 percent. The occupancy rate relates to the percentage of time that homeowners are present at home during commission of a burglary. Obviously burglars do not fear defenseless homeowners but defy them in those countries.[3]

As progressively stricter gun control laws were enacted in Great Britain, where citizens have no legal right to self-defense, much less to protect their property, crimes such as burglaries and auto theft, have escalated. For example, in England, people are nearly twice as likely to be robbed, assaulted, or have their vehicle stolen than in the United States. Home and business burglaries also continue to be a problem in all of Great Britain, while they declined in comparably small communities in the U.S., where criminals know that a large proportion of citizens are armed. Ditto for motor vehicle theft; it has risen in England because criminals know Britons are unarmed at home as well as in their cars.

In the early 1980s, Professors James D. Wright and Peter Rossi conducted a study funded by the U.S. Department of Justice that found that felons feared armed citizens more than the police.[4] We have already seen that since the 1990s, criminologists John Lott and Gary Kleck have substantiated and expanded on the earlier findings of Wright and Rossi, and have in fact provided mounds of additional data.

Promoting Family and Home Protection

According to government data, including the FBI Supplementary
Homicide Report, there are approximately 400 felons killed by police officers
or justifiable homicides yearly in the U.S. In 2012, for example, there were
426 such justifiable homicides.[5] Yearly, armed citizens shoot and kill more
criminals than do police, at least twice as many. Professor Gary Kleck found
that good citizens kill between 606 to 1527 attackers and violent criminals
in self-defense (or in justifiable homicides) every year. Citizens in fact have
a better track record than do the police in shooting the bad guys: "Only two
percent of civilian shootings involved an innocent person mistakenly identified as a criminal. The 'error rate' for the police, however, was 11 percent, more
than five times as high."[6] The reason citizens do a better job than the police
is because they are already on the scene. They witnessed what happened or
were the actual victims, so they know who the bad guys are, while the police
enter a scene in progress and must make judgments that occasionally turn
out to be wrong.

But sound data, even when analyzed by the foremost criminologist Gary
Kleck and corroborated by other investigators, pose no obstacle for anti-gun
propagandists. Facts are simply ignored and whatever contrary data they
attain are tortured until they confess. In 2012 the Violence Policy Center
(VPC) claimed, in an article published in one of their progressive allied media
outlets, the *Los Angeles Times*, that good citizens killed only 259 criminals
each year. To the VPC activists and the writer of the article, the 259 figure
of criminals killed by citizens in the commission of crimes or violent acts
was very small. In other words, the beneficial or defensive shooting deaths
in comparison with the 1.2 million violent crimes committed that same year
did not reflect much of a benefit in gun ownership.[6]

The *Los Angeles Times* writer suggested that, for a nation with over 300
million guns and one-third of citizens having guns in their homes, the number
of killings in self-defense were minuscule. He wrote, "This is also a nation
in which, in 2012, there were 1.2 million violent crimes, defined as murder,
forcible rape, robbery and aggravated assault. Or, put another way, 1.2 million
scenarios in which there was potential for someone to kill in self-defense."[6]

It is true that violent crimes are defined as murder, forcible rape, robbery
and aggravated assault, but that is about where the facts and in-depth analysis

end in that article. First, because the FBI Uniform Crime Report makes the assignation of "justifiable homicide" from the preliminary data of the reporting officer, and not from final determination, "justifiable homicides" are underreported. Up to 20 percent of the initially classified "homicides" are eventually judged to be "justifiable homicides" but they do not appear as such in the final data. Thus the correct figures, as we reported earlier, are that between 606 to 1,527 criminals are killed by good citizens in self-defense (or in justifiable homicides) every year. The 259 figure is way off the mark. Armed citizens killed at least twice and as many as three times the number of criminals as do police, as we discussed earlier.

Second, the assertion that only "one-third of citizens have guns in the home," is incorrect; in fact, it is double that percentage because it is under-estimated by another one-third, as we previously explained and documented in discussing gun surveys in Chapter 4. Third, the beneficial aspect of gun ownership, as a deterrent to crime, once again, was also vastly underestimated; to be sure, it's misrepresented. The VPC, the *Los Angeles Times* writer, and other anti-gun propagandists, forget that behind the scene, up to 2 million to 2.5 million defensive uses of firearms occur yearly, including criminal acts foiled by lawful citizens using guns to protect themselves, their families and their property. In over 90 percent of cases, there was no need for the firearms to be fired; merely displaying the weapon was enough to deter crime, although the citizen must be prepared to use the firearm if the need arises. Most of those instances of preventive gun uses go unreported, but we know about them from the work of criminologists Gary Kleck and John Lott, Professors James Wright and Peter Rossi, as well as the various studies carried out by the Department of Justice over the years. We have discussed the beneficial aspects of gun ownership at length in both Chapters 4 and 16 and at various points throughout this book.

The good guys (the cops and the armed citizens) do not kill unnec-essarily as violent criminals do, but only when they absolutely have to in self-defense or protecting others. Violent offenders, many of them repeat criminals, kill in the commission of crimes to get away with the criminal act and display little regard for human life. Some even kill for the sake of killing, so killings of innocent victims will always surpass the number of justifiable homicides when comparing body counts. As Kleck has shown, every 48 seconds a good citizen defends himself (or herself) against an attacker, even though the act of self-defense in most cases did not result in shooting the assailant or even firing the gun, but only in displaying the weapon to frighten away the attacker.[6] Thus, the counting of bodies of innocent victims versus those of the criminal element is unreliable as a measure of the protective benefits of firearms.

As we have said previously, when quoting Dr. Edgar Suter:

> *The true measure of the protective benefits of guns are the lives saved, the injuries prevented, the medical costs saved, and the property protected—not the burglar or rapist body count. Since only 0.1 percent to 0.2 percent of defensive gun usage involves the death of the criminal, any study, such as this, that counts criminal deaths as the only measure of the protective benefits of guns will expectedly underestimate the benefits of firearms by a factor of 500 to 1,000.*[7]

The *Los Angeles Times* writer also tried to play down Kleck's previously cited figure of up to 2 million to 2.5 million beneficial uses of firearms per year, instead citing a Federal Bureau of Justice Statistics' National Crime Victimization Survey (NCVS) that, according to the article, puts the number at a much lower figure of 67,740 times a year. We disagree on many counts with the *Los Angeles Times* article. First the NCVS is the only study to make such a claim, and Kleck and Suter among others have pointed out its unreliability because it is study of victimization and not about defensive gun use. To make matters worse, respondents in the NCVS are denied anonymity. As such, it vastly underestimates defensive uses of firearms by at least an order of magnitude.[6]

We have already cited various reports, including the one by the Department of Justice done at the time of the Clinton administration disclosing that up to 1.5 million beneficial gun uses take place every year. Yet, evasion and deliberate ignorance about defensive gun uses continue to the present. Another investigation that was not given the attention it deserved was a momentous study that was actually farmed out by the CDC to the Institute of Medicine and National Research Council. It found that while there were "about 300,000 violent crimes involving firearms in 2008," the estimated number of beneficial or defensive uses of firearms ranged, "from about 500,000 to more than 3 million per year."[7] This was a major study, this time during the Obama administration, which public health officials, the mainstream media, and Obama's Justice Department, all attempted to suppress, just as Clinton's Department of Justice study had been neglected and buried under layers of obfuscation and red tape.

Nevertheless, those seeking real answers uncovered and spoke the unpalatable truth that neither the Clinton nor the Obama administration wanted to hear. The Institute of Medicine study even cited the work of Kleck and Gertz (1995) as foundational research, underscoring the often ignored proposition that armed self-defense is an important deterrent to crime.[7] The mainstream liberal media, including *The Washington Post*, attempted to give the study deceptive spins, and when this did not work, they opted for ignoring the findings.

As far back as 1994, we explained the issue of surveys very clearly, and we still stand by Professor Kleck's original estimate of up to 2 million to 2.5 million beneficial gun uses per year because of the problems we have already discussed regarding survey questionnaires, understandable evasions, and underreporting, particularly when the questions concern guns used or present in the home, as discussed in Chapter 4. Evasive answers to survey questionnaires are given with good reason since knowledge of firearms in the home in certain states has resulted later in confiscation, as happened in cities like Washington, D.C., New York, and Detroit. In Chapter 21, we discussed gun confiscation at length not only in New York City and California but also in many other countries where this has taken place.

Some liberal states are presently banning different firearms, banning certain types of ammunition, trying to register guns, and presumably making preparations for confiscation when the Democrats gain power in the nation's capitol. So it's very understandable that the people are very leery of answering survey questionnaires truthfully when it comes to gun ownership. In the *JAMA* survey and in Prof. Kleck's studies, one-third of people will deny gun ownership when in fact they have guns in the home; and when no crime has been completed, most citizens will not report incidents in which they use guns to protect themselves and their property.

As if to justify their fears, in July 2017, the Democrat governor of Oregon signed into law a gun confiscation bill in that progressive state. According to GOA, the law calls for confiscation of property without due process or accusation; allows bureaucrats without mental health credentials to make determinations as to a gun owners' state of mind; and empowers judges to confiscate recently purchased firearms without cause.[8]

The point is that citizens in every state must remain vigilant. While gun rights activists have made considerable progress advancing a pro-Second Amendment agenda in many states, as well as on the national level, some states, like Massachusetts, New Jersey, Maryland, Oregon, and California, have become more restrictive. Californians should take notice; it is the state with the most mass-shooting incidents and one with the most restrictive gun laws. On July 4, 2016, just before getting on his plane for a European vacation, Governor Jerry Brown signed six sweeping gun control bills out of eleven prepared by the California legislature.[9]

Dr. Timothy Wheeler believes the people of California are not aware of their gradual loss of freedom, believing this incremental increase in gun restrictions is directed at criminals, merely crime control legislation. Because certain guns, magazines, and rifles have been criminalized by the stroke of the governor's pen, millions of Californians may have become instant criminals and they don't even know it. As if that were not enough, a rabid anti-gun California legislator even threatened to go door to door, make a sweep of every house, looking for illegal possession or unregistered weapons, lamenting only that they did not have the resources to do it. So much for liberty in California![9]

It should be reemphasized that despite the tremendous increase in gun sales and gun availability in the U.S., gun crime has steadily fallen in the last two decades. Because the truth is that guns in the hands of the law-abiding citizens deter crime and encourage a mutually respectful community. With the growing trend of concealed carry weapons (CCW) licensing, many states are now reaping the benefits. Criminals do not know who in the public is armed, and before considering commission of a crime, they must also consider whether they could be shot in the process. CCW based in most states on "shall issue" requirements is very beneficial legislation that will be discussed later in the chapter.

Hearing Protection Legislation

Another important issue that is gaining momentum and one strongly supported by Gun Owners of America (GOA) is hearing protection legislation by lifting the prohibition against firearm suppressors. The Hearing Protection Act is one such federal legislation aimed at allowing citizens to use firearms suppressors to protect their hearing when firing guns in sports shooting, hunting, or home protection. Existing laws lump suppressors with illegal machine guns and sawed-off shotguns as prohibited items that require difficult special exemptions. Under legislation proposed by Senator Mike Crapo (R-ID) and Congressman Jeff Duncan (R-SC), citizens who can lawfully buy firearms would be allowed to also buy suppressors.

Noise reduction is a safety issue that needs addressing, and suppressors may be the answer. But they have been erroneously referred to as "silencers" in the past, which is a misnomer because suppressors do not silence a firearm; they merely decrease the noise level to the same level as commonly used hearing protection devices. Suppressors are not at all like the fictional silencers so commonly depicted in Hollywood movies, where they are utilized by criminals in armed robberies or by professional hit men in assassinations. GOA emphasizes, "while suppressors protect the hearing of shooters, including the young and hearing-impaired, they are of almost no value to criminals."[10]

One would expect the AMA and other "organized medicine" groups to support the two bills now in Congress that would prevent permanent hearing loss in millions of Americans involved in shooting sports or hunting. But they are not supporting either the Hearing Protection Act or the Silencers Helping US Save Hearing Act (SHUSH). DRGO strongly supports the widespread use of firearm suppressors as a public health measure to prevent irreversible hearing loss. Dr. Timothy Wheeler, a retired head and neck surgeon, and founder and past director of DRGO, described the benefits of this legislation:

> *The Hearing Protection Act would remove Al Capone-era*
> *federal restrictions on firearm silencers or suppressors. The*
> *Act's repeal of the $200 transfer tax, the months-long wait,*
> *and the mountain of red tape would afford American hunters*
> *and sport shooters wider access to a safety device known to*
> *preserve hearing. SHUSH would go even further, defining*

*suppressors as just another firearm safety accessory, which
they are.*[11]

Dr. Wheeler expressed dismay at the position taken by "organized medicine" on the subject:

> *But the American Medical Association (AMA), the American
> College of Physicians (ACP), American College of Surgeons
> (ACS), and the American Academy of Pediatrics (AAP) not
> only refuse to support doing away with the outdated restric-
> tions. They won't even promote the use of suppressors as a
> valuable public health solution. Even the group representing
> ear doctors, the American Academy of Otolaryngology-Head
> and Neck Surgery, has decided officially to refuse their support
> of both this hearing-saving tool and the legislation that would
> make it widely available to their patients.*[11]

This stand is indeed as untenable as it is incredible. Once again "organized medicine" follows ideology and political expediency, joining the left
side of the political spectrum and opting against the medical aphorism that
patients come first. This is the opposite of the code of ethics of the conservative Association of American Physicians and Surgeons (AAPS), whose
motto remains *omnia pro aegroto*, "All for the patient," and still upholds the
Hippocratic dictum, *primum non nocere*, "First Do No Harm." As usual, the
medical politicians of the AMA chose the trappings of power and liberal
politics over science and the interests of their patients. The refusal of "organized medicine" to endorse this legislation is in Dr. Wheeler's view a moral
failure. In the view of many other physicians, it barely falls short of criminal.

Given our constitutional federalist system so marvelously conceived
by our Founding Fathers, several states on their own prerogative are leading
the way in experimenting with the application of good laws throughout the
Republic, laws that could benefit the public, even if the federal government
lags behind. We have seen this with "shall issue" concealed carry legislation and in allowing the carrying of firearms for self-protection on college

campuses, and we will eventually see it with hearing protection and other issues. Unfortunately, immediately after the Las Vegas shooting on October 1, 2017, House Republican leaders, after appropriately calling for unity and prayers, reported that the hearing protection bill that a House panel had supported the previous month to ease the regulations on suppressors, would be shelved indefinitely.[11]

In July 2018, the late Senator John McCain (R-AZ) sabotaged the effort to repeal ObamaCare, and the Republican-led Congress failed to come up with an alternative. GOA members and many citizens remain understandably concerned about the anti-gun provisions still in place in the health care law. It is therefore commendable that Senator Rand Paul (R-KY) introduced an amendment to the law. This amendment has provisions:

> *Which would prohibit insurance companies from asking about gun ownership or discriminating against gun owners; prohibit the government from forcing doctors to enter gun information into a federal database; prohibit the ATF from trolling the national health database for names of people with Post Traumatic Stress Disorder (PTSD), ADHD, Alzheimer's Disease, et cetera—for the purpose of sending their names to the national gun-ban list (which is essentially what has happened to more than 257,000 military veterans).[12]*

Unfortunately, most of the ObamaCare legislation that could affect gun owners remains intact, and Senator Paul's amendment has yet to be considered.

College Campus Concealed Carry

Carrying a concealed weapon on a college campus is another momentous issue for gun right proponents. When the topic was first brought up, gun control activists and their allies in the mainstream liberal media prognosticated that guns on campuses would increase gun violence and crime. The fact is that since the time campus carry took effect in Colorado in 2003, nearly 15 years ago, no campus concealed carry (CCW) holder has committed any crime or become a mass shooter, despite the dire predictions made by gun prohibitionists that CCW holders would turn campuses into Wild West shooting galleries.[13] Yet, despite the fact that the grim prognostication has not come true, the unfazed gun prohibitionists continue to augur dire predictions, as state after state passes concealed carry legislation. Eleven states, including my state of Georgia, now have legal provisions allowing concealed carry on their college campuses. And an additional 23 states allow their colleges to make the decision of whether or not to allow concealed carry by students and professors on their campuses.

University of West Georgia adjunct law professor Jason W. Swindle, Sr., a proponent of campus carry, discussed some of the concerns. To the complaint that "guns in the college lifestyle of drinking and partying would be a disaster," Professor Swindle replied, "First, it is unlawful for a licensed concealed permit holder to carry while under the influence of drugs or alcohol. Licensed holders went through the proper steps, underwent a background check, and were licensed by a probate judge. Logic would dictate that these class of gun owners possess the highest level of responsibility and thus would not carry while drinking."[13]

Swindle also demolished the argument that "gun-free zones" (GFZ) are safe. He pointed out that criminals prey on the weak and helpless, and that GFZs are areas where people are defenseless and not able to protect themselves from criminal predators. That is why they strike in those areas such as schools, some campuses, workplaces and other GFZs. He cites a study by the Crime Prevention Research Center that found that "92 percent of mass shootings in public places between 2009 and 2014 were in GFZs."[13] Dr. John Edeen, a pediatric orthopedic surgeon in San Antonio, Texas and DRGO member is active in seeking the right to carry for qualified hospital staff to prevent or stop mass-shooting incidents from taking place in the GFZ health care setting, where deranged gunmen or terrorists could kill the sick and vulnerable with impunity.

"Shall-Issue" CCW and "Constitutional Carry"

Liberalization of concealed carry and unrestricted carry are spreading through the states like wildfire, and gun control proponents are helpless to stop it. Despite millions of dollars spent by progressive foundations and gun prohibitionists, such as the notorious anti-gun billionaire Michael Bloomberg, CCW licensing continues to spread throughout the states and eventually we will have national CCW reciprocity, as we shall discuss shortly.

Several years ago, my state of Georgia enacted a "shall issue" concealed carry law. "Shall issue" refers to a legal requirement that a jurisdiction must issue a license to carry a concealed handgun to any applicant who meets a specified set of reasonable requirements. Implicit in "shall issue" is the understanding that an applicant need not demonstrate a specific need or "good cause." Thus, the jurisdiction does not have the power to exercise discretion in the awarding of licenses, but "shall issue" them because the permit holders are subject to only meeting specific criteria written in the law. Therefore most citizens should have concealed carry weapons (CCW) permits issued on demand.

The issue now in Georgia has gone beyond "shall issue" CCW to "con-stitutional carry" (CC), which means "unrestricted carry" or "permit-less carry"—e.g., "the ability of any law-abiding citizens to have in their posses-sion a handgun anywhere in public without a license," just as was intended by the Founders. The proposition that free citizens have the natural right to possess and carry firearms was expounded upon by Alexander Hamilton and James Madison in the *Federalist Papers,* not to mention most of the other Founding Fathers, most prominently perhaps by Thomas Jefferson and the Anti-Federalists in their writings and political speeches. While CC is a step forward in the direction of liberty, not all of those 16 states that have adopted "constitutional carry," really have fully unrestricted carrying. Some of the states have various restrictions such as "allowing the practice only outside of city limits, others limit the practice only to their own residents. Some require the firearm to be displayed or 'open-carried,' still others insist that it be concealed."[14]

Prior to 1990, there were very few states with "shall issue" concealed carry laws. Beginning with Florida in 1987 and over the next 30 years, states began to pass CCW legislation like wildfire,[15] and presently most states have approved either "shall issue" concealed carry weapons (CCW) licensing or laws for "constitutional carry," which as we have explained, means that a person can exercise their Second Amendment right openly and does not need a permit at all to carry a concealed, and in some states, a handgun openly. Twenty-nine states have CCW and eight states have "constitutional carry" freedom legislation.

There are 16 million concealed carry permit holders in the U.S. with eight percent of Americans having permits. California and New York have "may issue" licenses, where the citizens may apply for a license by expressing need, but the privilege is so stringent that, even after providing evidence of a pressing need, licenses are frequently delayed or denied, and citizens have been killed while waiting to obtain one, as we have seen in Chapter 16.

Before the American Civil War most states were "constitutional carry." After the Civil War, many states began to add gun control restrictions, and strict "may issue" gun licensing became the norm, presumably to keep guns away from minorities, particularly blacks after the civil war in the North and after reconstruction in the South.[16]

Following the lead of Florida in 1987 and its favorable experience, states began to opt for "shall issue." Today, states can remain "may issue" or take a step towards liberty and go for "shall issue" or "constitutional carry," depending on the politics of the state.[15,17] An important measure of personal freedom is the level of trust that each state places on its citizens' right to possess firearms—that relationship of freedom and trust increases substantially from "may issue" to "shall issue" and "constitutional carry."

All citizens should support either CCW or CC legislation, depending on the political possibilities of the state of residency. Let's now consider the problems that we mentioned at the beginning of this chapter—namely, what are lawful citizens to do when their lives are threatened by thugs in the streets and in their own homes?

The Castle Doctrine and Stand Your Ground

In Chapter 18 and thereafter, we discussed the ethics and moral principles bolstering the individual right to self-defense and how these principles were derived from the twin pillars of Western civilization—namely, our Judeo-Christian and Graeco-Roman legacies. We also discussed the 17th century contribution of the English philosopher and empiricist John Locke to the Anglo-American inheritance of freedom and the inalienable natural rights of the individual. We now proceed to discuss the principles of Anglo-American jurisprudence that bear on the legal right of citizens to protect themselves (and their families) at home or in public places.

The Castle Doctrine derives from the dictum of the great English states-man and jurist, Sir Edward Coke (1552—1634). A proponent of the English common law, Coke wrote, "The house of every one is to him as his castle and fortress, as well for his defense against injury and violence, as for his repose."[18] This tradition in English jurisprudence of a man's home being his castle and his natural right as a free man to keep and bear arms for his own protection and for the defense of the realm was reaffirmed by William Blackstone in England (1755). According to Blackstone:

> *And the law of England has so particular and tender a regard to the immunity of a man's house, that it stiles it his castle, and will never suffer it to be violated with immunity: agreeing herein with the sentiments of ancient Rome, as expressed in the works of Tully. For this reason no doors can in general be broken open to execute any civil process; though, in criminal causes, the public safety supersedes the private. Hence also in part arises the animadversion of the law upon eaves-droppers, nuisancers, and incendiaries: and to this principle it must be assigned, that a man may assemble people together lawfully without danger of raising a riot, rout, or unlawful assembly, in order to protect and defend his house; which he is not permit-ted to do in any other case.*[19]

That tradition of freedom was transferred to America with the English colonists and became the bedrock of Anglo-American jurisprudence. When the colonies became a nation and formed the United States, the freedom legacy was enshrined in our founding documents.[18,20,21]

At least 46 states have in place the Castle Doctrine that defines a man's home as his "castle," where no one can enter without his consent, and where he may use deadly force to protect it. The next important freedom legislation is "stand your ground."[22,23]

Georgia is one of the 24 states that has passed "stand your ground" legislation. According to Georgia statue, a person may use deadly force in defense of habitation and has a right to "stand his ground," with "no duty to retreat from the use of such force and shall not be held liable to the person against whom the use of force was justified or to any person acting as an accomplice..."[22] The law also carries the requisite that the person must be lawfully present where he is threatened and must not have been engaged in illegal conduct at the time.

Moreover, in Georgia an automobile is an extension of a person's home, an extension that he also has a right to defend. Again, self and family protection by law-abiding citizens is not vigilantism, but a duty of citizenship, and a desirable expedient for home and self protection against burglaries, forced entries, and potentially more dangerous crimes, such as home invasion, aggravated assault, and rape—serious, violent crimes, which are committed and which remain at endemic rates, too high for comfort.

Generally "stand your ground" refers to a situation wherever one happens to be legally, such as a street or public business; whereas the Castle Doctrine refers to one's own domicile, such as home, garage, yard, et cetera. Twenty-four states have "stand your ground" laws in place, while 17 states have imposed a duty to retreat. A duty to retreat means that a person can't resort to deadly force in self-defense, if he can avoid the risk of harm or death; this includes for example leaving one's home or place of business, escaping the assailant and running away. It may interest the reader to learn where his state stands on this issue and to familiarize himself with the law of the state where he resides, so he can either prepare himself to protect his home and family or to run for his life when danger presents itself uninvited at the door![23]

Unfortunately, many good citizens do not avail themselves of these favorable gun laws because the media and some politicians continue to demonize guns and associate crime rates with "easy gun availability," despite the accumulating evidence to the contrary. They are also not aware that the police, despite their motto "to protect and serve," cannot be everywhere at all times. They may be minutes away when seconds count. And in the final analysis, the courts have ruled the police do not have a legal obligation to protect individuals; the police owe a duty to protect the community at large (*Bowers v. DeVito*, 1982) but not individual persons, homes, or businesses.

One way to break the cycle of violence is for police and law enforcement officials to announce from time to time and publicize the availability of firearm training and gun safety courses offered by organizations or, even better, by the police departments. By inviting all interested citizens and business owners to take part in firearm training and safety classes, law enforcement can do their part to help law-abiding citizens more safely do their part toward home, self, and family protection.

A Brief Note on the Trayvon Martin-Zimmerman Affair

The shooting death of Trayvon Martin and the subsequent acquittal of George Zimmerman in Miami in 2012 was exploited by the Democrats into a race issue to re-energize a most reliable Democratic base for the November 2012 election, as well as—and a most important issue for us in this discussion—into a test of the Florida's "stand your ground" law.[23] The Democrats sided with the protesters and against the judicial system and the rule of law. At the expense of political strife and racial disharmony, the Democrats sought to ignite opposition against the state's "stand your ground" (also known as, "no duty to retreat") law not only in Florida but also in Georgia, Texas, and the rest of the West, mid-West, and South, and to stem the tide against the expansion of "shall issue" CCW and the whole concept of self-defense.[24] The tide could not be turned, and now the trend is in fact a step forward, for "constitutional carry," the expansion of open or concealed carry to more and all public places where guns can be carried legally, and the extension of the Castle Doctrine from homes to automobiles and businesses.

Concealed Carry Reciprocity

The extension of concealed carry reciprocity (CCR) legislation throughout the states, which is a momentous effort supported strongly by Gun Owners of America (GOA) and the National Rifle Association (NRA), would ensure that lawful citizens are not imprisoned for technicalities, such as traveling in another state while carrying firearms. This is not a hypothetical situation. Pennsylvania concealed carry holder Shaneen Allen was incarcerated for such an unfortunate incident.

The legal basis of CCW reciprocity is the application of Article IV, Section 1, of the U.S. Constitution requiring that states give "full faith and credit" to the "public acts, records and judicial proceedings of every other state. And the Congress may by general laws prescribe the manner in which such acts, records, and proceedings shall be proved, and the effect thereof." Two bills were introduced in Congress that would have moved forward national concealed carry reciprocity (CCR). Representative Richard Hudson (R-NC) and Senator John Cornyn (R-TX) each introduced one such bill early in 2017. Titled the Constitutional Concealed Carry Reciprocity Act of 2017 in the U.S. House of Representatives, the bill would have allowed individuals with concealed carry permits in their state of residence to exercise concealed carry in any other state while abiding by that state's laws, essentially functioning the same as a driver's license.[15]

Concealed carry reciprocity (CCR) refers to the policy of "mutual recognition," in which many jurisdictions recognize a permit or license issued by other jurisdictions. In most cases, this refers to states mutually honoring the licenses granted among them, but not always. Thirty-seven states now have reciprocity agreements with at least one other state, and several states, including Indiana, Kentucky, and Ohio, unilaterally recognize as legal all out-of-state concealed carry weapons (CCW) permits. Some states have special requirements such as undergoing training courses or passing safety examinations and do not honor permits from states without those requirements. In Georgia, we have partial or complete reciprocity with some other states but not with all states. Georgia has mutual reciprocity with Alabama, Florida, Tennessee, North Carolina, and South Carolina. State laws and reciprocity agreements change frequently. Concealed carry permit reciprocity maps are very helpful in determining which states have reciprocity with other states and under what requirements—vital information needed before traveling with firearms from one state to another.[25]

President Trump supported CCR but there remained a vociferous opposition not unexpectedly from California, Chicago, and New York.[17] Nevertheless, momentum gathered in the late summer of 2017 and the bill attained 208 co-sponsors.

As we stated in the prelude to this book, the heinous Las Vegas shooting of October 1, 2017 changed the dynamics of the gun control debate—from a favorable pro-gun atmosphere before the shooting, when the Republican

Congress was ready to take up the aforementioned pro-gun measures, to outright timidity. Suddenly measures such as National Concealed Carry Reciprocity (CCR) and Hearing Protection legislation for easing restrictions on gun suppressors were off the table indefinitely.[26] Instead, "bump stocks," which had been used in the Las Vegas shooting to simulate automatic gunfire, became the subject for discussion, and banning bump stocks became the order of the day.[27]

By mid-autumn, the issue had become intensely hot and some Republicans began to get cold feet about expanding gun rights. Newt Gingrich came out of the woodwork saying cryptically, "as technology changes, sometimes we have to change the rules," suggesting that some gun control was acceptable.[28] Paul Ryan (R-WI) wanted to surrender congressional responsibility for any gun legislation, attempting to drop the issue of bump stocks like a hot potato in the lap of the Bureau of Alcohol, Tobacco, Firearms, and Explosives (ATF), telling them that they could proceed on their own to restrict bump stocks. Senator John Cornyn (R-TX) quit talking about his own bill on national reciprocity. Even President Donald Trump momentarily hesitated and suggested that some other gun measures could be considered, apparently responding to the calls from the press and the usual vociferous Democrats.[26] Yet, it was not until the 2018 high school shooting in Parkland, Florida that President Trump formally directed the U.S. Attorney General to seek comments on a rule banning bump stocks.

In rapid succession came the Halloween truck massacre in New York City (October 31, 2017), where an Islamic terrorist plowed into a crowd, killing eight people and injuring 11 others, all in the name of jihad and ISIS. He was shot by police and hospitalized in critical condition. The shooting in the First Baptist Church in Sutherland Springs, Texas, followed on November 5, 2017. In the little church a madman opened fire, killing 26 and wounding 20 others. The gunman exchanged fire with armed bystander, Stephen Willeford, and then fled the scene apparently wounded. He was pursued by Willeford and another citizen, John Langendorff. Thankfully those two Texas heroes ended what could have been a series of massacres by another deranged malcontent. It was subsequently found that despite a domestic violence conviction and a bad conduct discharge from the military, the madman had been able to buy guns because the Air Force failed to report the guilty verdict to the FBI's National Instant Background Check System (NICS).[29]

Thus, fixing the problems of NICS and closing the alleged gaps in the system became a priority for Congress, including Senator Cornyn of Texas. This legislation, referred to as "Fix NICS" picked up steam in Congress and was added to the House version of the National Concealed Carry Reciprocity (CCR) Act. In the meantime, the gun prohibitionists proceeded with their usual scissor strategy, militating for drastic gun control measures capitalizing on the Las Vegas tragedy. The usual Democrats, including Hillary Clinton, Nancy Pelosi (D-CA), Dianne Feinstein (D-CA), John Lewis (D-GA), Kirsten Gillibrand (D-NY), and company, were on one side pushing for more gun restrictions; while on the other side, the progressivists public health officials and medical editors began clamoring once again for the application of the public health model to the problem of gun violence and justifying their proposals as "reasonable restrictions." At the same time, they were lobbying for more public money and the resumption of the politicized and discredited CDC gun violence research.[30] I responded in several commentaries to the medical editors pointing out not only factual errors but also errors of logic in their editorials and exposed their policy of censoring one side of the gun control debate. Pro-gun physicians continued to be silenced in the medical literature after more than two decades. My letters were not published in the medical journals, but full articles were posted in the *Telegraph* (Macon), *GOPUSA*, and other conservative outlets.[31,32]

Then suddenly, on December 6, 2017, as an anticipated Christmas present, the House of Representatives brought to the forefront and passed the National Concealed Carry Reciprocity (CCR) Act of 2017 that had been sponsored by Congressman Richard Hudson of North Carolina. The bill was approved with some bipartisan support in a 231 to 198 vote (six Democrats crossed over and voted with the GOP, while 14 Republicans joined with the rest of the Democrats to oppose it).[33] By this time Senator Cornyn had decided to withhold bringing up the old version of his bill until the Senate had passed separately the "Fix NICS" legislation. "Fix NICS" was also embraced by gun-prohibitionists Democrats and became the Cornyn-Schumer-Feinstein (S-2135) Bill in the Senate, raising questions as to what exactly this Pandora's box of legislation contained.

Gun Owners of America (GOA) opposed the bill because it would expand the "fugitives from justice" category (the second largest cause for denials) of the NICS and create "fugitives" out of anyone with minor offenses, such as unpaid traffic tickets. It would require states to search for and turn into the NICS names of individuals who are not violent. GOA raised additional objections to the expansion of the NICS, as discussed in Chapter 16, including that it would detrimentally affect military veterans, seniors, nonviolent offenders, and other gun owners, who would unfairly be thrown into the system and lose their gun rights.[34]

The National Rifle Association (NRA), on the other hand, fully backed "Fix NICS," so as to close the loopholes in the system and prevent the misreporting that took place with the shooter in Texas. The NRA denied that there would be "an expansion of disqualifications for gun ownership" or that law-abiding gun owners would be targeted.[35]

Be that as it may, the Fix NICS Act of 2017 passed both houses of Congress with bipartisan support and was signed into law by President Trump on March 23, 2018. Although the GOP garnered two additional U.S. Senate seats in the November 2018 mid-term election (gaining an advantage of 53 to 47), the fate of concealed carry reciprocity (CCR) remains uncertain because anti-gun Democrats attained control of the U.S. House of Representatives. Nancy Pelosi was re-elected Speaker of the House and some of the new Democrat House members are radical and vociferous anti-gun Democratic Socialists who will not compromise on the issue of expanding gun rights. On the other hand, a few Democrat senators may become vulnerable for re-election in 2020 if the CCR bill is brought to the Senate floor for a vote and they vote against it. If they cast anti-gun votes for states that already have CCW or CC in place, they would be denying the citizens of their own states the right to travel to other states with firearms. Moreover, in 2013, seven Democrats voted for a CCR bill.[33] Several of them are still in the Senate and may do so again. But for the next two years at least the U.S. House will remain an impediment for the expansion of gun rights. Only time will tell.

As I wrote at the beginning of this chapter, gun rights proponents must keep the politicians' feet to the fire, remembering that the best defense is a good active offense. Bringing National Concealed Carry Reciprocity to a vote would be the perfect tactic for Republicans to use, regardless of whether or not the GOP has the necessary votes. Bringing CCR to the Senate floor and requiring the members to vote and go on record as to how they stand, not only on the Second Amendment but also with the wishes of their constituents as reflected by the CCW laws of their own states, would be very interesting to watch!

EPILOGUE

*If I have seen further than others, it is by stand-
ing upon the shoulders of giants.*

—Sir Isaac Newton (1642—1727),
English mathematician and physicist

We have documented in this book and made several points about the flawed
gun control research promulgated by the public health establishment (PHE),
disseminated by the medical politicians via the major medical journals, and
then repeated as scientific truths by the mainstream liberal media. We hope
the reader can now reconsider and even rebut that propaganda with the factual
information contained in this book. Let's recapitulate some of those points.

The Public Health Model for Gun Control

The PHE's proposition that gun violence is a public health issue amenable
to study via the public health model has been proved erroneous and faulty. We
have shown how useless and biased studies were conducted by the PHE for
decades. The PHE studies, funded at taxpayer expense, failed to deliver verifiable
scientific information necessary to consider, deliberate, and formulate public
policy that would benefit Americans by reducing violence and crime in our
society. Another proposition, that guns are virulent pathogens is also erroneous.
Guns are not viruses that need to be eradicated from society, but inanimate
objects, useful tools used in sport shooting, hunting, as well as for self, family,
and home protection. It's also the ultimate tool against the inception of tyranny.

The gun research published by the PHE is self-serving, ideological propaganda, concocted to reach preordained conclusions. It is politicized, result-oriented research that can only be characterized as junk science or pseudoscience. Furthermore, over the years, public health investigators have disingenuously ignored the objections to their studies and rebuttals posed by criminologists, sociologists, physicians, and even economists. Instead, they have continued to propagate conclusions that have already been discredited. For these and other reasons as discussed in this book, particularly in Chapters 4 and 5, Congress acted wisely when it banned lobbying by public health officials and restricted gun (control) research conducted at taxpayer expense.

The sociological and criminological approaches to gun violence, on the other hand, have provided far more valuable information with a clear understanding of the problem and its solution—namely that the person who pulls the trigger is responsible and should be held accountable, not the gun, an inanimate tool that can be used to commit crime or to deter crime. In the liberal zeitgeist of our times, we tend to absolve the criminal offenders, who should be held accountable, and instead make excuses and blame society for their criminal actions. In fact, we have seen that Dr. Mark Rosenberg, a PHE figure, once claimed, "Most of the perpetrators of violence are not criminals by trade or profession. Indeed, in the area of domestic violence, most of the perpetrators are never accused of any crime. The victims and perpetrators are ourselves—ordinary citizens, students, professionals, and even public health workers." We have also seen how that claim is fallacious. According to the United States Department of Justice, *the typical murderer has had a prior criminal history of at least six years, with four felony arrests in his record, before he finally commits murder.* Federal Bureau of Investigation (FBI) statistics also reveal that *75 percent of all violent crimes for any locality are committed by six percent of hardened criminals and repeat offenders.* And *less than one to two percent of crimes committed with firearms are carried out by concealed carry weapons (CCW) permit holders.*

There are over 300 million guns approximately matching the U.S. population and kept within at least 50 to 60 percent of American homes. It would take a totalitarian State using police state tactics of banning and confiscation with persecution, informants, police raids, and a war on the citizenry to eradicate firearms from American society, thereby extinguishing liberty in the process and bringing about the death knell of the Republic.

Anti-Gun Propaganda by Omission or Commission

We have urged the mainstream liberal media and Hollywood to quit sensationalizing violence and cease granting celebrity status to criminals and madmen after mass shootings. The mainstream liberal media—either by omission, commission, or distortion—should also cease promulgating erroneous or misleading anti-gun propaganda that has already been rebutted by noted criminologists, sociologists and even physician investigators who presented contrarian and factual information debunking the usual public health propaganda masquerading as science.

An example of misleading propaganda by omission is the lack of coverage of the benefits of firearms; by commission, repeating the spurious claim that a homeowner has a greater chance of being injured by a firearm kept in the home than protecting him or herself from a criminal intruder. In Chapter 16 we reported the most effective method of self-protection, particularly for women, is the firearm. In several chapters, beginning with Chapter 4, we also documented that *the defensive uses of firearms by citizens amount to up to 2 million to 2.5 million uses per year and dwarf the offensive gun uses by criminals. Between 25 and 75 lives are saved by a gun for every life lost to a gun. Medical costs saved by guns in the hands of law-abiding citizens are 15 times greater than costs incurred by criminal uses of firearms. Guns also prevent injuries to good people and protect billions of dollars of property every year.*

Anti-Gun Propaganda by Deliberate Distortion

An example of a deliberate distortion is the claim that only 250 to 300 criminal predators are killed by homeowners or citizens acting in self-defense annually and since serious crimes exceed one million per year, the erroneous conclusion is drawn that guns in the hands of law-abiding citizens do not deter crime.

As pointed out by Dr. Edgar Suter quoted in Chapter 4:

> *The true measure of the protective benefits of guns are the lives saved, the injuries prevented, the medical costs saved, and the property protected—not the burglar or rapist body count.*

Since only 0.1 percent to 0.2 percent of defensive gun usage involves the death of the criminal, any study, such as this, that counts criminal deaths as the only measure of the protective benefits of guns will expectedly underestimate the benefits of firearms by a factor of 500 to 1,000.

Most of the cases where crimes have been foiled because lawful citizens used guns to protect themselves, their families and their property, go unreported. People fear giving information about guns in their home not only to researchers and pollsters but also in reporting gun uses to the police.

We know about these incidents from the work of Professor Gary Kleck, as well as various studies conducted by the Department of Justice over the years. In fact, we also know *that at least 760,000 and up to 2 million to 2.5 million times per year, beneficial uses of firearms take place and which in 90 percent of cases, there is not even the need to fire the defensive weapon*; and John Lott has corroborated the finding that in many instances just displaying the firearm was enough of a deterrence to avoid the commission of a crime, thus saving lives and property without violence and untoward consequences.

Public databases propounded by public health researchers and gun-grabbing politicians, as we inferred in Chapter 12, are not always innocuous, unbiased depositories of scientific data. They can be used as dangerous repositories of information that should be considered personal and private. Databases in the hands of corrupt and zealot government officials can be dangerous to one's health and in the case of gun data, as preliminary steps to banning and confiscation. After all, as we suggested in Chapter 21, even paranoids have enemies, and a government with infinite power can call any person, particularly political enemies or the more affluent, guilty whenever it wants, label him a tax evader, a veritable enemy of the State, and seize his property.

Myth: Gun Availability Means More Crime

Throughout the book, we also debunked the myth that gun availability is the cause of gun violence and crime. Suffice to say at least 50 to 60 percent of U.S. individuals and families have firearms in the home. In fact, we suggested the figure is closer to 66 percent. While the number of firearms in the hands of U.S. citizens has risen significantly from 200 million in 1991 to an excess of 300 million by 2017, the rates of serious crimes, including homicides with firearms and aggravated assaults, have continued to drop in the last 25 years. Despite the myth that more guns result in more crimes, the greatest drop in crimes have been in states where citizens have more guns and are allowed to have CCW licenses or live in constitutional carry states. The state with the most mass shootings (e.g., California) and the cities with the highest rates of serious crimes (Los Angeles, Chicago, Detroit, Baltimore, et cetera) are those with the strictest gun control laws.

Gun prohibitionists keep citing the high rate of gun violence in Washington, D.C., and blame the guns brought in from Virginia. That may be, but then why is the crime rate in Virginia, so much lower than in DC? Virginia has plenty of guns, yet Washington, D.C. has 30 times more gun crimes than Arlington, Virginia, just across the Potomac.[1]

Gun availability and firearms in the hands of the law-abiding, despite the assertion of PHE researchers, does not cause homicides or suicides, as we demonstrated in various chapters and most specifically in Chapters 9 and 10. The root causes of crime are complex and include socioeconomic issues in association with racial strife, general hatred, and the incitement of class envy by political demagogues; failures in the criminal justice and mental health systems; TV, cinema, and video game violence, particularly in idle and impressionable youth; failures in the schools to instruct in hard basic subjects, as well as civics and history, as to prepare students to confront an increasingly complex, technological and stressful future, as well as to prepare them to fulfill the civic duties of citizenship; and the failures in homes and churches to properly instruct the youth in ethics and morality to help them face the stress and uncertainty of life. We discussed these problems at length in Chapter 22.

America's "Gun Culture"—A Beacon of Hope to the World

We have faulted several anti-gun academicians for deliberate errors of omission and commission in many of their gun studies. We should also blame the mainstream liberal media for telling only one side of the story of guns and violence, and ignoring the American chronicles relating to the more encompassing story of guns and freedom. That is why the establishment's media joined with the academic world in praising Michael Bellesiles' fraudulent book, *Arming America*; yet, they tried to ignore—and when that tactic failed—find fault with the legitimate, scholarly books of criminologists Gary Kleck and John Lott, and civil rights attorney Dave Kopel. In the final chapters of this book, I have tried to relate the story that has not been told—that of America, guns, and freedom from the perspective of a personal journey into politics and the gun control movement of the public health establishment. As we close, let's just say that America, guns, and freedom are concepts inextricably entwined in our history and culture.

While those who do not really know America and the blessings of liberty may decry America's "gun culture," we should celebrate it. America's gun culture is not only a feature of American life, but also a beacon of hope and freedom to the world. Western Europeans have the privilege to criticize our "gun culture," lament "our love affair with firearms," while neglecting the fact that it was our guns, our treasure, and our military might that rescued them from the Nazis during World War II. Western Europe could not have rebuilt their countries as quickly as they did without America's protection, friendship, and the economic support generously provided by Americans through the Marshall Plan. It was Americans too who protected them from the Soviets during the Cold War.

Further protection and American generosity allowed them to build up the social safety net they so proudly proclaim. Yet, in the face of their citizens having their houses invaded and being confronted by criminals, their only undignified defense is the duty to shout and run, even from their own homes!

In this dangerous postmodern age of senseless violence, moral relativism, and terrorism, Europe should learn from America to entrust her citizens with liberty and full freedom with responsibilities. This includes the right to keep and bear arms, the right to self-defense, and the right to protect family and property. Even for those who envy America's spirit of innovation, free enterprise, and prosperity, America and her "gun culture" remain the ultimate beacons of hope and liberty for the world.

DRACONIAN GUN LAWS AND KNEE-JERK DEMOCRACY IN NEW ZEALAND

by Miguel A. Faria, M.D.

On April 10, 2019, New Zealand MPs voted almost unanimously to pass draconian gun control laws in the aftermath of the Christchurch mosque shooting. As a result, "military-style semiautomatic firearms" are now banned. New Zealand's Prime Minister Jacinda Ardem stated she would be signing the legislation into law, claiming "these weapons were designed to kill." The fact is these firearms were designed for civilian recreational shooting, and the original military version of these weapons that are fully automatic (true assault rifles) were designed to wound enemy soldiers in war, which tactically is better than killing because they tie up more enemy troops.

The facts surrounding the shooting have also been plagued by misinformation and deliberate media disinformation. Here is another view based on facts that have been hard to extract from the mainstream press.

On March 15, 2019 an Australian man suffering from the mass shooting derangement syndrome undertook a terrorist attack at two Islamic mosques in Christchurch, New Zealand, during Friday Prayer. The attack resulted in 50 dead and at least 40 wounded. Although the man has been described as a right-wing, white supremacist by the internationalist and mainstream liberal media, the reality is that the mass shooter could best be categorized as inhabiting the far left of the political spectrum.

The Islamophobic mass shooter described himself as an eco-fascist, which according to Wikipedia, places him among those who favor "totalitarian government requiring individuals to sacrifice their own interest to the 'organic whole of nature' and which would rely on militarism, expansionism, and possibly racism to defend the land." Obviously, this is far-left totalitarian stuff rather than traditional conservatism or right-wing libertarian philosophy. Two New Zealand nationalist, anti-immigration groups quickly condemned the attack. Nevertheless, MI5 in Great Britain is investigating possible links between the deranged killer and far-right British organizations.

The media have also made a lot out of the killer's alleged support for Donald Trump as a "symbol of white identity," but it neglected to follow through with the fact that the terrorist also admitted that he did not support Trump as a leader or his policies. Be that as it may, Trump was cited as somehow being responsible for the shooting. Moreover, in the terrorist's 73-page manifesto, the deranged killer stated that with the shooting he hoped to encourage drastic gun control laws and thereby cause a race war in America!

Returning to New Zealand, the new drastic gun control laws passed by its parliament represent a massive knee-jerk response to the shooting. New Zealand already has strict gun control laws. The single dissenter in parliament called the knee-jerk action "an exercise in political theater," but it is much worse than that: Thousands of citizens will have to surrender their semiautomatic firearms, a characterization that could be interpreted to include just about all firearms, except for single shot rifles and shotguns. Citizens have until September to comply with the new law or face penalties that include a two to ten-year incarceration.

The deranged madman wanted to promote incendiary gun control laws in America that would result in mayhem; instead he caused drastic gun laws to pass in New Zealand, and they passed without any opposition. We can thank our Founding Fathers for their foresight in drafting our constitution for our American Republic and warning us about the shortcomings of a mass democracy in which the passions of the majority can be aroused in the heat of the moment to pass draconian laws that trample individual rights and promote tyrannical government in the name of safety.

This article was published in haciendapublishing.com, GOPUSA.com, and DRGO in April 2019.

KNIFE CONTROL IN GREAT BRITAIN?

by Miguel A. Faria, MD

In a previous article, I described how news articles coming out of *BBC News* have become so biased and critical not only of President Donald Trump and Republicans but also of our judicial system and crime statistics. The pot I showed was calling the kettle black! In fact in that same article I responded exposing the deplorable crime statistics in Great Britain despite draconian gun control laws. I wrote:

"America has its share of crime, but at least in the U.S. it has been decreasing for decades, while in Great Britain it is increasing exponentially. London has become the crime capital of the world and not just for burglaries, but also for rapes and assaults with guns and knives. And remember knives are prohibited on the streets of London and handguns are prohibited in all of Great Britain."

Great Britain has been swamped with immigrants like much of Europe, many of them contributing not only to common crimes but also terrorism and ethnic strife. "Britain has also become the global capital for acid attacks." Acid attacks require a bit of an explanation. It refers to the horrible mutilating practice by immigrants from India and southeast Asian countries of throwing acid or other corrosive substances in the face of unwary victims, a practice that amounts to more than 800 per year.

Furthermore, I found:

"London has surpassed New York City in serious crimes and murders, something that has not happened in two hundred years, not even at the time of Jack the Ripper and the Whitechapel murders (1888-1891). In fact, the latest crime figures for England and Wales compiled in the fall of 2017 reveal an overall increase in violence and crime that astounded the United Kingdom—a 22 percent rise in rape, 26 percent rise in knife crimes, and a dramatic and even steeper rise in gun offenses—compounding the ascent that was noted in 2016."

And yet, in the past six months (from the time I wrote the article), progressive British Labor politicians are finally admitting the problem of increasing violence—never mind they continue to push for the same failed solutions of gun control and prohibition of self-defense. Incredibly they are now blaming Prime Minister Theresa May for their own failures at crime control in the large cities where their own Labour politicians control municipalities, particularly the industrial districts such as Liverpool and Manchester, not to mention London. Labour politicians recruited a former police official Lord Stevens (Metropolitan Commissioner, 2000-2005) to criticize Mrs. May for alleged "mishandling crime and policing as PM and when she was home secretary." This gives new meaning to the term finger-pointing and misallocation of responsibility.

Where was Lord Stevens when Labour officials and London's Muslim mayor, Sadiq Khan, launched their campaign against using "stop and search" on ethnic groups? Police officials have done nothing to oppose the soft-on-crime policies of Labour politicians in the metropolitan areas. The rank and file police officers are afraid to act. As I reported previously, "London police chief Cressida Dick has admitted, 'constables have become fearful of confronting suspects as they might get into trouble or might not be supported if they had a complaint.' " Now knife violence has become a growing concern in the capital; although knives, as we pointed out, are already prohibited on the streets of London.

This week a BBC article crowed, "Labour leader Jeremy Corbyn said Mrs. May was not doing enough to tackle the root causes of knife crime." Doesn't that sound familiar? Labour has even recruited a "conservative" politician and Home Secretary of the United Kingdom, Sajid Javid, who called for knife crime to be "treated like a disease." It seems gun control tactics from America are crossing the Atlantic to our British cousins to assist them in pushing for knife control as a public health issue in place of crime control. In the meantime, British citizens will have to barricade themselves in their homes, which are no longer their castles, and be prepared to run in the streets as there is no such thing as "stand your ground." Those accosted, mugged, or knifed would be lucky to find a constable when they need him, and one who would be willing to intercede.

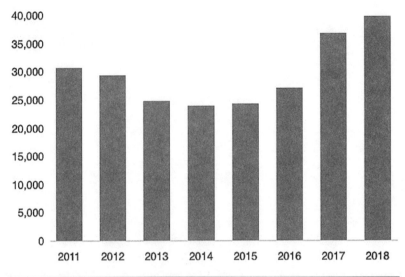

Total knife offences in England and Wales
Offences involving a knife or sharp instrument

Source: Home Office, year ending March except 2017 and 2018 which are year ending September. Figures exclude Greater Manchester. BBC

All the while, women will continue to become rape victims with no right to armed self-defense. When confronted by a rapist, British women have been instructed to run, and if outrun, to shout. The use of any type of weapon to fend off home invasion or to deter a rapist—knives, or God forbid, guns—are forbidden. If all else fails, the only item that a woman is permitted to use is a rape alarm!

So there you have it! This is the status, or rather the nadir, that human dignity has reached for law-abiding citizens in Great Britain, where criminals are coddled, while social and economic justifications are made for their crimes.

This article was published in haciendapublishing.com, GOPUSA.com, and by DRGO in March 2019.

ACKNOWLEDGMENTS

I want to thank my best friend and wife, Helen, for her continued encouragement, proofreading the manuscript, and making valuable suggestions, forcing me to write a better book. I also need to thank her for her research of certain topics that needed clarification and expansion. Nevertheless, any errors are my own. Words of appreciation go to Timothy Wheeler, M.D., founder and past director of Doctors for Responsible Gun Ownership (DRGO), for his support, encouragement, for reading the manuscript, and making valuable suggestions. Again, any errors are mine alone. I want to thank Erich Pratt, executive director of Gun Owners of America (GOA), for explaining to me how the NICS and the FBI databases work and the shortcomings thereof. I also wish to acknowledge Guy Smith, author of the e-book Gun Facts: Version 6.2, for sharing his graphic illustrations so generously. His graphs, compiled from data independent of my investigations, fit hand in glove with the compiled data—each graph depicting a thousand words of understanding. My appreciation is extended to my friend, Russell L. Blaylock, M.D., for using his considerable artistic talents to create the masterful drawings specifically for the book, and also to Miss Rozelle Mae Birador, R.N., for allowing me to use an essential comparative image from her PowerPoint presentation on head injuries in Chapter 18. She has become my good friend and advisor on the Philippines. My thanks and appreciation are also extended to my friend James I. Ausman, M.D., PhD, founder and editor emeritus of Surgical Neurology International (SNI), for graciously giving me full copyright ownership for all the material I had published in SNI for my new publication ventures "to use as I see fit." This was the case with text material previously used in Chapters 22, 23, and 24, as well as the idea for the title of this book. That material though was extensively revised and updated for this book. These friends and colleagues helped me document and write a better book, recognizing though that any errors that may have crept into this tome are totally my own.

REFERENCES/NOTES

PRELUDE

1. Seema Yasmin, "CDC isn't banned from studying gun violence; it's just too scared to do its job," *Dallas Morning News*, June 13, 2016, https://www.dallasnews.com/news/news/2016/06/13/the-cdc-isnt-banned-from-studying-gun-violence-its-just-too-scared-to-do-its-job.
2. "Gun deaths and the gun control debate in the USA," *Lancet*, (October 21) 2017:390:1812, http://www.thelancet.com/journals/lancet/article/PIIS0140-6736(17)32710-1/fulltext; Howard Bauchner, Frederick P. Rivara, Robert O. Bonow, et al. "Death by Gun Violence—A Public Health Crisis." *JAMA*. (October 9, 2017) 2017;318(18):1763-1764, https://jamanetwork.com/journals/jama/fullarticle/2657417.
3. Craig Schneider and Ernie Suggs, "CDC: Politics affected gun violence research," *Atlanta Journal-Constitution,* December 19, 2012, http://www.ajc.com/news/cdc-politics-affected-gun-violence-research/H1aKOO51fbkfMLOehRnyrK/.
4. Joyce Frieden and Molly Walker, "Calls Grow for CDC to Resume Gun Violence Research." *MedPage Today*, October 03, 2017, https://www.medpagetoday.com/publichealthpolicy/healthpolicy/68300.

PART I

CHAPTER 1

1. Daniel D. Polsby, "From the hip." *National Review*, March 24, 1997, p. 34.
2. Edgar A. Suter, "Guns in the medical literature—a failure of peer review," *J Med Assoc Ga* 1994;83(3):137-148.
3. Miguel A. Faria, Jr., "The perversion of science and medicine (Part I): On the nature of science," *Medical Sentinel* 1997;2(2):46-48; and Miguel A. Faria, Jr., "The perversion of science and medicine (Part II): Soviet science and gun control," *Medical Sentinel* 1997;2(2):49-53.
4. Miguel A. Faria, Jr., "Docs, guns, and the CDC," *The New American*, September 30, 1996, pp. 35-38.
5. Patrick W. O'Carroll, Acting Section Head of Division of Injury Control, CDC, quoted in Marsha F. Goldsmith, "Epidemiologists aim at new target: Health risk of handgun

proliferation," *Journal of the American Medical Association* 261, no. 5 (February 3, 1989): 675-676.

6. Patrick W. O'Carroll, "Correspondence: CDC's approach to firearms injuries," *JAMA* 1989;262:348-349.

7. Don B. Kates, Henry E. Schaffer, and William C. Waters IV, "How the CDC succumbed to the gun epidemic," *Reason*, April 1997, pp. 25-29; See also Don B. Kates, Henry E. Schaffer, John K. Lattimer, George B. Murray, Edwin H. Cassem, "Bad Medicine: Doctors and Guns" in *Guns: Who Should Have Them?* David B. Kopel, ed., (Amherst, NY: Prometheus Books, 1995), pp. 233-308.

8. Todd C. Frankel, "Why the CDC still isn't researching gun violence, despite the ban lifted two years ago," *Washington Post*, January 14, 2015, https://www.washingtonpost.com/news/storyline/wp/2015/01/14/why-the-cdc-still-isnt-researching-gun-violence-despite-the-ban-being-lifted-two-years-ago/?utm_term=.3d63ea9a94dc ; See also Emma Goldberg, "These are the U.S. billionaires who back gun control," *Forbes.com*, June 15, 2016, https://www.forbes.com/sites/emmagoldberg/2016/06/15/these-are-the-u-s-billionaires-who-back-gun-control/#335c3ccc7d9e.

9. Timothy Wheeler, "The AMA's Long March for gun control," *Doctors for Responsible Gun Ownership*, August 25, 2015, https://drgo.us/the-amas-long-march-for-gun-control/.

10. Don B. Kates, Henry E. Schaffer, John K. Lattimer, George B. Murray, and E.H. Cassem, "Guns and public health: Epidemic of violence or pandemic of propaganda?" *Tennessee Law Review* 1995;62:513-596. http://www.gunsandcrime.org/epidemic.pdf.

11. John H. Sloan, et al., "Handgun regulations, crime, assaults, and homicides: A tale of two cities." *N Engl J Med* 1988;319:1256-1262.

12. Brandon S. Centerwall, "Homicide and the prevalence of handguns: Canada and the United States, 1976 to 1980," *Am J Epidemiology* 1991;134:1245-1260.

13. Brandon S. Centerwall, "Exposure to television as a risk factor for violence," *Am J Epidemiology* 1989;129:643-652.

14. Brandon S. Centerwall, "Young adult suicide and exposure to television." *Soc Psy and Psychiatric Epid* 1990; 25:121.

15. Miguel A. Faria, Jr., "TV violence increases homicides," *NewsMax.com*, August 17, 2000, https://haciendapublishing.com/articles/TV-violence-increases-homicides.

CHAPTER 2

1. Miguel A. Faria, Jr., "Religious morality (and secular humanism) in Western civilization as precursors to medical ethics: A historic perspective," *Surg Neurol Int* 16-Jun-2015;6:105, http://surgicalneurologyint.com/surgicalint-articles/religious-morality-and-secular-humanism-in-western-civilization-as-precursors-to-medical-ethics-a-historic-perspective/.

2. Jane M. Orient, "Practice guidelines and outcomes research, part I: Insights from the Clinton health care task force," *Medical Sentinel* 1996;1(1):9-10.

3. Jane M. Orient, "Practice guidelines and outcomes research, part II: Scientific pitfalls," *Medical Sentinel* 1996;1(3):10-13.

4. AMA Council on Scientific Affairs, "Assault weapons as a public health hazard in the United States," *JAMA* (June 10)1992;267(22):3067-3070.

5. Edgar A. Suter, " 'Assault weapons' revisited—An analysis of the AMA report," *J Med Assoc Ga* 1994;83(5):281-289, http://rkba.org/research/suter/aw.html.

6. John H. Sloan, et al., "Firearm regulations and rates of suicide: A comparison of two metropolitan areas," *N Engl J Med* 1990:322:369.

7. Arthur L. Kellermann, Frederick P. Rivara, Grant Somes, et al., "Suicide in the home in relationship to gun ownership," *N Engl J Med* 1992;327:467-472.

8. Edgar A. Suter, "Guns in the medical literature—a failure of peer review," *J Med Assoc Ga* 1994;83(3):133-148.

9. Gary Kleck, *Point Blank: Guns and Violence in America* (New York: Aldine de Gruyter, 1991).

10. World Health Organization, "World Health Statistics (1989)," Geneva, Switzerland. More recent statistics are reported in: Vladeta Ajdacic-Gross, Mitchell G. Weiss, et al., "Methods of suicide: international suicide patterns derived from the WHO mortality database," *Bulletin of the World Health Organization* 2008;86:726-732, http://www.who. int/bulletin/volumes/86/9/07-043489/en/.

11. G. Marie Wilt, James D. Bannon, Ronald K. Breedlove, et al., *Domestic Violence and the Police: Studies in Detroit and Kansas City* (Washington DC, Police Foundation, 1977); See also Don B. Kates, Henry E. Schaffer, John K. Lattimer, George B. Murray, and Edwin H. Cassem, "Bad Medicine: Doctors and Guns" in *Guns: Who Should Have Them?* David B. Kopel, ed., (Amherst, NY: Prometheus Books, 1995), pp. 233-308.

12. Edgar A. Suter, William C. Waters IV, George B. Murray, et al., "Violence in America—effective solutions," *J Med Assoc Ga* 1995;84(6):253-264.

13. Miguel A. Faria, Jr., "On public health and gun control," *J Med Assoc Ga* 1995;84(6):251-252.

14. For the history of public health and gun control as written in a series of three articles by Timothy Wheeler, "Public health gun control: A brief history—Part I," *Doctors for Responsible Gun Ownership*, January 3, 2013, https://drgo.us/public-health-gun-control-a-brief-history-part-i/; Timothy Wheeler, "Public health gun control: A brief history—Part II," *Doctors for Responsible Gun Ownership*, January 18, 2013, https:// drgo.us/?p=285; and Timothy Wheeler, "Public health gun control: A brief history—Part III," *Doctors for Responsible Gun Ownership*, February 8, 2013, https://drgo.us/ public-health-gun-control-a-brief-history-part-iii/.

CHAPTER 3

1. Miguel A. Faria, Jr., *Cuba in Revolution: Escape From a Lost Paradise* (Macon, GA: Hacienda Publishing, Inc., 2002), pp. 192-194, 262-263; footnotes #48 and #79 for the systematic persecution and abuse of homosexuals in Cuba.

2. Miguel A. Faria, Jr., *Vandals at the Gates of Medicine: Historic Perspectives on the Battle Over Health Care Reform* (Macon, GA: Hacienda Publishing, Inc., 1994), pp. 242-244.

3. Miguel A. Faria, Jr., "Cuban Psychiatry—The Perversion of Medicine," *Medical Sentinel* Sept-Oct. 2000;5(5):160-162, https://haciendapublishing.com/medicalsentinel/cuban-psychiatry-perversion-medicine.

4. Miguel A. Faria, Jr., "Liberal orthodoxy and the squelching of political or scientific dissent," *HaciendaPublishing.com*, August 19, 2013, https://haciendapublishing.com/articles/liberal-orthodoxy-and-squelching-political-or-scientific-dissent-miguel-faria-jr-md.

5. Russell L. Blaylock, "When rejecting orthodoxy becomes a mental illness," *HaciendaPublishing.com*, August 15, 2013, https://haciendapublishing.com/articles/when-rejecting-orthodoxy-becomes-mental-illness-russell-l-blaylock-md.

6. Michael Fumento, *The Myth of Heterosexual AIDS: How a Tragedy Has Been Distorted by the Media and Partisan Politics* (New York: Basic Books, 1990).

7. David Horowitz, *Radical Son: A Generational Odyssey* (New York: Free Press, 1997), pp. 337-349 for details and description about how authorities in the San Francisco and Los Angeles areas caved in to the radical, gay community and refused to close the dirty, infective gay bathhouses as the death toll from AIDS continued to climb.

CHAPTER 4

1. Howard Wolinsky and Tom Brune, *The Serpent on the Staff: The Unhealthy Politics of the American Medical Association* (New York: G. P. Putnam's Sons, 1994).

2. Arthur L. Kellermann, Donald T. Reay, "Protection or peril? An analysis of firearm-related deaths in the home," *N Engl J Med* 1986;314:1557-1560.

3. Edgar A. Suter, "Guns in the medical literature—a failure of peer review," *J Med Assoc Ga* 1994;83(3):137-148.

4. Arthur L. Kellermann, Frederick P. Rivara, Norman B. Rushforth, et al., "Gun ownership as a risk factor for homicide in the home," *N Engl J Med* 1993;329(15):1084-1091.

5. Don B. Kates, Henry E. Schaffer, John K. Lattimer, George B. Murray, Edwin H. Cassem, "Guns and public health: epidemic of violence or pandemic of propaganda?" *Tennessee Law Review* 1995;62:513-596, http://www.gunsandcrime.org/epidemic.pdf.

6. As a result of the reluctance of some investigators, even those funded by taxpayer money, to share scientific data with other researchers, the *Medical Sentinel,* at the time the official, peer-reviewed journal of the Association of American Physicians and Surgeons (AAPS), established the open data policy for public review of research impacting on the formulation of public policy, see https://haciendapublishing.com/medicalsentinel/medical-sentinel-announces-new-open-data-policy; See also Dan Vergano, "Journal to Post Research Data Online—*Medical Sentinel* editor calls on other journals to follow suit," *Medical Tribune*, September 23, 1999;40(16):1,10.

7. Personal communication via e-mail, 09/21/99.

8. Gary Kleck, "Guns and self-protection," *J Med Assoc Ga* 1994;83(1):42.

9. Don B. Kates and Patricia T. Harris, "How to make their day," *National Review* 1991;43(19):30-32.

10. Gary Kleck, *Point Blank: Guns and Violence in America* (New York: Aldine de Gruyter, 1991).

11. Gary Kleck, *Targeting Guns: Firearms and Their Control* (New York: Aldine de Gruyter, 1997).

12. "*JAMA* 1996 Gun-Owners Survey" quoted in the *Medical Sentinel* 1999;3(2):40.

13. Edgar A. Suter, William C. Waters, George B. Murray, et al., "Violence in America—effective solutions. *J Med Assoc Ga* 1995;84(6):255. For the inflated health care costs of gun violence, see Philip J. Cook and Jens Ludwig, *Gun Violence: The Real Costs* (Studies in Crime and Public Policy, Oxford University Press, 2002). For the reply by gun rights proponents and the calculated savings from defensive gun uses (DGUs), see: Bruce W. Krafft, "Defensive gun uses save the U.S. one trillion dollars per year," *The Truth About Guns*, April 14, 2012, http://www.thetruthaboutguns.com/2012/04/bruce-w-krafft/defensive-gun-uses-save-the-u-s-one-trillion-dollars-per-year/; and Robert Farago, "NBC: 'gun violence' costs $2.8 billion per year (as opposed to $1 trillion saved by DGUs)," *The Truth About Guns*, November 16, 2017, http://www.thetruthaboutguns.com/2017/11/robert-farago/nbc-gun-violence-costs-2-8b-per-year-as-opposed-to-1t-saved-per-year-by-dgus/.

14. John R. Lott, Jr., *More Guns, Less Crime: Understanding Crime and Gun Control Laws* (Chicago: University of Chicago Press, 1998).

15. John R. Lott, Jr., *The Bias Against Guns: Why Almost Everything You've Heard About Gun Control is Wrong* (Washington DC: Regnery Publishing, Inc., 2003).

16. "US Department of Justice 1993 study" reported by *Washington Times*, September 7, 1997, http://www.usdoj.gov.

17. For the flaw *Los Angeles Times,* and VPC report see: Scott Martell, "Gun and self-defense statistics that might surprise you—and the NRA," *Los Angeles Times*, June 19, 2015, http://www.latimes.com/opinion/opinion-la/la-ol-guns-self-defense-charleston-20150619-story.html. For the contrary view, see: Gary Kleck, *Point Blank: Guns and Violence in America* (New York: Aldine de Gruyter, 1991), p.111-116, 148. For the armed citizen track record better than police, see: George F. Will, "Are We 'a Nation of Cowards'?," *Newsweek* (15 November 1993):93; and Edgar A. Suter, William C. Waters IV, George B. Murray, et al., "Violence in America—effective solutions," *J Med Assoc Ga* 1995;84(6):254-256. For the underreporting of justifiable homicides by 20%, see: Gary Kleck, "Crime control through the private use of armed force, *Social Problems*, 1988;35:1-21, and Edgar A. Suter, "Guns in the medical literature—a failure of peer review," *J Med Assoc Ga* 1994;83(3):137-148. For the critique of NCVS underreporting gun uses, see: Edgar A. Suter, William C. Waters IV, George B. Murray, et al., "Violence in America—effective solutions," *J Med Assoc Ga* 1995;84(6):254-256, and Gary Kleck, "Guns and self-protection," *J Med Assoc Ga* 1994;83(1):42.

18. AWR Hawkins, "Research Reaffirms: At Least 760,000 Defensive Gun Uses a year," https://www.ammoland.com/2015/02/researcher-reaffirms-at-least-760000-defensive-gun-uses-a-year/#ixzz4oM7Ua8Qu. Professor Gary Kleck's most recent findings were disclosed in Brian Doherty, "CDC, in surveys it never bothered

making public, provides more evidence that plenty of Americans innocently defend themselves with guns," *Reason*, April 20, 2018, https://reason.com/blog/2018/04/20/cdc-provides-more-evidence-that-plenty-o.

19. David C. Stolinsky and Timothy W. Wheeler, *Firearms—A Handbook for Health Professionals* (Claremont, California: The Claremont Institute, 1999). The California physicians cite as the best documented and corroborated study to be: Gary Kleck and Marc Gertz, "Armed Resistance to Crime: The Prevalence and Nature of Self-Defense With a Gun," *Journal of Criminal Law and Criminology* Fall 1995;86(1):182-183.

20. John R. Lott, Jr., *The War on Guns: Arming Yourself Against Gun Control Lies* (Washington DC: Regnery Publishing, 2016).

CHAPTER 5

1. Jerome P. Kassirer, "Guns in the household," *N Engl J Med* 1993;329(15):1117-1118.

2. William C. Waters IV, Miguel A. Faria Jr., Timothy Wheeler, Don B. Kates, "Testimony before the Subcommittee on Labor, Health and Human Services, Education, and Related Agencies," Washington DC, House Committee on Appropriations, March 6, 1996, Hearing Volume, Part 7:935-970, Archived edition, <http://archive.org/stream/departmentsoflab071996unit#page/944/mode/2up>. See also, Timothy Wheeler, "DRGO's 1996 Congressional Testimony: Defunding Gun Control Politics at the CDC," *Doctors for Responsible Gun Ownership*, April 7, 2016, https://drgo.us/drgos-1996-congressional-testimony-defunding-gun-control-politics-at-the-cdc/.

3. Katherine K. Christoffel, quoted in J. Somerville, "Gun control as immunization," *American Medical News*, January 3, 1994, p. 9.

4. Arthur Kellermann, "Letter to the editor," *J Med Assoc Ga* 1994;83(5):254-255.

5. Arthur Kellermann quoted in the *San Francisco Examiner*, April 3, 1994.

6. Department of Health and Human Services, Centers for Disease Control and Prevention, "Funding Opportunity Announcements, Additional Requirements—AR-13: Prohibition on Use of CDC Funds for Certain Gun Control Activities in DHS-CDC," 2003. Material included in instructions to grant reviewers (2003-2005) while I was a member of IRG of the CDC.

7. Mark Rosenberg quoted originally in *The Rolling Stone*, 1993, cited by Don B. Kates, Henry E. Schaffer, William C. Waters IV, "How the CDC succumbed to the gun epidemic," *Reason*, April 1997, pp. 25-29.

8. C. Kent, "AMA wants CDC gun research funds back," *American Medical News* 1997;40(1):8.

9. Craig Schneider and Ernie Suggs, "CDC: Politics affected gun violence research." *Atlanta Journal-Constitution*, December 19, 2012, http://www.ajc.com/news/cdc-politics-affected-gun-violence-research/H1aKOO51fbkfMLOehRnyrK/.

10. Seema Yasmin, "CDC isn't banned from studying gun violence; it's just too scared to do its job," *Dallas Morning News*, June 13, 2016, https://www.dallasnews.com/news/news/2016/06/13/the-cdc-isnt-banned-from-studying-gun-violence-its-just-too-scared-to-do-its-job.

11. Rebecca Shabad, "Democrats renew push to reverse gun violence research ban," *CBS News*, December 2, 2015, http://www.cbsnews.com/news/ democrats-renew-push-to-reverse-gun-violence-research-restriction/.

12. David Weigel, "Ben Carson open to letting CDC research gun violence." *Washington Post*, October 31, 2015.

13. Dan Good, "Jay Dickey wants law that stopped gun research repealed," *New York Daily News*, December 4, 2015.

PART II

CHAPTER 6

1. Bruce G. Charlton, "Statistical malpractice," *Journal of the Royal College of Physicians* March-April 1996:112-114.

2. Jerry C. Arnett, "Book review: *Junk Science Judo* by Steven J. Milloy," *Medical Sentinel* 2002;7(4):134-135, https://haciendapublishing.com/medicalsentinel/ junk-science-judo-steven-j-milloy.

3. James T. Bennett and Thomas J. DiLorenzo, *From Pathology to Politics: Public Health in America* (New Brunswick, NJ: Transaction Publishers, 2000), pp. 21-115.

4. Steven J. Milloy, *Junk Science Judo: Self-Defense Against Health Scares and Scams* (Washington DC: Cato Institute, 2001), pp. 41-114. I strongly recommend this very readable book for the busy clinician as well as the layman wanting to learn the basis of epidemiology.

5. Centers for Disease Control and Prevention, "Healthy People 2010," https://www.cdc. gov/nchs/healthy_people/hp2010.htm.

6. Thomas D. Brock, *Biology of Microorganisms* (Englewood Cliffs, NJ: Prentice Hall, Inc., 1970), pp. 9-12.

7. Miguel A. Faria, Jr., "The perversion of science and medicine (Part I): On the nature of science," *Medical Sentinel* 1997;2(2):46-48; Miguel A. Faria, Jr., "The perversion of science and medicine (Part II): Soviet science and gun control," *Medical Sentinel* 1997;2(2):49-53; Miguel A. Faria, Jr., "The perversion of science and medicine (Part III): Public health and gun control research," *Medical Sentinel* 1997;2(3):81-82; and Miguel A. Faria, Jr., "The perversion of science and medicine (Part IV): The battle continues," *Medical Sentinel* 1997;2(3):83-86.

CHAPTER 7

1. Steven J. Milloy, *Junk Science Judo: Self-Defense Against Health Scares and Scams* (Washington DC: Cato Institute, 2001), pp. 41-114.

2. Jerry C. Arnett, "Book review: *Junk Science Judo* by Steven J. Milloy," *Medical Sentinel* 2002;7(4):134-135, https://haciendapublishing.com/medicalsentinel/ junk-science-judo-steven-j-milloy.

3. James T. Bennett and Thomas J. DiLorenzo, *From Pathology to Politics: Public Health in America* (New Brunswick, NJ: Transaction Publishers, 2000), pp. 21-115.

4. Miguel A. Faria, Jr., "The perversion of science and medicine (Part I): On the nature of science," *Medical Sentinel* 1997;2(2):46-48; Miguel A. Faria, Jr., "The perversion of science and medicine (Part II): Soviet science and gun control," *Medical Sentinel* 1997;2(2):49-53; Miguel A. Faria, Jr., "The perversion of science and medicine (Part III): Public health and gun control research," *Medical Sentinel* 1997;2(3):81-82; and Miguel A. Faria, Jr., "The perversion of science and medicine (Part IV): The battle continues," *Medical Sentinel* 1997;2(3):83-86.

5. Miguel A. Faria, Jr., "Part 1: Public health, social science, and the scientific method," *Surgical Neurology* 2007;67(2):211-214. https://haciendapublishing.com/articles/public-health-social-science-and-scientific-method-part-i; and Miguel A. Faria, Jr., "Public health—from science to politics," *Medical Sentinel* 2001;6(2):46-49, https://haciendapublishing.com/medicalsentinel/public-health-science-politics.

6. Healthy People 2010, "Fact Sheet: Healthy People in Healthy Communities," pp. 1-5. Unfortunately, the material at the website Healthy People 2010 has been changed and updated to Healthy People 2020 and the language considerably toned down and altered in the ensuing years. http://www.health.gov/hpcomments/2010fctsht.htm.

7. Bruce G. Charlton, "Statistical malpractice," *Journal of the Royal College of Physicians* March-April 1996:112-114.

8. Johns Hopkins Bloomberg School of Public Health—Center for Gun Policy and Research, 2017, https://www.jhsph.edu/research/centers-and-institutes/johns-hopkins-center-for-gun-policy-and-research/index.html.

9. Miguel A. Faria, Jr., "The transformation of medical ethics through time (Part I): medical oaths and statist controls," *Medical Sentinel* 1998;3(1):19-24, https://haciendapublishing.com/medicalsentinel/transformation-medical-ethics-through-time-part-i-medical-ethics-and-statist-control.

10. Miguel A. Faria, Jr., "The transformation of medical ethics through time (Part II): medical ethics and organized medicine," *Medical Sentinel* 1998;3(2):53-56, https://haciendapublishing.com/medicalsentinel/transformation-medical-ethics-through-time-part-ii-medical-ethics-and-organized-medi.

11. Miguel A. Faria, Jr., "Managed care—corporate socialized medicine," *Medical Sentinel* 1998;3(2):45-46, https://haciendapublishing.com/medicalsentinel/managed-care-%E2%80%94-corporate-socialized-medicine.

12. Victor Robinson, *The Story of Medicine* (New York: New Home Library, 1943), pp. 371-520.

CHAPTER 8

1. James T. Bennett and Thomas J. DiLorenzo, *From Pathology to Politics: Public Health in America* (New Brunswick, NJ: Transaction Publishers, 2000), p. 136.

2. Ibid., pp. 80-85; For the asthma inhaler controversy, see pp. 84-85; See also Mark Hemingway, "Obama administration set to ban asthma inhalers over environmental concerns," *Weekly Standard*, September 23, 2011, http://www.weeklystandard.com/obama-administration-set-to-ban-asthma-inhalers-over-environmental-concerns/

article/594113; For the rise in costs of these inhalers causing hardship for families, see Alexander Gaffney, "FDA ban on CFCs in asthma inhalers raised costs for patients, new study finds," *Regulatory Affairs Professionals Society*, May 11, 2015, http://www.raps.org/Regulatory-Focus/News/2015/05/11/22139/ FDA-Ban-on-CFCs-in-Asthma-Inhalers-Raised-Costs-for-Patients-New-Study-Finds/.

3. Bennett and DiLorenzo, *From Pathology to Politics: Public Health in America*, p. 137.

4. Ibid., p. 33.

5. Ibid., p. 35.

6. Ibid., p. 37.

7. Ibid., p. 39.

8. Ibid., p. 124.

9. Ibid., p. 125.

10. American Public Health Association (APHA), "Transforming Health Systems," APHA.org, September 4, 2017, https://apha.org/topics-and-issues/health-reform/ transforming-health-systems.

11. Bennett and DiLorenzo, *From Pathology to Politics: Public Health in America*, p. 60.

12. American Public Health Association (APHA), "Tell Congress to pass common-sense measures to reduce gun violence," APHA.org, September 4, 2017. For lobbying Congress, see posted message at https://secure3.convio.net/apha/site/ Advocacy?cmd=display&page=UserAction&id=1205.

13. Bennett and DiLorenzo, *From Pathology to Politics: Public Health in America*, pp. 96-98.

14. Ibid., p. 99.

15. Ibid., p. 100.

16. Ibid., p. 102.

17. Ibid., p. 104.

18. Ibid., p. 138.

19. Ibid., p. 108.

20. Ibid., p. 105.

21. Ibid., p. 95.

PART III

CHAPTER 9

1. Miguel A. Faria, Jr., "Women, guns, and disinformation," *NewsMax.com*, February 21, 2001.

2. David B. Kopel, "The facts about gun shows," The Cato Institute, Jan. 10, 2000; See also Miguel A. Faria, Jr., "Gun shows under fire," *NewsMax.com*, April 27, 2001.

3. "AGS continues to lie to promote attacks on gun shows," *NRA/ILA* Fax Alert, Vol. 9, No. 4, January 25, 2002, p. 2.

4. "Americans for Gun Safety," *Third Way*, September 5, 2017, http://www.agsfoundation. com.

5. Bob Owens, "FAIL: Violence Policy Center is caught fabricating anti-gun data. Again. Still," *BearingArms.com*, April 29, 2014, https://bearingarms.com/bob-o/2014/04/29/ fail-violence-policy-center-is-caught-fabricating-anti-gun-data-again-still/; See also John Lott's Crime Prevention Research Center, https://crimeresearch.org/.

6. Matthew Miller, Deborah Azrael, David Hemenway, "Firearm availability and unintentional firearm deaths, suicide, and homicide among 5-14 year olds," *J Trauma* 2002;52(2):267-275.

7. "New Harvard University study shows direct link between gun availability and gun death among children," *Violence Policy Center*, press release, February 21, 2002.

8. For the number of criminals killed by both police and armed citizens see, Gary Kleck, *Point Blank: Guns and Violence in America* (New York: Aldine de Gruyter, 1991), p.111-116, 148, and Edgar A. Suter, William C. Waters IV, George B. Murray, et al., "Violence in America—effective solutions," *J Med Assoc Ga* 1995;84(6):254-256. For the homicides that turn out to be "justifiable homicides" of criminals by armed citizens, see: Gary Kleck, "Crime control through the private use of armed force, *Social Problems*, 1988;35:1-21, and for the benefits of firearms, wee: Edgar A. Suter, "Guns in the medical literature—a failure of peer review," *J Med Assoc Ga* 1994;83(3):137-148.

9. Brandon S. Centerwall, "Exposure to television as a risk factor for violence," *Am J Epidemiology* 1989;129:643-652.

10. Miguel A. Faria, Jr., "TV violence increases homicides," *NewsMax.com*, August 17, 2000, https://haciendapublishing.com/articles/TV-violence-increases-homicides.

11. Craig A. Anderson, Leonard Berkowitz, Edward Donnerstein, et. al., "The influence of media violence on youth," *Psychological Science in the Public Interest*, December 2003, Vol. 4, No. 3, pp. 81-110. http://journals.sagepub.com/doi/ abs/10.1111/j.1529-1006.2003.pspi_1433.x.

12. "Violence in the media: psychologists study potential harmful effects," *Psychology: Science in Action*, September 5, 2017. http://www.apa.org/action/resources/research-in-action/protect.aspx.

13. National Center for Education Statistics, *NCES Fast Facts, Table 16: Average proficiency in reading for 4th graders in public schools, by selected characteristics, region, and state, 1994*, https://nces.ed.gov/pubs98/98018/data/tab16.xls.

14. "Open-data, public review policy of the Medical Sentinel of the Association of American Physicians and Surgeons (AAPS)," *Medical Sentinel* 1999;4(6):193-195.

CHAPTER 10

1. Matthew Miller, Deborah Azrael, David Hemenway, "Firearm availability and unintentional firearm deaths, suicide, and homicide among 5-14 year olds," *J Trauma* 2002;52(2):267-275.

2. "New Harvard University study shows direct link between gun availability and gun death among children," *Violence Policy Center*, February 21, 2002, press release, http://www. vpc.org/press/0202study.htm.

3. Walter Williams, "An ugly conspiracy of silence," *World Net Daily*, August 18, 1999, http://www.wnd.com/1999/08/7517/. Writing in his syndicated column, Professor Williams of George Mason University analyzed the U.S. Department of Justice's National Crime Victimization Survey (NCVS) and found that in the category of interracial crimes (1997) there were "1,700,000 interracial crimes, of which 1,276,030 involved whites and blacks. In 90 percent of the cases, a white was the victim and a black was the perpetrator, while in 10 percent of the cases it was the reverse." Williams added, "Regardless of race, criminal violence is despicable and deserving of condemnation. But far more destructive are the official and unofficial attempts to mislead and conceal."

4. National Center for Education Statistics, *NAEP—State Education Data Profiles*, https://nces.ed.gov/programs/stateprofiles/.

5. *U.S. High School Graduation Rate Hits New Record High* (Washington DC: U.S. Department of Education, December 15, 2015), https://www.ed.gov/news/press-releases/us-high-school-graduation-rate-hits-new-record-high-0.

6. Cherrie Bucknor, *Young Black America. Part One: High School Completion Rates are at their Highest Ever* (Washington DC: Center for Economic and Policy Research, Issue Brief, March 2015), http://cepr.net/documents/black-hs-grad-rates-2015-03.pdf.

7. National Center for Education Statistics, *NCES Fast Facts. Scholastic Assessment Test (SAT) scores*, https://nces.ed.gov/fastfacts/display.asp?id=171.

8. National Center for Education Statistics, *NCES Fast Facts. Table 20: Household income and poverty rates, by state: 1990, 1995, and 1996*, https://nces.ed.gov/programs/digest/d97/d97t020.asp.

9. Edgar A. Suter, "Guns in the medical literature—a failure of peer review," *J Med Assoc Ga* 1994;83(3):137-148; for the *JAMA* survey, see: "*JAMA* 1996 Gun-Owners Survey" quoted in the *Medical Sentinel* 1999;3(2):40; Professor Gary Kleck discusses the unreliability of gun surveys in his books *Point Blank: Guns and Violence in America* (New York: Aldine de Gruyter, 1991) and *Targeting Guns: Firearms and Their Control* (New York: Aldine de Gruyter, 1997).

10. "Open-Data, Public Review policy of the *Medical Sentinel* of the Association of American Physicians and Surgeons (AAPS)," *Medical Sentinel* 1999;4(6):193-195. Roger Schlafly, personal communication with author, March 15, 2002.

11. Bruce C. Charlton, "Statistical malpractice," *Journal of the Royal College of Physicians* March-April 1996, pp. 112-114.

12. Steven J. Milloy, *Junk Science Judo: Self-Defense Against Health Scares and Scams* (Washington DC: Cato Institute, 2001), pp. 54-97; See also James T. Bennett and Thomas J. DiLorenzo, *From Pathology to Politics: Public Health in America* (New Brunswick, NJ: Transaction Publishers, 2000), pp. 80-83, 135-141.

13. Thomas D. Clark and Albert D. Kirwan, *The South Since Appomattox: A Century of Regional Change* (New York: Oxford University Press, 1967).

14. Miguel A. Faria, Jr., "The perversion of science and medicine (Part I): On the nature of science," *Medical Sentinel* 1997;2(2):46-48; Miguel A. Faria, Jr., "The perversion

of science and medicine (Part II): Soviet science and gun control," *Medical Sentinel*
1997;2(2):49-53; Miguel A. Faria, Jr., "The perversion of science and medicine (Part
III): Public health and gun control research," *Medical Sentinel* 1997;2(3):81-82; and
Miguel A. Faria, Jr., "The perversion of science and medicine (Part IV): The battle
continues," *Medical Sentinel* 1997;2(3):83-86.

15. Miguel A. Faria, Jr., "Public health and gun control—A review (Part I): The benefits
of firearms and (Part II): Gun violence and constitutional issues, *Medical Sentinel*
2001;6(1):11-18.

16. Don B. Kates, Henry E. Schaffer, John K. Lattimer, George B. Murray, Edwin H. Cassem,
"Guns and public health: epidemic of violence or pandemic of propaganda?" *Tennessee
Law Review* 1995;62:513-596, http://www.gunsandcrime.org/epidemic.pdf.

CHAPTER 11

1. Michael C. Monuteaux, Lois K. Lee, David Hemenway, Rebekah Mannix and Eric
W. Fleegler, "Firearm ownership and violent crime in the U.S.—an ecologic
study," *Am J Prev Med* 2015;49(2):207–214, http://www.ajpmonline.org/article/
S0749-3797(15)00072-0/fulltext.

2. Erica L. Smith and Alexia D. Cooper, *Homicide in the U.S. Known to Law Enforcement,
2011*, NCJ-243035 (Washington DC: Bureau of Justice Statistics, December 30, 2013),
https://www.bjs.gov/index.cfm?ty=pbdetail&iid=4863.

3. John R. Lott, Jr., *More Guns, Less Crime: Understanding Crime and Gun Control Laws*
(Chicago: University of Chicago Press, 1998).

4. Gary Kleck, *Targeting Guns: Firearms and Their Control* (New York: Aldine de Gruyter,
1997).

5. David C. Stolinsky, "America the most violent nation?" *Medical Sentinel* 2000;5(6):199-
201, https://haciendapublishing.com/medicalsentinel/america-most-violent-nation-0.

6. David C. Stolinsky, "Homicide and suicide in America, 1900-1998," *Medical
Sentinel* 2001;6(1):20-24, https://haciendapublishing.com/medicalsentinel/
homicide-and-suicide-america-1900-1998.

7. Miguel A. Faria, Jr., "America, guns, and freedom. Part I: A recapitulation of liberty,"
Surg Neurol Int 2012;3(1):133, http://surgicalneurologyint.com/surgicalint_articles/
america-guns-and-freedom-part-i-a-recapitulation-of-liberty/.

8. Miguel A. Faria, Jr., "America, guns and freedom: Part II—An international perspective,"
Surg Neurol Int 2012;3(1):135, http://surgicalneurologyint.com/surgicalint_articles/
america-guns-and-freedom-part-ii-an-international-perspective/.

9. Miguel A. Faria, Jr., "The American 'gun culture' that saved Europe," *GOPUSA.
com*, February 24, 2015, https://haciendapublishing.com/articles/
american-gun-culture-saved-europe.

10. Bruce C. Charlton, "Statistical malpractice," *Journal of the Royal College of Physicians*
March-April 1996, pp. 112-114.

11. Steven J. Milloy, *Junk Science Judo: Self-Defense Against Health Scares and Scams*
(Washington DC: Cato Institute, 2001), pp. 54-97.

12. Miguel A. Faria, Jr., "Shooting rampages, mental health, and the sensationalization of violence," *Surg Neurol Int* 2013;4(1):16, https://haciendapublishing.com/articles/shooting-rampages-mental-health-and-sensationalization-violence.

13. Cal Thomas, "Another signpost on the road to destruction," *Townhall*, April 27, 2015; For the deterioration of culture, not only with the media but also the popular culture of Hollywood, see: Russell L. Blaylock, "Contemporary popular culture and the antiheroes of the Hollywood left," *HaciendaPublishing. com*, March 10, 2016, https://haciendapublishing.com/articles/contemporary-popular-culture-and-antiheroes-hollywood-left-russell-l-blaylock-md; and Miguel A. Faria, Jr., "The Hollywood left, the antihero, and a dystopic future," *HaciendaPublishing.com*, March 13, 2016, https://haciendapublishing.com/articles/contemporary-popular-culture-and-antiheroes-hollywood-left-russell-l-blaylock-md.

14. Jane M. Orient, " 'Gun violence' as a public health issue: a physician's response," *J Am Phys Surg* 2013;18:77-83, http://www.jpands.org/vol18no3/orient.pdf.

15. Matthew Miller, Deborah Azrael, David Hemenway, "Firearm availability and unintentional firearm deaths, suicide, and homicide among 5-14 year olds," *J Trauma* 2002;52(2):267-275.

16. Miguel A. Faria, Jr., "Statistical malpractice—'Firearm Availability' and violence (Part II): Poverty, education and other socioeconomic factors. *HaciendaPublishing.com*, March 24, 2002, https://haciendapublishing.com/articles/statistical-malpractice-%C2%AD-firearm-availability-and-violence-part-ii-poverty-education-and-o.

17. Miguel A. Faria, Jr., "Gun Research 2013—an interview with Dr. Miguel A. Faria by Rebecca Trager of Research Europe." *HaciendaPublishing.com*, February 13, 2013, https://haciendapublishing.com/articles/gun-research-2013-%E2%80%94-interview-dr-miguel-faria-rebecca-trager-research-europe.

18. Miguel A. Faria, Jr., "Gun Research 2013—an interview with Dr. Miguel A. Faria by Craig Schneider of Atlanta Journal-Constitution," *HaciendaPublishing.com*, January 20, 2013, https://haciendapublishing.com/articles/gun-research-2013-%E2%80%94-interview-dr-miguel-faria-craig-schneider-reporter-atlanta-journal-cons.

19. Timothy Wheeler, "The history of public health gun control," *Doctors for Responsible Gun Ownership*, March 26, 2015, https://drgo.us/history-of-gun-control/.

20. Timothy Wheeler, "Private guns, public health—Hemenway is blindingly biased," *The Freeman*, July 12, 2010, http://fee.org/freeman/detail/private-guns-public-health.

21. Craig Schneider and Ernie Suggs, "CDC: Politics affected gun violence research." *Atlanta Journal-Constitution,* December 19, 2012, http://www.ajc.com/news/cdc-politics-affected-gun-violence-research/H1aKOO51fbkfMLOehRnyrK/.

22. Rebecca Trager, "In the line of fire," *Research Europe*, July 2, 2013, http://www.researchresearch.com/index.php?option=com_news&template=rr_2col&view=article&articleId=1290068.

23. Don B. Kates, Henry E. Schaffer, John K. Lattimer, George B. Murray, Edwin H. Cassem, "Guns and public health: epidemic of violence or pandemic of propaganda?" *Tennessee Law Review* 1995;62:513-596, http://www.gunsandcrime.org/epidemic.pdf.

CHAPTER 12

1. Michael Siegle and Molly Pahn, "New public database reveals striking differences in how guns are regulated from state to state," *The Telegraph* (Macon, GA), May 25, 2017.

2. Thomas Vaughan, "New public database reveals bias of gun control researchers," *Doctors for Responsible Gun Ownership*, May 25, 2017, https://drgo.us/new-public-database-reveals-bias-of-gun-control-researchers/; For the tremendous drop in crime in the last 25 years, see Matt Ford, "What caused the great crime decline in the US?" *The Atlantic*, April 15, 2016, https://www.theatlantic.com/politics/archive/2016/04/what-caused-the-crime-decline/477408/.

3. "FBI releases 2016 crime statistics" (Washington DC: FBI National Press Office, September 25, 2017), https://www.fbi.gov/news/pressrel/press-releases/fbi-releases-2016-crime-statistics; For further analysis of the 2014-2016 spike in violent crime, see Mark Herman, "Violent crimes and murders increased in 2016 for a second consecutive year, FBI says," *Washington Post*, September 25, 2017, https://www.washingtonpost.com/news/post-nation/wp/2017/09/25/violent-crime-increased-in-2016-for-a-second-consecutive-year-fbi-says/?utm_term=.6003bdf5dff3; For the militarization of police, see Miguel A. Faria, Jr., "Police shootings and the militarization of law enforcement," *HaciendaPublishing.com*, April 14, 2015, https://haciendapublishing.com/articles/police-shootings-and-militarization-law-enforcement.

4. Miguel A. Faria, Jr., "Looting and Burning—Trampling the Rule of Law," *HaciendaPublishing.com*, November 27, 2014, https://haciendapublishing.com/articles/looting-and-burning-%E2%80%94-trampling-rule-law.

5. Russell L. Blaylock, "The Dallas shooting of police officers: What it really means," *HaciendaPublishing.com*, July 17, 2016, https://haciendapublishing.com/articles/dallas-shooting-police-officers-what-it-really-means-russell-l-blaylock-md.

6. Miguel A. Faria, Jr., "Women, guns, and the medical literature—a raging debate," *Women and Guns*, October 1994, Vol. 6, No. 9, pp. 14-17, 52-53. https://haciendapublishing.com/articles/women-guns-and-medical-literature-raging-debate.

7. Michael R. Rand, *Guns and Crime: Handgun Victimization, Firearm Self-Defense, and Firearm Theft*, NCJ-147003 (Washington DC: Department of Justice, Bureau of Justice Statistics, April 1994); Federal Bureau of Investigation, *Uniform Crime Reports: Crime in the United States, 1992*, (Washington DC: Government Printing Office, 1993); See also Miguel A. Faria, Jr., "Public health and gun control—No deterrent to crime," *The New American*, Vol. 15, No. 24, November 22, 1999, pp. 2324, https://haciendapublishing.com/articles/public-health-and-gun-control-no-deterrent-crime.

8. Michael Planty and Jennifer L. Truman, *Firearm Violence, 1993-2011*, NCJ-241730 (Washington DC: Department of Justice, May 2013), https://www.bjs.gov/content/pub/pdf/fv9311.pdf.

9. Arthur Z. Przebinda, "The gun as talisman," *Doctors for Responsible Gun Ownership*, June 20, 2017, https://drgo.us/the-gun-as-talisman/.

10. Thomas E. Gift, "Firearms and 'rural' suicides," *Doctors for Responsible Gun Ownership*, August 24, 2017, https://drgo.us/firearms-and-rural-suicides/; For the original article, see Paul S. Nestadt, Patrick Tripplett, David R. Fowler, et al., "Urban-rural differences in suicide in the state of Maryland: The role of firearms," *American Journal of Public Health*, August 17, 2017, http://ajph.aphapublications.org/doi/abs/10.2105/AJPH.2017.303865.

PART IV

CHAPTER 13

1. "AMA joins gun grabbers," *NewsMax.com*, May 1, 2001, http://www.newsmax.com/Pre-2008/AMA-Joins-Gun-Grabbers/2001/04/30/id/661715/.

2. Don B. Kates, Henry E. Schaffer, John K. Lattimer, George B. Murray, Edwin H. Cassem, "Guns and public health: epidemic of violence or pandemic of propaganda?" *Tennessee Law Review* 1995;62:513-596, http://www.gunsandcrime.org/epidemic.pdf; See also Edgar A. Suter, "Guns in the medical literature—a failure of peer review," *J Med Assoc Ga* 1994;83(3):137-148.

3. Miguel A. Faria, Jr., *Medical Warrior: Fighting Corporate Socialized Medicine* (Macon, GA: Hacienda Publishing Inc., 1997), pp. 184-191.

4. Miguel A. Faria, Jr., "The medical sentinel—a breath of fresh air," *Medical Sentinel* 1999;4(3):94-99, https://haciendapublishing.com/medicalsentinel/medical-sentinel-breath-fresh-air.

5. William C. Waters IV, Miguel A. Faria Jr., Timothy Wheeler, Don B. Kates, "Testimony before the Subcommittee on Labor, Health and Human Services, Education, and Related Agencies," Washington DC, House Committee on Appropriations, March 6, 1996, Hearing Volume, Part 7:935-970, Archived edition, <http://archive.org/stream/departmentsoflab071996unit#page/944/mode/2up>; See also Miguel A. Faria, Jr., "The perversion of science and medicine (Parts III): Public health and gun control research, *Medical Sentinel* 1997;2(3):81-82, https://haciendapublishing.com/medicalsentinel/perversion-science-and-medicine-part-iii-public-health-and-gun-control-research; and Miguel A. Faria, Jr., "The perversion of science and medicine (Part IV): The battle continues," *Medical Sentinel* 1997;2(3):83-86, https://haciendapublishing.com/medicalsentinel/perversion-science-and-medicine-part-iv-battle-continues.

6. Timothy Wheeler, "Lab accident: How Congress stopped the CDC gun grabbers and saved science," *America's 1st Freedom*, February 2, 2016, https://drgo.us/lab-accident-how-congress-stopped-the-cdc-gun-grabbers-and-saved-science/.

7. Miguel A. Faria, Jr., "The transformation of medical ethics through time (Part II): medical ethics and organized medicine," *Medical Sentinel* 1998;3(2):53-56, https://haciendapublishing.com/medicalsentinel/transformation-medical-ethics-through-time-part-ii-medical-ethics-and-organized-medi; See also Miguel A. Faria, Jr., *Medical Warrior: Fighting Corporate Socialized Medicine*, pp. 184-191; The 1997 AMA reimbursement figures were cited in *Physicians Weekly*, July 21,1997.

8. Howard Wolinsky and Tom Brune, *The Serpent on the Staff: The Unhealthy Politics of the American Medical Association* (New York: G. P. Putnam's Sons, 1994); See also Miguel A. Faria, Jr., *Medical Warrior: Fighting Corporate Socialized Medicine,* pp. 142-146, 164-169.

9. Judith Graham, " 'Like a slap in the face': Dissent roils the AMA, the nation's largest doctor's group," *StatNews.com,* December 22, 2016, https://www.statnews.com/2016/12/22/american-medical-association-divisions/.

10. The 2012 figures were cited in, "Report of the House of Delegates Committee on Compensation of the Officers" by John H. Armstrong, Chair, June 2014 Annual Meeting, p. 399, https://www.ama-assn.org/sites/default/files/media-browser/public/hod/a14-hod-committee-compensation.pdf; The 1997 AMA reimbursement figures were cited in *Physicians Weekly,* July 21,1997; Miguel A. Faria, Jr., "The transformation of medical ethics through time (Part II): medical ethics and organized medicine," *Medical Sentinel* 1998;3(2):53-56, https://haciendapublishing.com/medicalsentinel/transformation-medical-ethics-through-time-part-ii-medical-ethics-and-organized-medi.

11. "AMA reimbursement figures, and financially for AMA, membership may be optional?" *Medical Sentinel* 1998;3(2):42.

12. Andy L. Schlafly, "AMA's secret pact with HCFA," *Medical Sentinel* 1998;3(4):149-150, https://haciendapublishing.com/medicalsentinel/amas-secret-pact-hcfa.

13. Miguel A. Faria, Jr., "The AMA, ethics and gun control—Part 2: Medical journalism and physician unionization," *NewsMax.com,* May 15, 2001, https://haciendapublishing.com/articles/ama-ethics-and-gun-control-part-ii.

14. Miguel A. Faria, Jr., "The AMA, ethics and gun control—Part 3: AMA, medical liability and HMO lawsuits," *NewsMax.com,* May 21, 2001, https://haciendapublishing.com/articles/ama-ethics-and-gun-control-part-iii.

CHAPTER 14

1. *Journal of the Medical Association of Georgia,* Special issue, March 1994, Volume 83, No. 13, pp. 133-159, see Edgar A. Suter, "Guns in the medical literature—a failure of peer review"; Larry Pratt, "Health care and firearms"; David B. Kopel, "The allure of foreign gun laws"; W.W. Carruth, III, "Guns: Health destroyer or protector." My plea was that both sides of the political debate affecting medicine or public health be heard. Since the AMA, the state medical journals, *JAMA,* and the *NEJM* had entered the debate on one side, then it would only be fair that at least one journal would present both sides of the debate. I did so in the *Journal of the Medical Association of Georgia (JMAG).*

2. Bill Hendrick, "Report: guns not to blame for murder epidemic—Georgia medical journal criticized for article," *Atlanta Journal-Constitution,* March 19, 1994.

3. Miguel A. Faria, Jr., *Medical Warrior: Fighting Corporate Socialized Medicine* (Macon, GA: Hacienda Publishing, Inc., 1997), pp. 107-120, 170-178.

4. Howard Wolinsky and Tom Brune, *The Serpent on the Staff: The Unhealthy Politics of the American Medical Association* (New York: G. P. Putnam's Sons, 1994). pp. 19-20, 24,

35. The examples of opportunism and political expediency by the AMA are peppered throughout the book.

5. Nancy Dickey, "A special message regarding *JAMA* from the president of the AMA," January 1999; See also E.R. Anderson, "AMA statement," January 15, 1999.

6. Michael Fumento, "Medical journals give new meaning to political science," *Wall Street Journal*, January 21, 1999.

7. Timothy Wheeler, "Sex, lies, and JAMA's headache," *The Claremont Institute*, 1999.

8. George D. Lundberg. "House of Delegates reaffirms editorial independence for AMA's scientific journals," *JAMA* 1993; 270(10):1248-1249.

9. "*JAMA's* Mission and Objectives, 1994," www.ama-assn.org; *JAMA's* mission and objectives were rewritten after Dr. George Lundberg's dismissal. The subsequent report replaced the old standard: "*JAMA* and Editorial Independence," *JAMA* 1999;281(5):460, http://jamanetwork.com/journals/jama/article-abstract/188727.

10. Miguel A. Faria, Jr., "Corporate socialized medicine," *Medical Sentinel* 1998;3(2):45-46.

11. Don McCane. "AMA position on single payer," October 31, 2008, http://pnhp.org/blog/2008/10/31/ama-position-on-single-payer/

12. Joshua Holland, "Medicare-for-all isn't the solution for universal health care: The health-care debate is moving to the left. But if progressives don't start sweating the details, we're going to fail yet again," *The Nation*, August 2, 2017, https://www.thenation.com/article/medicare-for-all-isnt-the-solution-for-universal-health-care/.

13. Judith Graham, " 'Like a slap in the face': Dissent roils the AMA, the nation's largest doctor's group," *StatNews.com*, December 22, 2016, https://www.statnews.com/2016/12/22/american-medical-association-divisions/.

14. George D. Lundberg, "National health care reform—the aura of inevitability intensifies," *JAMA* 1992;267(18):2521-2522; For other issues, see: George D. Lundberg, "*JAMA*, abortion and editorial responsibility," *JAMA* 1998;280(8):740; and George D. Lundberg, "Perspective from the editor of *JAMA*," *Bull Med Libr Assoc* 1992; 80(2):110-114.

15. Miguel A. Faria, Jr., *Vandals at the Gates of Medicine: Historic Perspectives on the Battle Over Health Care Reform* (Macon, GA: Hacienda Publishing, Inc., 1994), pp. 195-197.

16. Michael Fumento, *The Myth of Heterosexual AIDS: How a Tragedy Has Been Distorted by the Media and Partisan Politics* (New York: Basic Books, 1990); See also Miguel A. Faria, Jr., *Medical Warrior*, pp. 130-134.

17. Miguel A. Faria, Jr., "The perversion of science and medicine (Part I): On the nature of science," *Medical Sentinel* 1997;2(2):46-48; Miguel A. Faria, Jr., "The perversion of science and medicine (Part II): Soviet science and gun control," *Medical Sentinel* 1997;2(2):49-53; Miguel A. Faria, Jr., "The perversion of science and medicine (Part III): Public health and gun control research," *Medical Sentinel* 1997;2(3):81-82; and Miguel A. Faria, Jr., "The perversion of science and medicine (Part IV): The battle continues," *Medical Sentinel* 1997;2(3):83-86.

18. Edgar A. Suter, "Guns in the medical literature—a failure of peer review," *J Med Assoc Ga* 1994;83(3):144-145.

19. C. Everett Koop, George D. Lundberg, "Violence in America: a public health emergency," *JAMA* 1992;267(22):3075-3076.

20. Jerome P. Kassirer, "A partisan assault on science—the threat to the CDC," *New Engl J Med* 1995;333(12):793-798. Dr. Kassirer was also critical of *JMAG* and my editorship and wrote an editorial after my resignation in 1995 supporting the "science" of public health and gun control. A year before that he had to rectify his assertion that *JMAG* was an "obscure journal" by the fact the journal was a peer-reviewed, official state medical journal read even by out-of-state physicians (correspondence on file). Kassirer lost his job in a dispute, supposedly over administrative issues, with the Massachusetts Medical Society six months after Lundberg. Kassirer's associate, Marcia Angell, took over as interim editor-in-chief until 2000, when she resigned, reportedly to write a book on alternative medicine. Regarding censorship of contrary views, particularly in the *NEJM*, see: Miguel A. Faria, Jr., "Junk science of public health and gun control" (correspondence), *Medical Sentinel* July/August 2000;5(4), https://haciendapublishing. com/medicalsentinel/junk-science-public-health-and-gun-control; and J.E. Dyer, "Surgeon General-gate and the double standard for mixing health, guns, and politics," *Liberty Unyielding*, March 21, 2014, http://libertyunyielding.com/2014/03/21/ surgeon-general-gate-double-standard-mixing-health-guns-politics/.

21. Miguel A. Faria, Jr., *Vandals*, pp. 294-299.

22. Russell L. Blaylock, "Running for cover—The herd instinct among physicians," *Medical Sentinel* 1996;1(2):14-17.

23. Miguel A. Faria, Jr., "Physician unions not the answer to managed care," *NewsMax.com*, September 1, 2000.

CHAPTER 15

1. Miguel A. Faria, Jr., "Doctors warn of grave risk to your medical records. AAPS: It's time to draw the line in the sand on medical privacy," *NewsMax.com*, March 22, 2001.

2. "Testimony of the American Psychiatric Association on H.R. 4585, the Medical Financial Privacy Protection Act" before the Committee on Banking and Financial Services, U.S. House of Representatives, June 14, 2000.

3. Josh Benson, "Medical Machers ask: Should guns be part of patient profile?" *The New York Observer*, March 15, 2001.

4. Timothy Wheeler. "Boundary violation: Gun politics in the doctor's office," *Medical Sentinel* 1999;4(2):60-61, https://haciendapublishing.com/medicalsentinel/ boundary-violations-gun-politics-doctors-office.

5. Timothy Wheeler, "The AMA's Long March for gun control," *Doctors for Responsible Gun Ownership*, August 25, 2015, https://drgo.us/the-amas-long-march-for-gun-control/, for the 15% AMA membership figure; See also "AMA joins gun grabbers," *NewsMax.com*, May 1, 2001, http://www.newsmax.com/Pre-2008/AMA-Joins-Gun-Grabbers/2001/04/30/id/661715/; Miguel A. Faria, Jr., "The perversion of science and medicine (Part I): On the nature of science," *Medical Sentinel* 1997;2(2):46-48; Miguel A. Faria, Jr., "The perversion of science and medicine (Part II): Soviet science and

gun control," *Medical Sentinel* 1997;2(2):49-53; Miguel A. Faria, Jr., "The perversion of science and medicine (Part III): Public health and gun control research," *Medical Sentinel* 1997;2(3):81-82; and Miguel A. Faria, Jr., "The perversion of science and medicine (Part IV): The battle continues," *Medical Sentinel* 1997;2(3):83-86; See also Miguel A. Faria, Jr., "Public health and gun control—A review (Part I): The benefits of firearms and (Part II): Gun violence and constitutional issues, *Medical Sentinel* 2001;6(1):11-18.

6. American Psychiatric Association (APA), "Position Statement on Homicide prevention and gun control," *Am J Psychiatry* 1994;151(4):630.

7. Miguel A. Faria, Jr., "To the tune of Washington's pied pipers," *Medical Sentinel* 1996;1(3):8-9, https://haciendapublishing.com/medicalsentinel/ tune-washingtons-pied-pipers.

8. Oath of Hippocrates quoted in full with explanation for modern reader, see *Miguel A. Faria, Jr., "Transformation of medical ethics through time (Part I): Medical ethics and statist controls," Medical Sentinel 1998;3(1):19-24,* https://haciendapublishing. com/medicalsentinel/transformation-medical-ethics-through-time-part-i- medical-ethics-and-statist-control. For the 2Adoc.com *referral service, see:* Arthur Z Przebinda, "2Adoc.com will connect patients with gun-friendly providers," *Doctors for Responsible Gun Ownership*, September 5, 2017, https://drgo. us/2adoc-com-will-connect-patients-and-providers/.

9. Robert B. Young, "Wollschlaeger (FOPA) again," *Doctors for Responsible Gun Ownership*, February 21, 2017. https://drgo.us/wollschlaeger-fopa-again/; See also "Official DRGO Statement Regarding the *en banc* 11th Circuit Court Wollschlaeger (FOPA) Decision," *Doctors for Responsible Gun Ownership*, February 21, 2017, https://drgo.us/drgo- statement-regarding-the-en-banc-11th-circuit-court-wollschlaeger-fopa-decision/.

10. Vladimir Bukobsky, Alexis Klimoff (ed.), and Denise H. Wood (trans.), *To Choose Freedom* (Stanford, CA: Hoover Institution, October 1987); For medical abuses in other egalitarian socialist bloc nations, see: Miguel A. Faria, Jr., *Vandals at the Gates of Medicine: Historic Perspectives on the Battle Over Health Care Reform* (Macon, GA: Hacienda Publishing Inc., 1995), pp. 235-244.

11. Charles J. Brown and Armando M. Lago, *The Politics of Psychiatry in Revolutionary Cuba* (New York: Freedom House, 1991); For an extensive review of this book, see: Miguel A. Faria, Jr., "Cuban psychiatry—The perversion of medicine," *Medical Sentinel* 2000;5(5):160-162, https://haciendapublishing.com/medicalsentinel/ cuban-psychiatry-perversion-medicine.

12. Robert J. Lifton, *The Nazi Doctors: Medical Killing and the Psychology of Genocide* (New York: Basic Books, 1986).

13. Leo Alexander, "Medical science under dictatorship," *New England Journal of Medicine*, July 14, 1949; For a summarization of this now very difficult to obtain article, see: Miguel A. Faria, Jr., "Euthanasia, medical science, and the road to genocide," *Medical Sentinel* 1998;3(3):79-83, https://haciendapublishing.com/medicalsentinel/ euthanasia-medical-science-and-road-genocide.

PART V

CHAPTER 16

1. Karl P. Adler, Jeremiah A. Barondess, et al., "Firearm violence and public health—
limiting the availability of guns," *JAMA* 1994;271 (16):1281-1283.

2. Arthur L. Kellermann, Frederick P. Rivara, Norman B. Rushforth, et al., "Gun ownership
as a risk factor for homicide in the home," *N Engl J Med* 1993;329(15):1084-1091.

3. Gary Kleck, "Guns and self-protection," *J Med Assoc Ga* 1994;83(1):42.

4. Don B. Kates and Patricia T. Harris, "How to make their day," *National Review*
1991;43(19):30-32.

5. Gary Kleck and Marc Gertz, "Armed Resistance to Crime: The Prevalence and
Nature of Self-Defense With a Gun," *Journal of Criminal Law and Criminology* Fall
1995;86(1):164-185; See also Gary Kleck, *Point Blank: Guns and Violence in America*
(New York: Aldine de Gruyter, 1991), p.111-116, 148, for criminals killed by citizens
and police and p. 132 for the phrase "the police cannot be everywhere."

6. Miguel A. Faria, Jr., "On guns and violence," *J Med Assoc Ga* 1993;82(7):317-320.

7. Alan M. Gottlieb, *Gun Rights Fact Book* (Bellevue, WA: Merril Press, 1988); See also
Robert W. Lee, "Going for our guns," *The New American* 1990;6(9):21-28; For the
Florida alligators versus CCW holders unusual analogy, consider that "from 1988
through 1997, there were 146 documented alligator attacks on human beings in
Florida. This does not include any unreported encounters," interview with Mark
Trainor, Public Information Specialist for the Office of Information Services, Florida
Game and Fresh Water Fish Commission, Tallahassee, Florida, December 14, 1998;
By contrast, there were only 88 CCW holders who used their guns during the same
period to commit a crime, see "GOA Resources—1999 Firearms Fact Sheet," *Gun
Owners of America*, December 24, 2008.

8. U.S. Court of Appeals for the Seventh Circuit, *Bowers v. DeVito* cited in Robert W. Lee in
"Police protection or self-defense?" *The New American* 1992;8(8):16-17; See also Court
of Appeals ruling *Riss v. City of New York* (1968) and Superior Court ruling *Warren v.
District of Columbia* (1981).

9. For armed protection during the 1992 Los Angeles riots, see "Koreans make armed
stand to protect shops from looters," *Roanoke Times & World-News*, May 3, 1992; For
the Ferguson (MO) riots, see Bob Owens, "Armed business owners thwart mobs in
Ferguson riots," *Bearing Arms*, November 25, 2014, https://bearingarms.com/bob-
o/2014/11/25/armed-business-owners-thwart-mobs-ferguson-riots/; For causes and
development of the Ferguson riots, see Miguel A. Faria, Jr., "Looting and burning—
trampling the rule of law," *HaciendaPublishing.com*, November 27, 2014, https://
haciendapublishing.com/articles/looting-and-burning-%E2%80%94-trampling-
rule-law; See also Miguel A. Faria, Jr., "Let's not make any more excuses," *The Macon
Telegraph*, September 17, 2014, https://haciendapublishing.com/randomnotes/
let%E2%80%99s-not-make-any-more-excuses.

10. Mary T. Schmich, "After Hugo: 'Quicksand and snakes everywhere," *Chicago Tribune*, September 24, 1989, http://articles.chicagotribune.com/1989-09-24/ news/8901150712_1_looters-sullivans-island-palms.

11. Mark Silva, Charles Strouse and John Donnelly, "Destruction at dawn: What Hurricane Andrew did to South Florida 25 years ago," *Miami Herald*, August 24, 2015, http:// www.miamiherald.com/news/weather/hurricane/article32006499.html.

12. For armed citizens protecting their property during Hurricane Andrew see: "Andrew picks up speed as it races across gulf," *Detroit Free Press*, August 27, 1992, http:// www.nhc.noaa.gov/archive/storm_wallets/atlantic/atl1992/andrew/news/dn0827p2. gif; See also Dan Fesperman, "Andrew's little wonder: No looters are dead yet," *The Baltimore Sun*, September 3, 1992, http://articles.baltimoresun.com/1992-09-03/ news/1992247087_1_gun-dealers-andrew-dade-county; For other civilian uses of "assault weapons," see Edgar A. Suter, " 'Assault weapons' revisited—An analysis of the AMA report," *J Med Assoc Ga* 1994;83(5):281-289, http://rkba.org/research/suter/ aw.html.

13. Liz Fabian, "Looters set fire to Macon store without power since tropical storm Irma," *The Telegraph* (Macon), September 13, 2017; and "9 arrested in Florida for looting sneakers during Irma," *Associated Press*, September 10, 2017.

14. For an excellent discussion on the differences between "assault weapons" and "assault rifles," and the passage of the Assault Weapons Ban of 1994, see *Guns: Who Should Have Them?* David B. Kopel, ed., (Amherst, NY: Prometheus Books, 1995), pp.159-232; For gun crime statistics, see Alan Beck et al., *Survey of State Prison Inmates, 1991*, NCJ-136949 (Washington DC: Department of Justice, Bureau of Justice Statistics, March 1993), p.18; and FBI, "Crime in the United States," (1994):18; See also Caroline Wolf Harlow, *Firearm Use by Offenders*, NCJ-189369 (Washington DC: Department of Justice, Bureau of Justice Statistics, November 4, 2001); Edgar A. Suter, " 'Assault weapons' revisited—An analysis of the AMA report," *J Med Assoc Ga* 1994;83(5):281-289, http://rkba.org/research/suter/aw.html; For general information and additional references, see "GOA Resources—1999 Firearms Fact Sheet," *Gun Owners of America*, December 24, 2008, https://www.gunowners.org/fs9901.htm; For the most recent data corroborating what gun rights proponents had advocated, see Lois Beckett, "The assault weapons myth," *The New York Times*. September 12, 2014. For the mischaracterization of assault rifles as assault weapons, see Christopher Ingraham, "Assault rifles are becoming mass shooters' weapons of choice," *Washington Post*, June 12, 2016. For Maryland's assault weapons ban, see: Lydia Wheeler, "Supreme Court refuses to take up Maryland's assault weapons ban," November 27, 2017, http://thehill. com/regulation/court-battles/361969-supreme-court-refuses-to-take-up-marylands-assault-weapons-ban. *United States v. Miller*, 307 U.S. 174 (1938).

15. James D. Wright, and Peter H. Rossi, *The Armed Criminal in America: A Survey of Incarcerated Felons*, NCJ-097099 (Washington DC: Department of Justice, National Institute of Justice, July 1985), p. 27; See also James Wright and Peter H. Rossi, *Armed and Considered Dangerous: A Survey of Felons and Their Firearms* (New York: Aldine

de Gruyter, 1986); See also Paul H. Blackman, *The Armed Criminal in America*, cited in Don Feder, "Gun control doesn't work," *New Dimensions* 1991;5(4):44- 45; Gary Kleck, *Targeting Guns: Firearms and Their Control* (New York: Aldine de Gruyter, 1997).

16. Edgar A. Suter, "Guns in the medical literature—a failure of peer review," *J Med Assoc Ga* 1994;83(3):133-148; For the Militia Act of 1790, see: "The right to keep and bear arms: Report of the Subcommittee on the Constitution of the Committee on the Judiciary, United States Senate, Ninety-seventh Congress, second session," (Washington DC: U.S. Government Printing Office, February 1982), p. 7; and *United States v. Miller*, 307 U.S. 174 (1938).

17. Paxton Quigley, *Armed and Female*, cited in Robert W. Lee, "Gun report—ladies in waiting," *The New American* 1992;8(7).

18. David B. Kopel, "Guns on university campuses: The Colorado experience," *Washington Post*, April 20, 2015, https://www.washingtonpost.com/news/volokh-conspiracy/ wp/2015/04/20/guns-on-university-campuses-the-colorado-experience/?utm_term=. d34aad771db8; and Robert Kukla cited in Robert W. Lee, "The right that secures all others," *The New American* 1992;8(19):20; The primary data on the Orlando, Florida, gun training for women (1966-67) came from Gary Kleck, "Crime control through the private use of armed force," *Social Problems*, February 1988;(35):13-15. For Australian domestic violence and the experience of women and guns, see: David B. Kopel, *The Samurai, the Mountie, and the Cowboy: Should America Adopt the Gun Controls of Other Democracies?* (Amherst, NY: Prometheus Books, 1992), pp. 210-214.

19. The original study is M. Joan McDermott, *Rape Victimization in 26 American Cities: Applications of the National Crime Survey Victimization and Attitude Data*, 1979, NCJ-55878 (Washington DC: Department of Justice, Law Enforcement Assistance Administration, 1979), p. 31; See also Larry Pratt, "Health care and firearms," *J Med Assoc Ga* 1994;83(3): 149-151.

20. "Guns and violence against women: America's uniquely lethal domestic violence problem," *Everytown for Gun Safety*, https://everytownresearch.org/reports/ guns-and-violence-against-women.

21. Jacqueline C. Campbell, Daniel Webster, Jane Koziol-McLain, et al., "Risk factors for femicide in abusive relationships: Results from a multisite case control study," *Am J Public Health* 2003 July; 93(7): 1089-1097, https://www.ncbi.nlm.nih.gov/pmc/articles/ PMC1447915/.

22. Timothy W. Wheeler and E. John Wipfler, III, *Keeping Your Family Safe: The Responsibilities of Firearm Ownership* (Bellevue, WA: Merrill Press, 2009), pp. 27-31. For the Detroit and Kansas City study, see: G. Marie Wilt, James D. Bannon, Ronald K. Breedlove, et al., *Domestic Violence and the Police: Studies in Detroit and Kansas City* (Washington DC, Police Foundation, 1977); See also Don B. Kates cited in Robert W. Lee, "Going for our guns," *The New American* 1990;6(9):21-28.

23. Articles supportive of the individual rights view include: William Van Alstyne, "The second amendment and the personal right to arms," *Duke Law Journal* 1994; 43(6):

1236-55; Akhil Reed Amar, "The bill of rights and the fourteenth amendment," *Yale Law Journal* 1992; 101: 1193-1284; Don B. Kates, "The second amendment and the ideology of self-protection," *Constitutional Commentary* Winter 1992; 9: 87-104; Elaine Scarry, "War and the social contract: the right to bear arms," *Univ Penn Law Rev* 1991; 139(5): 1257-1316; David C. Williams, "Civic republicanism and the citizen militia: the terrifying second amendment," *Yale Law Journal* 1991; 101:551-616; Robert J. Cottrol and Raymond T. Diamond, "The second amendment: toward an Afro-Americanist reconsideration," *The Georgetown Law Journal*, December 1991: 80; 309-61; Akhil Reed Amar, "The bill of rights as a constitution," *Yale Law Journal* 1991; 100 (5): 1131-1210; Sanford Levinson, "The embarrassing second amendment," *Yale Law Journal* 1989; 99:637-659; Don B. Kates, "The second amendment: a dialogue," *Law and Contemporary Problems* 1986; 49:143; Joyce L. Malcolm, "Essay review," *George Washington Univ Law Review* 1986; 54: 452-464; F.S. Fussner, "Essay review," *Constitutional Commentary* 1986; 3: 582-8; Robert E. Shalhope, "The armed citizen in the early republic," *Law and Contemporary Problems* 1986; 49:125-141; Stephen P. Halbrook, "What the framers intended: a linguistic interpretation of the second amendment," *Law and Contemporary Problems* 1986; 49:151-162.; Don B. Kates, "Handgun prohibition and the original meaning of the second amendment," *Michigan Law Review* 1983; 82:203-73; Stephen P. Halbrook, "The right to bear arms in the first state bills of rights: Pennsylvania, North Carolina, Vermont, and Massachusetts," *Vermont Law Review* 1985; 10: 255-320; Stephen P. Halbrook, "The right of the people or the power of the state: bearing arms, arming militias, and the second amendment," *Valparaiso Law Review* 1991; 26:131-207; Stefan B. Tahmassebi, "Gun control and racism," *George Mason Univ Civil Rights Law Journal* Winter 1991; 2(1):67-99; Glenn Harlan Reynolds, "The right to keep and bear arms under the Tennessee Constitution," *Tennessee Law Review* Winter 1994; 61:2; T.M. Bordenet, "The right to possess arms: the intent of the Framers of the second amendment," *UWLA L Review* 1990; 21:1-30; Thomas M. Moncure Jr., "Who is the militia—the Virginia ratifying convention and the right to bear arms," *Lincoln Law Review* 1990; 19:1-25; Nelson Lund, "The second amendment, political liberty and the right to self-preservation," *Alabama Law Review* 1987; 39:103-130; Eric C. Morgan, "Assault rifle legislation: unwise and unconstitutional," *American Journal of Criminal Law* 1990; 17:143-174; Robert Dowlut, "Federal and state constitutional guarantees to arms," *Univ Dayton Law Review* 1989; 15(1):59-89; Stephen P. Halbrook, "Encroachments of the crown on the liberty of the subject: pre-revolutionary origins of the second amendment," *Univ Dayton Law Review* 1989; 15(1):91-124; David T. Hardy, "The second amendment and the historiography of the Bill of Rights," *Journal of Law and Politics* Summer 1987; 4(1):1-62; David T. Hardy, "Armed citizens, citizen armies: toward a jurisprudence of the second amendment," *Harvard Journal of Law and Public Policy* 1986; 9:559-638; Robert Dowlut, "The current relevancy of keeping and bearing arms," *Univ Baltimore Law Forum* 1984; 15:30-32; Joyce L. Malcolm, "The right of the people to keep and bear arms: The Common Law tradition," *Hastings Constitutional Law Quarterly*

Winter 1983; 10(2):285-314; Robert Dowlut, "The right to arms: does the Constitution or the predilection of judges reign?" *Oklahoma Law Review* 1983; 36:65-105; D.I. Caplan, "The right of the individual to keep and bear arms: a recent judicial trend," *Detroit College of Law Review* 1982; 789-823; Stephen P. Halbrook, "To keep and bear their private arms: The adoption of the Second Amendment, 1787-1791," *Northern Kentucky Law Review* 1982; 10(1):13-39; Alan M. Gottlieb, "Gun ownership: a constitutional right," *Northern Kentucky Law Review* 1982; 10:113-40; R. Gardiner, "To preserve liberty—a look at the right to keep and bear arms," *Northern Kentucky Law Review* 1982; 10(1):63-96; K.E. Kluin, "Note. Gun control: is it a legal and effective means of controlling firearms in the United States?" *Washburn Law Journal* 1982; 21:244-264; Stephen P. Halbrook, "The jurisprudence of the second and fourteenth amendments," *George Mason U Civil Rights Law Review* 1981; 4:1-69; Jay R. Wagner, "Comment: Gun control legislation and the intent of the second amendment: To what extent is there an individual right to keep and bear arms?" *Villanova Law Review* 1992; 37:1407-1459. The following opinions in book form also affirm that the individual right position is correct: Joyce L. Malcolm, *To Keep and Bear Arms: The Origins of an Anglo-American Right* (Cambridge MA: Harvard University Press, 1994); Robert Cottrol, *Gun Control and the Constitution, 3 volume set* (New York: Garland, 1993); Clayton E. Cramer, *For the Defense of Themselves and the State: The Original Intent and Judicial Interpretation of the Right to Keep and Bear Arms* (Westport CT: Praeger Publishers, 1994); Robert Cottrol and Raymond T. Diamond, "Public Safety and the Right to Bear Arms" in David J. Bodenhamer and James W. Ely (editors), *The Bill of Rights in Modern America: After 200 Years* (Bloomington, IN: Indiana University Press, 1993); *Oxford Companion to the United States Supreme Court* (New York: Oxford University Press, 1992) for entry on the Second Amendment; Eric Foner and John Garrity, *Reader's Companion to American History* (New York: Houghton Mifflin, 1991), pp. 477-478 for entry on "Guns and Gun Control"; Don B. Kates, "Minimalist interpretation of the Second Amendment" in Eugene W. Hickok Jr. (editor), *The Bill of Rights: Original Meaning and Current Understanding* (Charlottesville: University Press of Virginia, 1991); Stephen P. Halbrook, "The original understanding of the second amendment," in Eugene W. Hickok Jr. (editor), *The Bill of Rights: Original Meaning and Current Understanding* (Charlottesville: University Press of Virginia, 1991); David E. Young (editor). *The Origin of the Second Amendment: A Documentary History of the Bill of Rights in Commentaries on Liberty, Free Government & an Armed Populace, 1787-1792* (Ontonagon, MI: Golden Oak Books, 1991); Stephen P. Halbrook, *A Right to Bear Arms: State and Federal Bills of Rights and Constitutional Guarantees* (Westport, CT: Greenwood Press, 1989); Leonard Levy, *Original Intent and the Framers' Constitution* (New York: Macmillan, 1988); David T. Hardy, *Origins and Development of the Second Amendment* (Chino Valley, AZ: Blacksmith Corporation, 1986); Leonard Levy (editor), *Encyclopedia of the American Constitution* (New York: Macmillan, 1986) for entry on the Second Amendment; Stephen P. Halbrook, *That Every Man Be Armed: The Evolution of a Constitutional Right* (Albuquerque, NM:

University of New Mexico Press, 1984); William J. Marina, "Weapons, Technology and Legitimacy: The Second Amendment in Global Perspective" and Stephen P. Halbrook, "The Second Amendment as a phenomenon of classical political philosophy" cited in Don B. Kates (editor), *Firearms and Violence* (San Francisco: Pacific Research Institute, 1984); See also Joyce L. Malcolm, *To Keep and Bear Arms: The Origins of an Anglo-American Right* (Cambridge, MA: Harvard University Press, 1994). Professor Malcolm explains how the individual right to keep and bear arms evolved and was "secured by the Englishmen and bequeathed to their American colonists." An excellent introductory tome is Les Adams, *The Second Amendment Primer* (Birmingham, AL: Palladium Press, 1996). Regarding incorporation of the Second Amendment, see: "The right to keep and bear arms: Report of the Subcommittee on the Constitution of the Committee on the Judiciary, United States Senate, Ninety-seventh Congress, second session," (Washington DC: U.S. Government Printing Office, February 1982); Richard L. Aynes, "On misreading John Bingham and the fourteenth amendment," *Yale Law Journal* 1993; 103:57-104.

24. Edgar A. Suter, William C. Waters, George B. Murray, et al., "Violence in America— effective solutions. *J Med Assoc Ga* 1995;84(6):253-264.

25. The minority supporting a collective right only view: Keith A. Ehrman and Dennis A. Henigan, "The second amendment in the 20th century: Have you seen your militia lately?" *Univ Dayton Law Review* 1989; 15:5-58; Dennis A. Henigan, "Arms, anarchy and the second amendment," *Valparaiso University Law Review* Fall 1991; 26: 107-129; S. Fields, "Guns, crime and the negligent gun owner," *Northern Kentucky Law Review* 1982; 10(1): 141-162; and W. Spannaus, "State firearms regulation and the second amendment," *Hamline Law Review* 1983; 6:383-408.

26. Tony Mauro, "Scholar's shift in thinking angers liberals—the federal government may not disarm individual citizens without some unusually strong justification," *USA Today*, August 27, 1999, https://www.tysknews.com/Depts/2nd_Amend/scholar_angers_liberals.htm.

27. Elizabeth J. Swasey, "Mission creep in the war on crime," *American Guardian*, September 1998, p. 10.

28. Richard Willing, "Case should shape future of gun control," *USA Today*, August 27, 1999.

29. Michael R. Rand, *Guns and Crime: Handgun Victimization, Firearm Self-Defense, and Firearm Theft*, NCJ-147003 (Washington DC: Department of Justice, Bureau of Justice Statistics, April 1994); Federal Bureau of Investigation, *Uniform Crime Reports: Crime in the United States, 1992*, (Washington DC: Government Printing Office, 1993); See also Don B. Kates and Patricia T. Harris, "How to make their day," *National Review* 1991;43(19):30-32.

30. "GOA Resources—1999 Firearms Fact Sheet," *Gun Owners of America*, December 24, 2008, https://www.gunowners.org/fs9901.htm; See also Guy Smith, *Gun Facts. Version 6.2.* (CreateSpace Independent Publishing Platform, 1st edition, February 26, 2013), http://www.gunfacts.info/.

31. "GOA Resources—Background checks: Ineffective, unconstitutional and dangerous," *Gun Owners of America*, August 11, 2016, https://www.gunowners.org/fs08112016. htm; See also Larry Pratt, "We don't need no stinkin' background checks," *Gun Owners of America*, January 25, 2016, https://www.gunowners.org/news01252016.htm; and "GOA Resources—Problems with background checks," *Gun Owners of America*, February 22, 2011, https://www.gunowners.org/fs2011b.htm; See also John Lott, "Why background checks couldn't stop Dylan Roof," *The Daily Caller*, July 5, 2015, http:// dailycaller.com/2015/07/10/why-background-checks-couldnt-stop-dylan-roof/2/; On the ATF illegal database, see Sam Rolley, "ATF forgot to comply with policy, accidentally creating gun owner database," *Gun Owners of America*, August 2, 2016, https://www.gunowners.org/oped08092016b.htm.

32. U.S. Department of Justice, Federal Bureau of Investigation, *National Instant Criminal Background Check System (NICS) Operations 2010 Report,* https:// www.fbi.gov/file-repository/2010-nics-ops-report-4-19-11-1.pdf/view; Erich Pratt comments on the FBI 2010 Report via personal communication on file. Pratt's analysis is supported by Matt Stroud citing the work of John R. Lott, Jr. of the Crime Prevention Research Center in "CRPC in the Associated Press on background checks," December 9, 2014, https://crimeresearch.org/2014/12/ cprc-in-the-associated-press-on-background-checks/.

33. Becket Adams, "Vietnam vet barred from owning a gun because of a teenage misdemeanor 45 years ago," *The Blaze*, February 26, 2013.

34. "Newsletters 1994-2001: 6/98 Lautenberg gun ban racking up the horror stories," *Gun Owners of America*, October 10, 2008, http://www.gunowners.org/nws9806-htm.htm.

35. "Driving Laws: How can I learn if I have a warrant for traffic tickets," *NOLO*, http://www.drivinglaws.org/resources/traffic-tickets/traffic-laws/ how-can-i-find-out-i-have-a-warrant-unpaid-traffic-tickets.

36. Dean Weingarten, "Federal government spends $1 billion a year on gun law enforcement," *The Truth About Guns*, August 8, 2016.

37. Larry Buchanan, Josh Keller, Richard A. Oppel Jr., and Daniel Victor, "How they got their guns," *The New York Times*, June 12, 2016, https://www.nytimes.com/ interactive/2015/10/03/us/how-mass-shooters-got-their-guns.html?mcubz=1.

38. Elizabeth Chuck, "More than 80% of guns used in mass shootings obtained legally," *NBC News*, December 5, 1015, http:// www.nbcnews.com/storyline/san-bernardino-shooting/ more-80-percent-guns-used-mass-shootings-obtained-legally-n474441.

39. Eyder Peralta, "Study: Most gun deaths happen outside of mass shootings," *NPR*, February 1, 2013, http://www.npr.org/sections/thetwo-way/2013/02/01/170872321/ study-most-gun-deaths-happen-outside-of-mass-shootings.

40. "Background checks for guns," *NRA-ILA*, the NRA Institute for Legislative Action, August 8, 2016, https://www.nraila.org/issues/background-checks-nics/.

CHAPTER 17

1. Don B. Kates, Henry E. Schaffer, John K. Lattimer, George B. Murray, Edwin H. Cassem, "Bad Medicine: Doctors and Guns" in *Guns: Who Should Have Them?* David B. Kopel, ed., (Amherst, NY: Prometheus Books, 1995), pp. 233-308.

2. Michael R. Rand, *Guns and Crime: Handgun Victimization, Firearm Self-Defense, and Firearm Theft*, NCJ-147003 (Washington DC: Department of Justice, Bureau of Justice Statistics, April 1994).

3. Federal Bureau of Investigation, *Uniform Crime Reports: Crime in the United States, 1992*, (Washington DC: Government Printing Office, 1993).

4. Gary Kleck, *Point Blank: Guns and Violence in America* (New York: Aldine de Gruyter, 1991).

5. "Uniform Crime Reports: Crimes in the United States, 1991," (Washington, DC: U.S. Government Printing Office, 1992), p. 12. For more recent data consult the Uniform Crime Reports and Guy Smith, "Concealed Carry and Violent Crime" in *Gun Facts. Version 6.2.* (CreateSpace Independent Publishing Platform, 1st edition, February 26, 2013), http://www.gunfacts.info/.

6. "20th Century U.S. Homicide and Suicide Rates per 100,000 population" adopted from Robert D. Grove and Alice M. Hetzel, *Vital Statistics Rates in the United States 1940-1960*, (Washington DC: National Center for Health Statistics, 1968) and *Vital Statistics of the United States*, (Hyattsville MD: National Center for Health Statistics, individual volumes for 1961 through 1991); and Guy Smith, "U.S. Homicide Rate per 100,000 Population," in *Gun Facts. Version 6.2.* (CreateSpace Independent Publishing Platform, 1st edition, February 26, 2013), http://www.gunfacts.info/.

7. John R. Lott, Jr., *More Guns, Less Crime: Understanding Crime and Gun Control Laws* (Chicago: University of Chicago Press, 1998) For CDC statistics see, Tom Vaughan, "The Illusion of Safety," *Doctors for Responsible Gun Ownership*, July 10, 2017, https://drgo.us/the-illusion-of-safety/.

8. National Safety Council, "Accident Facts 1991," (Chicago: National Safety Council, 1992).

9. David B. Kopel, "Children and Guns" in *Guns: Who Should Have Them?* (Amherst, NY: Prometheus Books, 1995), pp. 309-406.

10. National Safety Council, "Accident Facts 1992," (Chicago: National Safety Council, 1993).

11. "Eddie Eagle is not Joe Camel," *Medical Sentinel* 1998;3(3):76 and "Guns and safety," *Medical Sentinel* 1998;3(1):7; For a critical view of Eddie Eagle program and gun safety training, see Tara Halle, "Gun safety programs won't save your child, but this question might," *Forbes*, June 21, 2017, https://www.forbes.com/sites/tarahaelle/2017/06/21/gun-safety-programs-wont-save-your-child-but-this-question-might/#16127f3755b8; Contrary to the *Forbes* article and with statistics that support it, the NRA believes the Eddie Eagle program is effective and has even set up a new website. The NRA New Eddie Eagle program is Eddie Eagle GunSafe® Program and the website is https://eddieeagle.nra.org/.

12. David B. Kopel, "Children and Guns" in *Guns: Who Should Have Them?* (Amherst, NY: Prometheus Books, 1995), pp. 309-406.

13. For the tremendous drop in crime in the last 25 years, see Matt Ford, "What caused the great crime decline in the US?" *The Atlantic*, April 15, 2016, https://www.theatlantic. com/politics/archive/2016/04/what-caused-the-crime-decline/477408/; See also Anne Gearan, "Violent crime hits 25-year low," *Associated Press*, December 28, 1998; Michael J. Sniffen, "Murder rate reaches 30-year low," *Associated Press*, November 23, 1998; "Serious crimes drops in early 1998," *Associated Press*, December 14, 1998; "Juvenile Justice and Delinquency Prevention," FBI website, December 14, 1998.

14. James Alan Fox, *Multiple Homicide: Patterns of Serial and Mass Murder*. (Chicago: University of Chicago Press, 1998), quoted by Tanya Metaska in "Vicious media feeding frenzy," *World Net Daily*, August 19, 1999.

15. For the difficulty with what constitutes a mass shooting incident and for Professor James A. Fox's discussion on the FBI's "active shooter" report, see Gwyneth Kelly, "Here's why no one can agree on the number of mass shootings," *The New Republic*, October 3, 2015, https://newrepublic.com/article/123027/heres-why-no-one-can-agree-number-mass-shootings; See also James Alan Fox, "Umpqua shooting—a tragedy, not a trend," *USA Today*, October 2, 2015, https://www.usatoday.com/story/opinion/2015/10/02/umpqua-community-college-shooting-oregon-mass-shooting-fbi-statistics-column/73199052/.

16. "UPDATED: France had more casualties from mass public shootings in 2015 than the U.S. suffered during Obama's entire presidency (532 to 527)," *Crime Prevention Research Center*, February 22, 2017, https://crimeresearch.org/2017/02/france-suffered-more-casualties-murders-and-injuries-from-mass-public-shootings-in-2015-than-the-us-has-suffered-during-obamas-entire-presidency-508-to-424-2/. For mass shooting comparison between U.S and other countries see, "Sorry, despite gun-control advocate's claims, U.S. isn't the worst country for mass shootings." *Investor's Business Daily*, February 21, 2018, https://www.investors.com/politics/editorials/sorry-despite-gun-control-advocates-claims-u-s-isnt-the-worst-country-for-mass-shootings/. For Israel's experience, see, David Th. Schiller, "Israel's answer to eliminating school terrorism," *The Libertarian Enterprise*, No. 45, May 1, 1999, http://www.ncc-1776.org/tle1999/libe45-19990501-03.html.

17. For the California statistic, see Bonnie Berkowitz, Lazaro Gamio, Denise Lu, Kevin Uhrmacher, Todd Lindeman, "The math of mass shootings," *Washington Post*, June 6, 2017, https://www.washingtonpost.com/graphics/national/mass-shootings-in-america/; and for the FBI report, see *A Study of Active Shooter Incidents in the United States Between 2000 and 2013*, (Washington DC: Department of Justice, Federal Bureau of Investigation, September 16, 2013), https://www.fbi.gov/file-repository/active-shooter-study-2000-2013-1.pdf/view.

18. Brandon S. Centerwall, "Exposure to television as a risk factor for violence," *Am J Epidemiology* 1989; 129: 643-52; Brandon S. Centerwall, "Young adult suicide and exposure to television," *Soc Psy and Psychiatric Epid* 1990; 25:121;

Miguel A. Faria, Jr., "TV violence increases homicides," *NewsMax.com*, August 17, 2000, https://haciendapublishing.com/articles/tv-violence-increases-homicides; For a more recent and comprehensive article on the relationship of media sensationalism, violence and rampant shootings, see Miguel A. Faria, Jr., "Shooting rampages, mental health, and the sensationalization of violence," *Surg Neurol Int* 2013;4:16, https://haciendapublishing.com/articles/shooting-rampages-mental-health-and-sensationalization-violence.

19. For the critique of the study in *Pediatrics* (2017), see Jacob Sullum, "Report on 'children' killed by guns hypes accidents, which are rare and declining—Most gun-related deaths among minors are homicides, and four-fifths involve teenagers," *Reason*, June 20, 2017, http://reason.com/blog/2017/06/20/cnn-report-on-children-killed-by-guns-em). For the actual study, see Katherine A. Fowler, Linda L. Dahlberg, Tadesse Haileyesus, Carmen Gutierrez and Sarah Bacon, "Childhood firearm injuries in the United States," *Pediatrics*, June 15, 2017, http://pediatrics.aappublications.org/content/early/2017/06/15/peds.2016-3486.

20. *Urban Delinquency and Substance Abuse*, NCJ-143454 (Washington DC: Department of Justice, National Institute of Justice, Office of Juvenile Justice and Delinquency Prevention, August 1995); See also "Urban Delinquency and Substance Abuse," (Washington DC: Department of Justice, National Institute of Justice, Office of Juvenile Justice and Delinquency Prevention, 1999), p. 18; The study was cited also in "Juvenile Delinquency—Children and Guns," *Medical Sentinel* 1999;4(5):160.

21. Robert B. Young, "How to make friends and influence people—about guns," Doctors for Responsible Gun Ownership, September 7, 2017, https://drgo.us/how-to-make-friends-and-influence-people-about-guns/.

CHAPTER 18

1. Miguel A. Faria, Jr., "Religious morality (and secular humanism) in Western civilization as precursors to medical ethics: A historic perspective," *Surg Neurol Int* 16-Jun-2015;6:105, http://surgicalneurologyint.com/surgicalint-articles/religious-morality-and-secular-humanism-in-western-civilization-as-precursors-to-medical-ethics-a-historic-perspective/.

2. Larry Pratt, *Safeguarding Liberty: The Constitution & Citizen Militias*. (Franklin, TN: Legacy Communications, 1995).

3. Thomas Hobbes, *Leviathan* (The Great Books of the Western World, "Chapter XIII: Of the Natural Condition of Mankind As Concerning Their Felicity, and Misery." The Franklin Library, Pennsylvania, 1983), pp. 149-152.

4. Saint Thomas Aquinas, *Summa Theologica*, II, Ch. 64, Art. 7. And Aristotle, *On Man in the Universe*. (Metaphysics. Roslyn, NY: Walter J. Black, Inc., 1943), p. 86-142.

5. Cicero. *Selected Political Speeches*. Michael Grant, translator, (Penguin Classics, 1969), p. 222.

6. Catechism of the Catholic Church. Article 5: the Fifth Commandment. Legitimate defense, #2265, http://www.vatican.va/archive/ccc_css/archive/catechism/p3s2c2a5.htm; and Pope John Paul II, Encyclical Letter, EVANGELIUM VITAE, 1995.

7. John Locke. *Two Treatises on Government*, (Delanco, New Jersey, Special Edition, The Classics of Liberty Library, 1992), pp. 221-223. See also: Timothy W. Wheeler and E. John Wipfler, III. *Keeping Your Family Safe: The Responsibilities of Firearm Ownership*. (Bellevue, WA: Merrill Press, 2009), pp. 70-81.

8. Michael Brown, "The ethics of armed self defense," *Doctors for Responsible Gun Ownership*, February 18, 2016, https://drgo.us/the-ethics-of-armed-self-defense/.

9. "Understanding blunt force trauma lethality: An interview with Dr. Robert Margulies (Part 2)" for the Armed Citizens Legal Defense Network's ejournal, *Doctors for Responsible Gun Ownership*, March 30, 2017, https://drgo.us/understanding-blunt-force-trauma-lethality-an-interview-with-dr-robert-margulies-part-2/.

10. David C. Stolinsky, "America: The most violence nation?" *Medical Sentinel* 2000;5(6):199-201, https://haciendapublishing.com/medicalsentinel/america-most-violent-nation-0.

11. Miguel A. Faria, Jr., "Guns and violence," *Medical Sentinel* 2002;7(4):112-115, 118, https://haciendapublishing.com/medicalsentinel/guns-and-violence. For the "knockout game," see: Michael Gartland, "I was a victim of the knockout game," *New York Post*, November 23, 2013. For the fatal assault on the deputy sheriff and the surveillance video, see: Brian Rokos and Beatriz E. Valenzuela, "Suspect charged with murder in San Bernardino deputy's death," *Daily bulletin*, January 3, 2018, https://www.dailybulletin.com/2018/01/03/suspect-named-murder-charges-brought-in-attack-on-off-duty-san-bernardino-county-sheriffs-deputy/

12. Miguel A. Faria, Jr. and George T. Tindall, "Evacuation of subdural hematoma," in *The Medical Management of the Surgical Patient,* eds. Lubin, Walker, and Smith (Boston, MA: Butterworth Inc., 1982).

13. Don B. Kates and Patricia T. Harris, "How to make their day," *National Review* 1991;43(19):30-32.

14. Gary Kleck and Marc Gertz, "Armed Resistance to Crime: The Prevalence and Nature of Self-Defense With a Gun," *Journal of Criminal Law and Criminology* Fall 1995;86(1):164-185; See also Gary Kleck, *Point Blank: Guns and Violence in America* (New York: Aldine de Gruyter, 1991).

15. John R. Lott, Jr., *More Guns, Less Crime: Understanding Crime and Gun Control Laws* (Chicago: University of Chicago Press, 1998).

16. James Wright and Peter H. Rossi, *Armed and Considered Dangerous: A Survey of Felons and Their Firearms* (New York: Aldine de Gruyter, 1986)

PART VI

CHAPTER 19

1. For the "victim," see Geraldine Parker, "Invasion of Privacy," Letter to the Editor, *The Telegraph* (Macon), February 9, 2015, http://www.macon.com/opinion/letters-to-the-editor/article30171885.html; For those who believe there is nothing to hide, see Jim Huber, "Privacy," Letter to the Editor, *The Telegraph* (Macon), February 9, 2015; and Michael Collins, "Move to Macon." Letter to the Editor, *The Telegraph* (Macon), February 9, 2015, http://www.macon.com/opinion/letters-to-the-editor/article30172479.html. For the chastising citizen and others, see Bob White, "Obstinate Naïveté!" February 27, 2015, https://haciendapublishing.com/randomnotes/faria-american-na%C3%AFvet%C3%A9-part-2-if-you-have-nothing-hide.

2. For references on the Waco tragedy, see: David B. Kopel and Paul H. Blackman, *No More Wacos: What's Wrong With Federal Law Enforcement and How to Fix It* (Amherst, NY: Prometheus Books, 1997); and watch the film and video documentary, *WACO: The Rules of Engagement* by Dan Gifford, Amy Gifford, and William Gazecki (Los Angeles, CA: Somford Entertainment, 1997); For the saga of Carl Drega, see Vin Suprynowicz, *The Ballad of Carl Drega: Essays on the Freedom Movement 1994 to 2001* (Reno, Nevada: Mountain Media, 2002); For the stories of John Gerald Quinn, Bruce Abramski, and the many lawful American gun owners, who over the years have been victimized by the federal government for technical gun violations or errors, particularly the ATF, see *Gun Owners of America* (GOA) website, https://www.gunowners.org.

3. James W. Harris, "Privacy: You DO have something to hide," *Liberator Online*, June 26, 2013, https://www.theadvocates.org/tag/united-states-code/

4. "Clackamas mall shooter faced man with concealed weapon," *KGW.com*, Portland, http://www.kgw.com/news/clackamas-mall-shooter-faced-man-with-concealed-weapon_20160307101447700/71624413.

5. Wayne LaPierre, "Fugitive from injustice," *America's 1st Freedom*, October 2003, pp. 36-39, 54-55; See also Miguel A. Faria, Jr., "A nation of thieves," *World Net Daily*, October 17, 2003, https://haciendapublishing.com/articles/nation-thieves.

6. Miguel A. Faria, Jr., "Russia's invasion of the Ukraine—Tsarism or Stalinism anew?" *HaciendaPublishing.com*, March 5, 2014, https://haciendapublishing.com/articles/russias-invasion-ukraine-%E2%80%94-tsarism-or-stalinism-anew; For the fuss about NATO spending and payments, see Miguel A. Faria, Jr., "A glance at Trump's tough foreign policy!" *HaciendaPublishing.com*, July 22, 2016, https://haciendapublishing.com/articles/glance-trumps-tough-foreign-policy.

7. Miguel A. Faria, Jr., "A nation of Elois," *HaciendaPublishing.com*, October 1, 2014, https://haciendapublishing.com/articles/nation-elois.

8. Miguel A. Faria, Jr., "American naïveté—European social democracies and gun control," *HaciendaPublishing.com*, April 14, 2015, https://haciendapublishing.com/articles/

american-na%C3%AFvet%C3%A9-%E2%80%94-european-social-democracies-and-gun-control.

9. Miguel A. Faria, Jr., "The American 'gun culture' that saved Europe," *GOPUSA.com*, February 24, 2015, https://haciendapublishing.com/articles/american-gun-culture-saved-europe.

10. Miguel A. Faria, Jr., "The political spectrum (Part 1): The totalitarian left from communism to social democracy," *HaciendaPublishing.com*, September 28, 2011, https://haciendapublishing.com/articles/political-spectrum-part-i-totalitarian-left-communism-social-democracy.

11. Miguel A. Faria, Jr., "America, guns, and freedom. Part I: A recapitulation of liberty," *Surg Neurol Int* 2012;3:133, https://haciendapublishing.com/articles/america-guns-and-freedom-part-i-recapitulation-liberty.

12. Miguel A. Faria, Jr., "America, guns and freedom. Part II—An international perspective," *Surg Neurol Int* 2012;3:135, https://haciendapublishing.com/articles/america-guns-and-freedom-part-ii-%E2%80%94-international-perspective.

13. Midge Gillies, "Defending their realm," *The Guardian*, June 18, 2006, https://www.theguardian.com/world/2006/jun/19/secondworldwar.gender; see also: Mark A. Keefe, IV, "Send a gun to defend a British home, pistols, rifles, revolvers, shotguns, binoculars," *American Rifleman*, April 2002, http://www.freerepublic.com/focus/news/650257/posts.

14. The story of Sergeant Alvin York comes entirely from David B. Kopel, *The Morality of Self-Defense and Military Action: The Judeo-Christian Tradition* (Santa Barbara, CA: Praeger, 2017), pp. 353-355.

15. *Hogs Gone Wild*. Discovery Channel documentary, https://www.youtube.com/watch?v=5dxIVUfn-y8.

16. Wallace Schwam, "Gun control: A passivity disorder?" *Doctors for Responsible Gun Ownership*, June 8, 2017, https://drgo.us/gun-control-a-passivity-disorder/.

17. Miguel A. Faria, Jr., "Wild hogs—hunt (or trap), shoot—and let's make excellent barbecue!" *HaciendaPublishing.com*, March 12, 2016, https://haciendapublishing.com/articles/wild-hogs-%E2%80%94-hunt-or-trap-shoot-%E2%80%94-and-let%E2%80%99s-make-excellent-barbecue. I first read the story by Dr. J. G. McDaniel about the wild hogs of Horse-Shoe Bend in a pamphlet printed by the Association of American Physicians and Surgeons (AAPS).

CHAPTER 20

1. David B. Kopel, *The Samurai, the Mountie, and the Cowboy: Should America Adopt the Gun Controls of Other Democracies?* (Amherst, NY: Prometheus Books, 1992). For the gun control experience in Japan, see pages 20-58; for Great Britain, see pages 59-135; for Canada, see pages 136-192; for Australia, see pages 193-232.

2. For the Crocodile Dundee story, see: Rory Carroll and Helen O'Neill, "Real Crocodile Dundee shot dead after rampage," *The Guardian*, August 4, 1999, https://www.theguardian.com/world/1999/aug/05/rorycarroll. For what happened after the

Tasmanian resort, see: H.L. Richardson, "The Gun Owners," newsletter for *Gun Owners of America*, January 31, 2000.

3. Robert Wainwright, "Gun laws fall short in war on crime," *The Sydney Morning Herald*, October 29, 2005, http://www.smh.com.au/news/national/gun-laws-fall-short-in-war-on-crime/2005/10/28/1130400366681.html.

4. "Australia: There will be blood," *America's 1st Freedom*, July 9, 2015, https://www.americas1stfreedom.org/articles/2015/7/9/australia-there-will-be-blood/. "Decades after firearm confiscation, Australia announces new amnesty program," *NRA-ILA*, Institute for Legislative Action, March 10, 2017, https://www.nraila.org/articles/20170310/decades-after-firearm-confiscation-australia-announces-new-amnesty-program.

5. For the Australian criminal justice system and the New South Wales figures, see: David B. Kopel, *The Samurai, the Mountie, and the Cowboy: Should America Adopt the Gun Controls of Other Democracies?* (Amherst, NY: Prometheus Books, 1992), pages 211-216, and for the U.S. convictions and jail terms, in comparison, see pages 375-376.

6. For those who still dispute what has happened in Australia and claimed that the ban did not increase crime and mayhem while restricting liberty Down Under, watch the video at https://www.youtube.com/watch_popup?v=fGaDAThOHhA.

7. Miguel A. Faria, Jr., "A nation of thieves," *World Net Daily*, October 17, 2003.

8. Wayne LaPierre, "Fugitive from injustice," *America's 1st Freedom*, October 2003, pp. 36-39, 54-55.

9. See "Tony Martin, 15 years on: I don't want to go back there because it could happen again," *Telegraph.co.uk*, http://www.telegraph.co.uk/news/uknews/crime/11044022/Tony-Martin-15-years-on-I-dont-want-to-go-back-there-because-it-could-happen-again.html; "Tony Martin held over gun possession," *BBC News*, December 31, 2015, http://www.bbc.co.uk/news/uk-england-35206113.

10. Patrick Henry, Speech to the Second Virginia convention at St. John's Church in Richmond, Virginia, March 23, 1775.

11. Miguel A. Faria, Jr., "England and gun control—moral decline of an empire," *Medical Sentinel* March/April 1999, pp. 52-55; See also Miguel A. Faria, Jr., "More gun control, more crime," *Human Events*, July 9, 1999.

12. T. Marshall, "Is Times Square safer than Piccadilly Circus?" *Washington Times*, National Weekly Edition, October 19-25, 1998.

13. David B. Kopel, *Gun Control in Great Britain: Saving Lives or Constricting Liberty?* (Chicago: Office of International Criminal Justice at the University of Illinois at Chicago, 1992), p. 46, quoted by Murphy C. Current in "Theory and reality of self-defense in Great Britain," *Gun News Digest*, Spring 1997, pp. 22-23, 45.

14. Michael J. Sniffen, "Murder rate reaches 30-year low," *Associated Press*, November 23, 1998. For how the UK uses misleading data, see Daily Staff, "How the UK covers up murder stats," *America's 1st Freedom*, July 17, 2015, https://www.americas1stfreedom.org/articles/2015/7/17/how-the-uk-covers-up-murder-stats/?utm_source=newsletter&utm_medium=insider&utm_campaign=1217; and for

the "sham" British figures, see David Kopel, Paul Gallant and Joanne D. Eisen, "Fear in Britain: They have no guns—so they have a lot of crime," *National Review Online*, July 18, 2000, http://www.davekopel.org/NRO/2000/Fear-in-Britain.htm.

15. J. Ungoed-Thomas, "A nation of thieves," *London Sunday Times*, January 11, 1998; See also Joseph Tartaro, "Great Britain—a nation of thieves," *Gun News Digest*, Fall 1998, p. 27. For the more recent statistics, especially England and Wales and London, see: Oliver JJ Lane, "London is falling: UK capital now more dangerous than NYC… more rape, more robbery, more violence," *Breitbart.com*, October 21, 2017, http://www.breitbart.com/london/2017/10/21/london-falling-uk-capital-now-dangerous-nyc-rape-robbery-violence/; Jack Montgomery, "Murders in London overtake New York for first time since 1800 under Sadiq Khan," *Breitbart.com*, April 1, 2018, http://www.breitbart.com/london/2018/04/01/murders-london-overtake-new-york-first-time-since-1800-sadiq-khan/; Virginia Hale, "Police say Britain now a global capital for acid attacks, *Breitbart.com*, December 8, 2017, http://www.breitbart.com/london/2017/12/08/uk-global-capital-acid-attacks/

16. John R. Lott, Jr., *More Guns, Less Crime: Understanding Crime and Gun Control Laws* (Chicago: University of Chicago Press, 1998); See also John R. Lott, Jr., *The Bias Against Guns: Why Almost Everything You've Heard About Gun Control is Wrong* (Washington DC: Regnery Publishing, Inc., 2003).

17. Aleksandr Solzhenitsyn, "Chapter 16: The socially friendly" in *The Gulag Archipelago 1918-1956: An Experiment in Literary Investigation III-IV*. (New York: Harper & Row Publisher), pp. 425-446.

18. Solzhenitsyn, "Chapter 13: Hand over your second skin too!" in *The Gulag Archipelago*, pp. 375-390.

19. Miguel A. Faria, Jr., *Cuba in Revolution: Escape From a Lost Paradise*. (Macon, GA: Hacienda Publishing, Inc., 2002), pp. 62-64; The Russian *druzhina* were the counterpart for the Cuban communist, *milicianos*, "the militia" used to fight bandits or other "enemies of the people."

20. "UK police tell subjects not to harm their attackers, get a rape alarm," *Daily Caller*, May 31, 2015, http://dailycaller.com/2015/05/31/uk-police-tell-subjects-not-to-harm-their-attackers-get-a-rape-alarm/.

CHAPTER 21

1. Miguel A. Faria, Jr., "Mass shootings and the mental health—At what cost?" *GOPUSA.com*, December 17, 2012.

2. Miguel A. Faria, Jr., "Shooting rampages, mental health, and the sensationalization of violence," *Surg Neurol Int* 2013;4:16, https://haciendapublishing.com/articles/shooting-rampages-mental-health-and-sensationalization-violence.

3. Miguel A. Faria, Jr., "National gun registration: The road to tyranny," *The Freeman*, March 1, 2001; For evidence of registration leading to confiscation in New York, California, and foreign countries, see "GOA resources—Problems with background checks," *Gun Owners of America*, February 22, 2011, https://www.gunowners.org/fs2011b.htm.

4. For the illegal databases and the Fast and Furious scandal, see Larry Pratt, "We don't need no stinkin' background checks," *Gun Owners of America*, January 25, 2016, https://www.gunowners.org/news01252016.htm; and Miguel A. Faria, Jr., "Gunrunning ATF runs amok!" *HaciendaPublishing.com*, July 18, 2011, https://haciendapublishing.com/articles/faria-gunrunning-atf-runs-amok; For the excesses of the ATF, the reader will find a fountain of information at "The Gun Owners," newsletter for *Gun Owners of America* (GOA), https://www.gunowners.org; For the infamy of the Waco tragedy, I refer the reader to David B. Kopel and Paul H. Blackman, *No More Wacos: What's Wrong With Federal Law Enforcement and How to Fix It.* (Amherst, NY: Prometheus Books, 1997).

5. Deroy Murdock, "Trump haters call for presidential assassination," *National Review Online*, March 25, 2017, http://www.nationalreview.com/article/446110/trump-assassination-threats-investigate-prosecute.

6. Cliff Kincaid, "America's elected government hangs in the balance," *GOPUSA.com*, May 19, 2017, http://www.gopusa.com/americas-elected-government-hangs-in-the-balance/; See also Miguel A. Faria, Jr., "Donald Trump president elect—One man's view of the 2016 election coverage!" *HaciendaPublishing.com*, November 9, 2016, https://haciendapublishing.com/articles/donald-trump-president-elect-%E2%80%94-one-man%E2%80%99s-view-2016-election-coverage.

7. Miguel A. Faria, Jr., "Wishful thinking and divining Donald Trump," *HaciendaPublishing.com*, April 30, 2017, https://haciendapublishing.com/articles/wishful-thinking-and-divining-donald-trump-miguel-faria-md.

8. Miguel A. Faria, Jr., "The dog and pony show of year round electioneering and the mainstream media," *GOPUSA.com*, May 12, 2015, https://haciendapublishing.com/articles/dog-and-pony-show-year-round-electioneering-and-mainstream-media.

9. Russell L. Blaylock, "Managed truth: The great danger to our republic," *Medical Sentinel* 1998;3(6):92-93, https://haciendapublishing.com/medicalsentinel/managed-truth-great-danger-our-republic; See also Russell L. Blaylock, *"The use of propaganda and psychological warfare by the left,"* *HaciendaPublishing.com, August 8, 2016, https://haciendapublishing.com/articles/use-propaganda-and-psychological-warfare-left-russell-l-blaylock-md.*

10. Miguel A. Faria, Jr., *Cuba in Revolution: Escape From a Lost Paradise.* (Macon, GA: Hacienda Publishing, Inc., 2002), pp. 256-281.

11. Ibid., pp. 215-228.

12. Brian McNicoll, "Violent leftist extremists' new intellectual champion becomes media darling," *Accuracy in Media* (AIM), August 22, 2017, http://www.aim.org/aim-column/violent-leftist-extremists-new-intellectual-champion-becomes-media-darling/.

13. The directive was cited in *People's Daily World*, the official newspaper of the Communist Party USA, February 25, 1961.

14. Miguel A. Faria, Jr., "The political spectrum (Part 1): The totalitarian left from communism to social democracy," *HaciendaPublishing.com*, September 28, 2011,

https://haciendapublishing.com/articles/political-spectrum-part-i-totalitarian-left-communism-social-democracy.

15. Miguel A. Faria, Jr., "Liberal intolerance—Tearing down monuments, rejecting history," *HaciendaPublishing.com*, August 17, 2017, https://haciendapublishing.com/articles/liberal-intolerance-%E2%80%94-tearing-down-monuments-rejecting-history-miguel-faria-md.

16. Miguel A. Faria, Jr., "Millennials—Anti-capitalist, socialist American youth?" *HaciendaPublishing.com*, May 11, 2016, https://haciendapublishing.com/articles/millennials-%E2%80%94-anti-capitalist-progressive-socialist-american-youth.

17. David Horowitz, *Radical Son: A Generational Odyssey*. (New York: Free Press, 1997).

18. Miguel A. Faria, Jr., "America guns and freedom: Part 1—A recapitulation of liberty," *Surg Neurol Int* 2012, https://haciendapublishing.com/articles/america-guns-and-freedom-part-i-recapitulation-liberty.

19. Miguel A. Faria, Jr., "America, guns and freedom: Part II—An international perspective," *Surg Neurol Int* 2012;3:135, https://haciendapublishing.com/articles/america-guns-and-freedom-part-ii-%E2%80%94-international-perspective.

20. Larry Pratt, "Trump signs GOA-supported repeal of Social Security gun ban," *The Gun Owners*, newsletter for *Gun Owners of America* (GOA), March 31, 2017, p. 8.

21. John Marzulli, "Weapons ban defied: S.I. man, arsenal seized," *Daily News*, September 5 1992; See also "GOA Resources—1999 Firearms Fact Sheet," *Gun Owners of America*, December 24, 2008, https://www.gunowners.org/fs9901.htm.

22. "Gun confiscation begins: Gun law victim holds press conference and turns in gun to local officials," *National Rifle Association*, press release, January 28, 1998. For an update, see: Charles C.W. Cooke, "In California, confiscation is no longer a threat. It's the Law," *America's 1st Freedom*, August 31, 2017, https://www.americas1stfreedom.org/articles/2017/8/31/in-california-confiscation-is-no-longer-a-threat-it-s-the-law/?

23. David B. Kopel, "Trust the people: The case against gun control," *Cato Institute*, Policy Analysis 109, July 11, 1988:25.

24. Don B. Kates, Henry E. Schaffer, John K. Lattimer, George B. Murray, Edwin H. Cassem, "Guns and public health: epidemic of violence or pandemic of propaganda?" *Tennessee Law Review* 1995;62:513-596.

25. Timothy Wheeler, "Public health gun control: A brief history—Part 1," *DRGO News*, January 3, 2013.

26. Timothy Wheeler, "Obama directs his executive power at American gun owners," *National Review Online*, January 16, 2013.

27. "Feinstein goes for broke with new gun-ban bill," *NRA-ILA*, December 27, 2012.

28. Lorne Gunter, "Shot in the foot by their gun registry: Auditor general confirms liberal boondoggle has cost us at least $1B," *Edmonton Journal*, December 4, 2002, p. A18.

29. Jay Simkin, Aaron S. Zelman, Alan M. Rice, *Lethal Laws: Gun Control is the Key to Genocide.* (Milwaukee, WI: Jews for the Preservation of Firearm Ownership, 1994), http://www.jpfo.org.

30. Albert Jay Nock, *Our Enemy the State* (1935). (San Francisco: Fox and Wilkes, 5th edition, 1994).

31. Rudolph J. Rummel, *Death by Government: Genocide and Mass Murder Since 1900.* (Piscataway, NJ: Transaction Publishers, 1994); Stéphane Courtois, Nicolas Werth, Jean-Louis Panne, et al., *The Black Book of Communism: Crimes, Terror, Repression.* (Cambridge, MA: Harvard University Press, 1999).

32. Don B. Kates (editor), *Firearms and Violence.* (San Francisco: Pacific Research Institute, 1984), pp. 14-22.

33. Thomas Jefferson to Edward Carrington, May 27, 1788, in *PTJ*, 13:208-9. Letterpress copy available online at the Library of Congress. Transcription available at Founders Online, http://founders.archives.gov/documents/Jefferson/01-13-02-0120.

34. John Locke, *Second Treatise of Civil Government, 1690.* Internet edition, https://www.marxists.org/reference/subject/politics/locke/ch03.htm.

PART VII

CHAPTER 22

1. Miguel A. Faria, Jr., "The tragedy in Arizona—A mental health challenge failure," *GOPUSA.com*, http://www.gopusa.com/commentary/2011/01/12/faria-the-tragedy-in-arizona-a-mental-healthchallenge-failure/.

2. Miguel A. Faria, Jr., "America, guns and freedom: Part II—An international perspective," *Surg Neurol Int* 2012; 3:135, https://haciendapublishing.com/articles/america-guns-and-freedom-part-ii-%E2%80%94-international-perspective.

3. P. Solomon Banda, "Suspect in Aurora, Colo. church shooting had been in prison," *CBS Denver*, April 24, 2012, http://denver.cbslocal.com/2012/04/24/suspect-in-aurora-church-shooting-had-been-in-prison/.

4. Miguel A. Faria, Jr., "Women, guns, and the medical literature—a raging debate," *Women and Guns*, October 1994, Vol. 6, No. 9, pp. 14-17, 52-53. https://haciendapublishing.com/articles/women-guns-and-medical-literature-raging-debate; See also James Wright and Peter H. Rossi, *Armed and Considered Dangerous: A Survey of Felons and Their Firearms* (New York: Aldine de Gruyter, 1986). This 247-page hardbound book was the analysis of extensive data collected from over 1,800 convicted felons in American state prisons; Gary Kleck, *Targeting Guns: Firearms and Their Control* (New York: Aldine de Gruyter, 1997); and Don B. Kates, Henry E. Schaffer, John K. Lattimer, George B. Murray, Edwin H. Cassem, "Guns and public health: epidemic of violence or pandemic of propaganda?" *Tennessee Law Review* 1995;62:513-596.

5. Miguel A. Faria, Jr., "Public health and gun control—A review (Part I): The benefits of firearms," *Medical Sentinel* 2001;6:11-13, https://haciendapublishing.com/articles/public-health-and-gun-control-review-part-i-benefits-firearms.

6. For the number of criminals killed by both police and armed citizens see, Gary Kleck, *Point Blank: Guns and Violence in America* (New York: Aldine de Gruyter, 1991), p.111-116, 148, and Edgar A. Suter, William C. Waters IV, George B. Murray, et al., "Violence in America—effective solutions," *J Med Assoc Ga* 1995;84(6):254-256. For the homicides that turn out to be "justifiable homicides" of criminals by armed citizens, see: Gary Kleck, "Crime control through the private use of armed force, *Social Problems*, 1988;35:1-21, and Edgar A. Suter, "Guns in the medical literature—a failure of peer review," *J Med Assoc Ga* 1994;83(3):137-148, http://www.rkba.org/research/suter/med-lit.html.

7. Robert A. Waters, *The Best Defense: True Stories of Intended Victims Who Defended Themselves With a Firearm.* (Nashville, TN: Cumberland House; 1998).

8. Ford Fessenden, William Glaberson, Laurie Goodstein, "They threaten, seethe and unhinge, then kill in quantity," *The New York Times*, April 9, 2000, http://www.nytimes.com/2000/04/09/us/they-threaten-seethe-and-unhinge-then-kill-in-quantity.html?pagewanted=allandsrc=pm.

9. Mark Follman, "More guns, more mass shootings—coincidence?" *Mother Jones*, September 26, 2012, http://m.motherjones.com/politics/2012/09/mass-shootings-investigation?page=1 [Last accessed on 2012 Sept 26].

10. Claude Fischer, "A crime puzzle: Violent crime declines in America," *UC Berkeley News Center, The Berkeley Blog*, June 16, 2010, http://blogs.berkeley.edu/2010/06/16/a-crime-puzzle-violent-crime-declines-in-america/.

11. Erica L. Smith and Alexia D. Cooper, *Homicide in the U.S. Known to Law Enforcement, 2011*, NCJ-243035 (Washington DC: Bureau of Justice Statistics, December 30, 2013), https://www.bjs.gov/index.cfm?ty=pbdetail&iid=4863.

12. "Criminal Victimization, 2013," (Washington DC: Bureau of Justice Statistics, September 18, 2014), http://www.bjs.gov/index.cfm?ty=pbdetail&iid=5113; see also: "United States Crime Rates 1960-2016," *FBI Uniform Crime Reports*, http://www.disastercenter.com/crime/uscrime.htm.

13. Daniel Webster, "Gun owners and Republicans don't really want concealed carry reciprocity bill," *The Hill*, December 20, 2017. The book cited by Webster is Louis Klarevas, *Rampage Nation: Securing America from Mass Shootings*, (Amherst NY: Prometheus Books, 2016).

14. Personal communication and interview with Brian Rigsby, 1996; See also Brian Rigsby cited in Robert A. Waters, *The Best Defense: True Stories of Intended Victims Who Defended Themselves With a Firearm.* (Nashville, TN: Cumberland House; 1998), pp. 125-128.

15. John R. Lott, Jr., *The Bias Against Guns: Why Almost Everything You've Heard About Gun Control is Wrong* (Washington DC: Regnery Publishing, Inc., 2003), pp. 24-27.

16. Katie Pavlich, "Mass murder prevented by off-duty cop," *Townhall.com*, December 18, 2012, http://townhall.com/tipsheet/katiepavlich/2012/12/18/mass-murder-prevented-by-offduty-cop-n1469380; See also: David B. Kopel, "Guns, mental illness and

Newtown," *Wall Street Journal*, December 17, 2012, http://online.wsj.com/article/SB10
0014241278873237231045781852718571857424036.html.

17. Madison Park and Holly Yan, "Texas church shooting leaves 26 dead, including 8
members of one family," *CNN*, November 6, 2017, http://www.cnn.com/2017/11/06/
us/texas-church-shooting/index.html; and Saeed Ahmed, Doug Criss, and
Emanuella Grinberg, " 'Hero' exchanged fire with gunman, then helped chase
him down," *CNN*, November 7, 2017, http://www.cnn.com/2017/11/05/us/texas-
church-shooting-resident-action/index.html; and Nomaan Merchant, Jim Vertuno,
Will Weissert, "Texas church gunman once escaped from mental health center,"
Associated Press, November 8, 2017, http://www.windstream.net/news/read/article/
the_associated_press-air_force_admits_fault_in_reporting_shooters_past-ap.

18. John Fund, "Facts about mass shootings: It's time to address mental health and gun-free
zones," *National Review Online*, December 16, 2012, http://www.nationalreview.com/
article/335739/facts-about-mass-shootings-john-fund.

19. Tracy Connor, "Dylann Roof indicted for murder in Charleston church
massacre," *NBC News*, July 7, 2015, http://www.nbcnews.com/storyline/
charleston-church-shooting/dylann-roof-indicted-murder-church-
massacre-n388066; For the Charleston, S.C., restaurant shooting, see Russ
Bynum, "Witness: Charleston gunman declared 'There's a new boss,' " *Associated
Press*, August 24, 2017, http://www.windstream.net/news/read/article/
the_associated_press-witness_charleston_gunman_declared_theres_a_new_bo-ap.

20. Columbine High School Shootings, *History Channel*, Internet edition, http://www.
history.com/topics/columbine-high-school-shootings.

21. Michael S. Schmidt and Richard Perez-Pena, "FBI treating San Bernardino
attack as terrorism case," *The New York Times*, December 4, 2015, https://
www.nytimes.com/2015/12/05/us/tashfeen-malik-islamic-state.html. See also,
Timothy Wheeler, "Active shooter seminar: Jihad comes to the inland empire,"
Doctors for Responsible Gun Ownership, October 13, 2016, https://drgo.us/
active-shooter-seminar-jihad-comes-to-the-inland-empire/.

22. Cliff Kincaid, "Blaming conservatives for Muslim terrorism," *GOPUSA.com*, June 14,
2016, http://www.gopusa.com/blaming-conservatives-for-muslim-terrorism/.

23. Larry Elder, "Obama on Orlando: It's all about the guns," *GOPUSA.com*, June 16,
2016, http://www.gopusa.com/obama-on-orlando-its-all-about-the-guns/. For the
recent jihad-inspired truck attack in New York City, see: Larry Celona, "Terror
Suspect in NYC truck attack pledged allegiance to ISIS," *New York Post*, October
31, 2017, http://nypost.com/2017/10/31/terror-suspect-in-nyc-truck-attack-
had-pledged-allegiance-to-isis/. For President Trump's attempted immigration
ban, see: Miguel A. Faria, Jr., "Media duplicity, activist judges, and the attack on
Trump's immigration ban," *HaciendaPublishing.com*, February 12, 2017, https://
haciendapublishing.com/articles/media-duplicity-activist-judges-and-attack-
trump%E2%80%99s-immigration-ban-miguel-faria-md. As for the NYT columnist
and NYC politicians peddling gun control, see Matt Vespa, "NYT columnists gets

ripped for peddling gun control talking points after NYC terror attack," *Gun Owners of America*, November 1, 2017, https://gunowners.org/nyt-columnist-gets-ripped-for-peddling-gun-control-talking-points-after-nyc-terror-attack.htm; and Brenda Kirby, "New York Dems Push Gun Control After Truck Attack—Gov. Andrew Cuomo and New York City Mayor Bill de Blasio talked firearms, avoiding the real cause of terror." *Polizette*, November 2, 2017, http://www.lifezette.com/polizette/in-wake-of-pickup-truck-attack-new-york-pols-decry-guns/

24. "Nebraska Democrat removed from party position after wishing Steve Scalise had died," *GOPUSA.com*, June 24, 2017, http://www.gopusa.com/nebraska-democrat-removed-from-party-position-after-wishing-steve-scalise-had-died/.

25. Ryan W. Miller, "Pressure mounts for state senator to resign after Trump assassination comment," *USA Today*, August 18, 2017, https://www.usatoday.com/story/news/politics/onpolitics/2017/08/18/maria-chappelle-nadal-eric-greitens-call-resignation-after-trump-assassination-comment/582468001/.

26. Susan Cornwell and David Morgan, "U.S. congressman in critical condition after surgery," *Reuters*, June 15, 2017), https://www.reuters.com/article/us-virginia-shooting-idUSKBN1961W8.

27. Michael Haberluck, "After Scalise shooting congress wants to pack heat," *GOPUSA.com*, June 19, 2017.

28. Robert B. Young, "Executive Action, gun control and mental illness: Too little still too much," *Doctors for Responsible Gun Ownership*, January 14, 2016, https://drgo.us/executive-action-gun-control-and-mental-illness-too-little-is-still-too-much/. For the U.S. Secret Service and the U.S. Department of Education, see: "The final report and findings of the safe school initiative: Implications for the prevention of school attacks in the United States," 2004, https://www2.ed.gov/admins/lead/safety/preventingattacksreport.pdf. Regarding gun-violence restraining order, see David French, "A gun-control measure conservatives should consider," *NationalReview.com*, February 16, 2018, https://www.nationalreview.com/2018/02/gun-control-republicans-consider-grvo/?utm_source=Facebook&utm_medium=Social&utm_campaign=French

29. Miguel A. Faria, Jr., "California: Another lesson about children and guns," *Newsmax.com*, March 12, 2001, https://haciendapublishing.com/articles/california-another-lesson-about-children-and-guns.

30. Michael S. Brown, "The Smear: A review of Sharyl Attkinson's book," *Doctors for Responsible Gun Ownership*, July 26, 2017, https://drgo.us/the-smear-a-book-review/.

31. Miguel A. Faria, Jr., "TV violence increases homicides," *Newsmax.com*, August 17, 2000, https://haciendapublishing.com/articles/tv-violence-increases-homicides.

32. "Newtown shootings: Democrats Malloy and Feinstein seek gun controls," *BBC News*, December 16, 2012, http://www.bbc.co.uk/news/world-us-canada-20749167.

33. Timothy Wheeler, "Heal the sick and stop the shootings," *The GunMag*, December 17, 2012, http://www.thegunmag.com/heal-the-sick-and-stop-the-shootings/.

34. Richard Simon, "Senate votes down Feinstein's assault weapons ban," *Los Angeles Times*, April 12, 2013.

35. Stacy Washington, "U.S. Virgin Islands politician uses hurricane to order gun confiscation," *America's 1st Freedom*, September 7, 2017, https://www.americas1stfreedom.org/articles/2017/9/7/us-virgin-islands-politician-uses-hurricane-to-order-gun-confiscation/.

36. U.S. & Texas Law Shield, Legal Defense for Self Defense, "Can the government confiscate my firearms during a disaster?" *USLawShield.com*, September 6, 2017, https://blog.uslawshield.com/can-government-confiscate-guns-disaster/; For the mayhem in the Virgin Islands, see John Farnam, "Chaos and looting of the Caribbean after Hurricane Irma, residents defenseless," *Ammoland*, September 16, 2017, https://www.ammoland.com/2017/09/chaos-looting-caribbean-after-hurricane-irma/#ixzz4tnY5wU66.

37. Charlton Heston, 'Arming America,' Letter, *The New York Times*, October 1, 2000, http://www.nytimes.com/2000/10/01/books/l-arming-america-266906.html; and Clayton E. Cramer, "What Clayton Cramer saw and (nearly) everyone else missed," *History News Network*, 2002, http://historynewsnetwork.org/article/1185; See also Clayton Cramer, "Shots in the Dark: Bellesiles' Arming America is novel in both senses," *National Review*, September 23, 2000.

38. Roger D. McGrath, *Gunfighters, Highwaymen and Vigilantes: Violence on the Frontier*, (Berkeley: University of California Press, 1984). For a summary of the experience of other frontier towns, see: David B. Kopel, *The Samurai, the Mountie, and the Cowboy: Should America Adopt the Gun Controls of Other Democracies?* (Amherst, NY: Prometheus Books, 1992), pp. 327-329.

39. Russell L. Blaylock, "Contemporary popular culture and the antiheroes of the Hollywood left," *HaciendaPublishing.com*, March 10, 2016, https://haciendapublishing.com/articles/contemporary-popular-culture-and-antiheroes-hollywood-left-russell-l-blaylock-md.

40. Miguel A. Faria, Jr., "The Hollywood left, the antihero, and a dystopic future," *HaciendaPublishing.com*, March 13, 2016, https://haciendapublishing.com/articles/contemporary-popular-culture-and-antiheroes-hollywood-left-russell-l-blaylock-md.

41. Cristina Marcos, "Scalise; Shooting 'fortified' my view on gun rights," *The Hill*, October 3, 2017, http://thehill.com/homenews/house/353714-scalise-shooting-fortified-view-on-gun-rights.

42. Andrew Blankstein, Pete Williams, Rachel Elbaum and Elizabeth Chuck, "Las Vegas shooting: 59 killed and more than 500 hurt near Mandalay Bay," *NBC News*, October 2, 2017, https://www.nbcnews.com/storyline/las-vegas-shooting/las-vegas-police-investigating-shooting-mandalay-bay-n806461.

43. Marlee Macleod, "Charles Whitman: The Texas tower sniper," *Crime Library: Criminal minds and methods*, https://web.archive.org/web/20120701063429/http://www.trutv.com/library/crime/notorious_murders/mass/whitman/charlie_2.html.

44. "Who is Stephen Paddock? Las Vegas gunman's father was 'psychopathic' bank robber on FBI most wanted list," *National Post*, October 2, 2017, http://nationalpost.com/news/world/who-is-stephen-paddock-nothing-secret-or-strange-about-retiree-behind-las-vegas-shooting.

45. Miguel A. Faria, Jr., "Violence, mental illness, and the brain—A brief history of psychosurgery: Part 2—From the limbic system and cingulotomy to deep brain stimulation," *Surg Neurol Int* 2013;4(1):75, http://surgicalneurologyint.com/surgicalint_articles/violence-mental-illness-and-the-brain-a-brief-history-of-psychosurgery-part-2-from-the-limbic-system-and-cingulotomy-to-deep-brain-stimulation/.

46. Miguel A. Faria, Jr., "Violence, mental illness, and the brain—A brief history of psychosurgery: Part 3—From deep brain stimulation to amygdalotomy for violent behavior, seizures, and pathological aggression in humans," *Surg Neurol Int* 2013;4(1):91, https://haciendapublishing.com/articles/violence-mental-illness-and-brain-%E2%80%93-brief-history-psychosurgery-part-3-%E2%80%93-deep-brain-stimula.

PART VIII

CHAPTER 23

1. Abraham Lincoln, "The Perpetuation of Our Political Institutions," an oration delivered to the Young Men's Lyceum of Springfield, Illinois, 1839.

2. Marek Edelman, *The Ghetto Fights: Warsaw, 1941–43* (London: Bookmarks Publications, 1990).

3. Stanley Blejwas, "A heroic uprising in Poland," *The Polish American Journal*, August 2004, http://www.polamjournal.com/Library/APHistory/Warsaw_Uprising/warsaw_uprising.html; and Apolonja Kojder and Mark Wegierski, "The Role of Poland and the Poles in World War II," *The Polish American Journal*, August 2004, http://www.polamjournal.com/Library/APHistory/Warsaw_Uprising/warsaw_uprising.html.

4. David Wdowiński, *And We Are Not Saved: The Jewish Military Organization in the Warsaw Ghetto* (New York: Philosophical Library, 1963).

5. Holocaust Encyclopedia, "Hungary after the German occupation," *United States Holocaust Memorial Museum*, Washington, DC, http://www.ushmm.org/wlc/en/article.php?ModuleId=10005458.

6. Miguel A. Faria, Jr., *Cuba in Revolution: Escape From a Lost Paradise.* (Macon, GA: Hacienda Publishing, Inc., 2002), https://haciendapublishing.com/articles/interview-dr-miguel-faria-part-i-myles-b-kantor. For the most updated figures of non-combat victims of Fidel and Raúl Castro's regime, visit the Cuba Archive, www.CubaArchive.org.

7. Juan Clark, Cuba, *Mito y Realidad: Testimonios de un Pueblo* (Miami, FL: Saeta Ediciones, 2nd edition, 1992).

8. Enrique Encinosa, *Cuba en Guerra: Historia de la Oposicion AntiCastrista 19591993* (Miami, FL: The Endowment for Cuban American Studies, 1994).

9. Les Adams, *The Second Amendment Primer: A Citizen's Guidebook to the History, Sources, and Authorities for the Constitutional Guarantee of the Right to Keep and Bear Arms* (Birmingham, AL: Palladium Press, 1996).

10. Stephen P. Halbrook, *That Every Man Be Armed: The Evolution of a Constitutional Right* (Albuquerque, NM: University of New Mexico Press, 1984).

11. Larry Pratt, *Safeguarding Liberty: The Constitution and Citizen Militias* (Franklin, TN; Legacy Communications, 1995).

12. Albert Jay Nock, *Our Enemy the State* (1935). (San Francisco: Fox and Wilkes, 5th edition, 1994).

13. Joseph Story, *Commentaries on the Constitution of the United States (1830)* quoted in Les Adams, *The Second Amendment Primer: A Citizen's Guidebook to the History, Sources, and Authorities for the Constitutional Guarantee of the Right to Keep and Bear Arms* (Birmingham, AL: Palladium Press, 1996).

14. Elizabeth Slattery, "Another gun rights victory: Fed appeals court strikes down concealed carry restriction," *CNS News*, July 26, 2017, http://www.cnsnews.com/commentary/elizabeth-slattery/another-dc-gun-rights-victory-fed-appeals-court-strikes-down-concealed; See also, Brandon Carter, "Supreme Court declines to hear two Second Amendment cases," June 26, 2017, http://thehill.com/regulation/court-battles/339455-supreme-court-refuses-to-hear-two-second-amendment-cases; and Ann E. Marimow, "Appeals court blocks enforcement of District's strict concealed-carry law," *Washington Post*, July 25, 2017, https://www.washingtonpost.com/local/public-safety/appeals-court-blocks-enforcement-of-districts-strict-concealed-carry-law/2017/07/25/29bcbdfc-7146-11e7-9eac-d56bd5568db8_story.html?utm_term=.a49a36c94d9c.

15. "U.S. Supreme Court refuses to take up Florida gun case that banned open-carry," *The News Service of Florida*, November 27, 2017, http://www.news-press.com/story/news/2017/11/27/u-s-supreme-court-refuses-take-up-florida-gun-case-banned-open-carry/898047001/. Lydia Wheeler, "Supreme Court refuses to take up Maryland's assault weapons ban," November 27, 2017, http://thehill.com/regulation/court-battles/361969-supreme-court-refuses-to-take-up-marylands-assault-weapons-ban.

16. "Help Gun Owners of America stop the UN's continuous attempts to destroy the 2nd Amendment," *Gun Owners of America*, July 31, 2012, http://www.gunowners.org/a07312012.htm.

17. Larry Pratt, "We don't need no stinkin' background checks," *Gun Owners of America*, January 25, 2016, https://www.gunowners.org/news01252016.htm; and Miguel A. Faria, Jr., "Gunrunning ATF runs amok!" *HaciendaPublishing.com*, July 18, 2011, https://haciendapublishing.com/articles/faria-gunrunning-atf-runs-amok.

18. "Czechs file suit challenging EU gun controls," *NRA-ILA*, Institute for Legislative Action, August 11, 2017, https://www.nraila.org/articles/20170811/czechs-file-suit-challenging-eu-gun-controls.

19. Edgar A. Suter, "Guns in the medical literature—a failure of peer review," *J Med Assoc Ga* 1994;83(3):13748, http://rkba.org/research/suter/med-lit.html.

20. Gary Kleck, *Point Blank: Guns and Violence in America* (New York: Aldine de Gruyter, 1991).

21. Gary Kleck, *Targeting Guns: Firearms and Their Control* (New York: Aldine de Gruyter, 1997).

22. Edgar A. Suter, William C. Waters, George B. Murray, et al., "Violence in America— effective solutions," *J Med Assoc Ga* 1995;84(6):25363, http://www.rkba.org/research/ suter/violence.html. For the 2015 "gun violence" costs statistics, see: Mark Follman, Julie Lurie, Jaeah Lee, and James West, "The true cost of gun violence in America," *Mother Jones*, April 15, 2015. For the economic savings of guns, see: Robert B. Young, "Guns save lives (and money)." *Doctors for Responsible Gun Ownership*, June 5, 2018, https://drgo.us/guns-save-lives-and-money/.

23. Criminal histories of murder victims are based on statistics from the city of Chicago, see Matt L. Rodriguez, Superintendent of Police for the City of Chicago, *1997 Murder Analysis*, *1996 Murder Analysis*, and *1995 Murder Analysis*. For criminal histories of murderers nationwide, see Bureau of Justice Statistics, *National Update*, October 1991: 4.

24. Arthur L. Kellermann and Donald T. Reay, "Protection or peril? An analysis of firearm-related deaths in the home," *N Engl J Med* 1986;314:1557-1560.

25. James T. Bennett and Thomas J. DiLorenzo, *From Pathology to Politics: Public Health in America* (New Brunswick, NJ: Transaction Publishers, 2000).

26. Miguel A. Faria, Jr., "Public health—from science to politics," *Medical Sentinel* 2001;6(2):46-49, https://haciendapublishing.com/medicalsentinel/ public-health-science-politics.

27. Miguel A. Faria, Jr., "The perversion of science and medicine (Part II): Soviet science and gun control," *Medical Sentinel* 1997;2:4953, https://haciendapublishing.com/medicalsentinel/ perversion-science-and-medicine-part-ii-soviet-science-and-gun-control.

28. Miguel A. Faria, Jr., "Statistical malpractice—'Firearm availability' and violence (Part I): Politics or science?" *Medical Sentinel* 2002;7:132133, https://haciendapublishing.com/medicalsentinel/ statistical-malpractice-firearm-availability-and-violence-part-i-politics-or-science.

29. Miguel A. Faria, Jr., "Statistical malpractice—'Firearm availability' and violence (Part II): Poverty, education and other socioeconomic factors," *HaciendaPublishing.com*, March 25, 2002, https://haciendapublishing.com/articles/statistical-malpractice-%C2%AD-firearm-availability-and-violence-part-ii-poverty-education-and-other-socioeconomic-factors.

30. Miguel A. Faria, Jr., "Part 1: Public health, social science, and the scientific method," *Surgical Neurology* 2007;67(2):211-214. https://haciendapublishing.com/articles/ public-health-social-science-and-scientific-method-part-i.

31. Miguel A. Faria, Jr., "Part II: Public health, social science, and the scientific method," *Surgical Neurology* 2007;67:31822, https://haciendapublishing.com/articles/ public-health-social-science-and-scientific-method-part-ii.

32. Don B. Kates, Henry E. Schaffer, John K. Lattimer, George B. Murray, Edwin H. Cassem, "Guns and public health: epidemic of violence or pandemic of propaganda?" *Tennessee Law Review* 1995;62:513-596.

33. Timothy Wheeler. "Boundary violation: Gun politics in the doctor's office," *Medical Sentinel* 1999;4(2):60-61, https://haciendapublishing.com/medicalsentinel/boundary-violations-gun-politics-doctors-office.

34. John R. Lott, Jr., *More Guns, Less Crime: Understanding Crime and Gun Control Laws* (Chicago: University of Chicago Press, 1998); See also John R. Lott, Jr., *The Bias Against Guns: Why Almost Everything You've Heard About Gun Control is Wrong* (Washington DC: Regnery Publishing, Inc., 2003); and the summation of Lott's work in David C. Stolinsky and Timothy W. Wheeler, *Firearms—A Handbook for Health Professionals* (Claremont, California: The Claremont Institute, 1999).

35. David B. Kopel, *Guns: Who Should Have Them?* (Amherst, NY: Prometheus Books, 1995), p. 309-379; See also Jacob Sullum, "Report on 'children' killed by guns hypes accidents, which are rare and declining—Most gun-related deaths among minors are homicides, and four-fifths involve teenagers," *Reason*, June 20, 2017, http://reason.com/blog/2017/06/20/cnn-report-on-children-killed-by-guns-em).

CHAPTER 24

1. David B. Kopel, *The Samurai, the Mountie, and the Cowboy: Should America Adopt the Gun Controls of Other Democracies?* (Amherst, NY: Prometheus Books, 1992).

2. Miguel A. Faria, Jr., "The tragedy in Arizona—A mental health challenge failure, *GOPUSA.com*, http://www.gopusa.com/commentary/2011/01/12/faria-the-tragedy-in-arizona-a-mental-healthchallenge-failure/; See also Miguel A. Faria, Jr., "Shooting rampages, mental health, and the sensationalization of violence," *Surg Neurol Int* 2013;4(1):16.

3. Erich Pratt, "Colorado shooting shows the failure of gun control laws," *U.S. News and World Report*, July 26, 2012, https://www.usnews.com/debate-club/does-the-colorado-shooting-prove-the-need-for-more-gun-control-laws/colorado-shooting-shows-the-failure-of-gun-control-laws.

4. "Prosecutors in Norway call for Breivik insanity verdict," *BBC News*, June 21, 2012, http://www.bbc.co.uk/news/world-europe-18530670

5. Don B. Kates, Henry E. Schaffer, John K. Lattimer, George B. Murray, Edwin H. Cassem, "Guns and public health: epidemic of violence or pandemic of propaganda?" *Tennessee Law Review* 1995;62:513-596.

6. Don B. Kates and Patricia T. Harris, "How to make their day," *National Review* 1991;43(19):30-32.

7. Michael R. Rand, *Guns and Crime: Handgun Victimization, Firearm Self-Defense, and Firearm Theft*, NCJ-147003 (Washington DC: Department of Justice, Bureau of Justice Statistics, April 1994).

8. Federal Bureau of Investigation, *Uniform Crime Reports: Crime in the United States, 1992*, (Washington DC: Government Printing Office, 1993).

9. Miguel A. Faria, Jr., "Public health and gun control—A review (Part I): The benefits of firearms," *Medical Sentinel* 2001;6:14-18, https://haciendapublishing.com/medicalsentinel/public-health-and-gun-control-review-part-i-benefits-firearms.

10. Gary Kleck, *Point Blank: Guns and Violence in America* (New York: Aldine de Gruyter, 1991).

11. John R. Lott, Jr., *More Guns, Less Crime: Understanding Crime and Gun Control Laws* (Chicago: University of Chicago Press, 1998).

12. G. Marie Wilt, James D. Bannon, Ronald K. Breedlove, et al., *Domestic Violence and the Police: Studies in Detroit and Kansas City* (Washington DC, Police Foundation, 1977).

13. *Thomas E. Gift, "Firearms and 'rural' suicides," Doctors for Responsible Gun Ownership, August 24, 2017,* https://drgo.us/firearms-and-rural-suicides/.

14. Gary Kleck, *Targeting Guns: Firearms and Their Control* (New York: Aldine de Gruyter, 1997).

15. "20th Century U.S. Homicide and Suicide Rates per 100,000 population" adopted from Robert D. Grove and Alice M. Hetzel, *Vital Statistics Rates in the United States 1940-1960*, (Washington DC: National Center for Health Statistics, 1968) and *Vital Statistics of the United States*, (Hyattsville MD: National Center for Health Statistics, individual volumes for 1961 through 1991); and Guy Smith, "U.S. Homicide Rate per 100,000 Population," in *Gun Facts. Version 6.2.* (CreateSpace Independent Publishing Platform, 1st edition, February 26, 2013), http://www.gunfacts.info/.

16. Edgar A. Suter, "Guns in the medical literature—a failure of peer review," *J Med Assoc Ga* 1994;83(3):137-148; See also Edgar A. Suter, William C. Waters, George B. Murray, et al., "Violence in America—effective solutions. *J Med Assoc Ga* 1995;84(6):253264, http://rkba.org/research/suter/violence.html.

17. Richard Poe, *The Seven Myths of Gun Control: The Truth about Guns, Crime, and the Second Amendment* (Roseville, CA: Prima Publishing, 2001).

18. Robert A. Waters, *The Best Defense: True Stories of Intended Victims Who Defended Themselves With a Firearm.* (Nashville, TN: Cumberland House; 1998).

19. Miguel A. Faria, Jr., "Public health and gun control—No deterrent to crime," *The New American*, Vol. 15, No. 24, November 22, 1999, pp. 2324, https://haciendapublishing.com/articles/public-health-and-gun-control-no-deterrent-crime; The Maalot incident is described in the June 13, 1998, *Wyoming Star Tribune*. Charles Curley observed: "[After the Maalot incident] teachers and kindergarten nurses now started to carry guns. Schools were protected by parents (and often grandparents) guarding them in voluntary shifts. No school group went on a hike or a trip without armed guards. The police involved the citizens in a voluntary civil guard project Mishmar Esrachi that even had its own sniper teams. The army taught firearm safety and shooting techniques."

20. Stephen P. Halbrook, "Armed to the teeth and free," *Wall Street Journal*, Europe edition, June 4, 1999.

21. Miguel A. Faria, Jr., "Public health and gun control—A review (Part II): Gun violence
    and constitutional issues, *Medical Sentinel* 2001;6:1113, https://haciendapublishing
    .com/medicalsentinel/public-health-and-gun-control-review-part-ii-gun-violence-
    and-constitutional-issues.

22. Miguel A. Faria, Jr., "Gun control in Australia—chaos down under," *Medical Sentinel*
    2000;5:107; For more statistics and perspective, see H.L. Richardson, "The Gun
    Owners," newsletter for *Gun Owners of America* (GOA), January 31, 2000; Robert
    Wainwright, "Gun laws fall short in war on crime," *The Sydney Morning Herald*,
    October 29, 2005, http://www.smh.com.au/news/national/gun-laws-fall-short-in-war-
    on-crime/2005/10/28/1130400366681.html; "Australia: There will be blood," *America's
    1st Freedom*, July 9, 2015, https://www.americas1stfreedom.org/articles/2015/7/9/
    australia-there-will-be-blood/; "Decades after firearm confiscation, Australia
    announces new amnesty program," *NRA-ILA*, Institute for Legislative Action,
    March 10, 2017, https://www.nraila.org/articles/20170310/decades-after-firearm-
    confiscation-australia-announces-new-amnesty-program; and for those who still
    dispute what has happened in Australia and claimed that the ban did not increase
    crime and mayhem while restricting liberty Down Under, watch the video at https://
    www.youtube.com/watch_popup?v=fGaDAThOHhA.

23. Miguel A. Faria, Jr., "A nation of thieves," *World Net Daily*, October 17, 2003, http://
    www.wnd.com/index.php?fa=PAGE.view&pageId=21323. For further references
    to the title and the associated increase in crime in Great Britain in the 1990s, see
    J. Ungoed-Thomas, "A nation of thieves," *London Sunday Times*, January 11, 1998;
    Joseph Tartaro, "Great Britain—a nation of thieves," *Gun News Digest*, Fall 1998, p.
    27; Wayne LaPierre, "Fugitive from injustice," *America's 1st Freedom*, October 2003,
    pp. 36-39, 54-55; "Tony Martin, 15 years on: I don't want to go back there because
    it could happen again," *Telegraph.co.uk,* http://www.telegraph.co.uk/news/uknews/
    crime/11044022/Tony-Martin-15-years-on-I-dont-want-to-go-back-there-because-
    it-could-happen-again.html; "Tony Martin held over gun possession," *BBC News*,
    December 31, 2015, http://www.bbc.co.uk/news/uk-england-35206113.

24. Phillip Ramati, " 'I carry a gun all the time' says woman who thwarted Macon holdup
    attempt," *Macon Telegraph*, April 23, 2012, http://www.macon.com/news/local/crime/
    article30104844.html.

25. John H. Sloan, et al., "Firearm regulations and rates of suicide: A comparison of two
    metropolitan areas," *N Engl J Med* 1990:322:369373. More recently *Lancet* has entered
    the fray with a misleading and inflammatory editorial: "Gun deaths and the gun
    control debate in the USA," *Lancet*, (October 21) 2017:390:1812, http://www.thelancet.
    com/journals/lancet/article/PIIS0140-6736(17)32710-1/fulltext.

26. World Health Organization, "Mental health—suicide data," Geneva, Switzerland,
    2017, http://www.who.int/mental_health/prevention/suicide/suicideprevent/en/
    See also: Vladeta Ajdacic-Gross, Mitchell G. Weiss, et al., "Methods of suicide:
    international suicide patterns derived from the WHO mortality database," *Bulletin
    of the World Health Organization* 2008;86:726-732, http://www.who.int/bulletin/

volumes/86/9/07-043489/en/. For the misuse of statistics by the mainstream media (in this case CNN), including suicide data misinterpretation, see Miguel A Faria, Jr., "Gun statistics—Should they be tortured or gently cross-examined?" *HaciendaPublishing. com*, October 17, 2017, https://haciendapublishing.com/articles/gun-statistics-%E2%80%94-should-they-be-tortured-or-gently-cross-examined-miguel-faria-md

27. For the figures and discussion on children's death, see: David B. Kopel, *Guns: Who Should Have Them?* (Amherst, NY: Prometheus Books, 1995), pp. 309-379. For the critique of the study in *Pediatrics* (2017), see Jacob Sullen, "Report on 'children' killed by guns hypes accidents, which are rare and declining—Most gun-related deaths among minors are homicides, and four-fifths involve teenagers," *Reason*, June 20, 2017, http://reason.com/blog/2017/06/20/cnn-report-on-children-killed-by-guns-em). For the actual study, see Katherine A. Fowler, Linda L. Dahlberg, Tadesse Haileyesus, Carmen Gutierrez and Sarah Bacon, "Childhood firearm injuries in the United States," *Pediatrics*, June 15, 2017, http://pediatrics.aappublications.org/content/early/2017/06/15/peds.2016-3486.

28. Not everyone agrees that safe storage rules are followed and produce good results. See: Christen Smith, "Study: Safe storage programs produce mixed results." *Guns.com*, October 20, 2017. http://www.guns.com/2017/10/20/study-safe-storage-programs-produce-mixed-results/. That same article updates CDC statistics for 2015, including children's gun injuries and death. For documentation of the decline in serious crimes, including homicides, in previous decades, see: Anne Gearan, "Violent crime hits 25-year low," *Associated Press*, December 28, 1998; Michael J. Sniffen, "Murder rate reaches 30-year low," *Associated Press*, November 23, 1998; "Serious crimes drops in early 1998," *Associated Press*, December 14, 1998; "Juvenile Justice and Delinquency Prevention," FBI website, December 14, 1998. For the latest crime statistics and discussion of why serious crime has dropped in the last 25 years, see Matt Ford, "What caused the great crime decline in the U.S.?" *The Atlantic*, April 15, 2016, https://www.theatlantic.com/politics/archive/2016/04/what-caused-the-crime-decline/477408/. As for the serious crime increase in the U.S. in the past two years, see: "FBI releases 2016 crime statistics" (Washington DC: FBI National Press Office, September 25, 2017), https://www.fbi.gov/news/pressrel/press-releases/fbi-releases-2016-crime-statistics; For further analysis of the 2014-2016 spike in violent crime, see Mark Herman, "Violent crimes and murders increased in 2016 for a second consecutive year, FBI says," *Washington Post*, September 25, 2017, https://www.washingtonpost.com/news/post-nation/wp/2017/09/25/violent-crime-increased-in-2016-for-a-second-consecutive-year-fbi-says/?utm_term=.6003bdf5dff3

29. The dismal statistics that demonstrated the dramatic increase in Australian crime rates following the gun ban are no longer posted or were deliberately removed. Australian officials have even denied posting these data, even though they were documented at the time by the NRA and other sources. The truth is coming out despite the denials, see J. Schneider, "Australia's lesson for US gun owners," *Gun News Digest* 1996;2:2425,2831; J. Coochey, "Under handed statistics from 'Down Under,' " *Gun*

News Digest 1999;4:423; and J. Coochey, "Australia's antigun officials have no statistics to wear," *Gun News Digest* 2000;5:346. The graphs compiled from multiple sources in this book illustrate and tell the story. See also, Guy Smith, "Australia Violent Crime" and "Australia Homicide Rate," in *Gun Facts. Version 6.2.* (CreateSpace Independent Publishing Platform, 1st edition, February 26, 2013), http://www.gunfacts.info/.

30. *Urban Delinquency and Substance Abuse*, NCJ-143454 (Washington DC: Department of Justice, National Institute of Justice, Office of Juvenile Justice and Delinquency Prevention, August 1995); See also "Urban Delinquency and Substance Abuse," (Washington DC: Department of Justice, National Institute of Justice, Office of Juvenile Justice and Delinquency Prevention, 1999), p. 18.

31. Rudolph J. Rummel, *Death by Government: Genocide and Mass Murder Since 1900.* (Piscataway, NJ: Transaction Publishers, 1994).

32. Miguel A. Faria, Jr., "America, guns and freedom: Part II—An international perspective," *Surg Neurol Int* 2012;3(1):135, http://surgicalneurologyint.com/ surgicalint_articles/america-guns-and-freedom-part-ii-an-international-perspective/.

33. Jay Simkin, Aaron S. Zelman, Alan M. Rice, *Lethal Laws: Gun Control is the Key to Genocide.* (Milwaukee, WI: Jews for the Preservation of Firearm Ownership, 1994), http://www.jpfo.org.

34. Miguel A. Faria, Jr., "The perversion of science and medicine (Part II): Soviet science and gun control," *Medical Sentinel* 1997;2:4953, https://haciendapublishing.com/ medicalsentinel/perversion-science-and-medicine-part-ii-soviet-science-and-gun-control.

35. James Bovard, *Lost Rights: The Destruction of American Liberty* (New York: St. Martin's Griffin, 1995).

36. Stéphane Courtois, Nicolas Werth, Jean-Louis Panne, et al., *The Black Book of Communism: Crimes, Terror, Repression.* (Cambridge, MA: Harvard University Press, 1999).

37. Stephen P. Halbrook, *Target Switzerland: Swiss Armed Neutrality in World War II* (Boston: Da Capo Press; 1998).

38. Stephen P. Halbrook, *That Every Man Be Armed: The Evolution of a Constitutional Right* (Albuquerque, NM: University of New Mexico Press, 1984).

39. David T. Hardy, *Origins and Development of the Second Amendment* (Chino Valley, AZ: Blacksmith Corporation, 1986).

40. Larry Pratt, *Armed People Victorious* (Springfield, VA: Gun Owners Foundation, 1990). Hollie McKay, "Venezuelans regret gun ban, 'a declaration of war against an unarmed population,'" *Fox News*, December 14, 2018, https://www.foxnews.com/world/ venezuelans-regret-gun-prohibition-we-could-have-defended-ourselves.

41. Miguel A. Faria, Jr., "America, guns, and freedom. Part I: A recapitulation of liberty," *Surg Neurol Int* 2012;3(1):133, http://surgicalneurologyint.com/surgicalint_articles/ america-guns-and-freedom-part-i-a-recapitulation-of-liberty/.

42. Miguel A. Faria, Jr., "The perversion of science and medicine (Part I): On the nature of science," *Medical Sentinel* 1997;2(2):46-48; and Miguel A. Faria, Jr., "The perversion

of science and medicine (Part II): Soviet science and gun control," *Medical Sentinel* 1997;2(2):49-53.

43. Charles J. Brown and Armando M. Lago, *The Politics of Psychiatry in Revolutionary Cuba* (New York: Freedom House, 1991); For an extensive review of this difficult to obtain book, see Miguel A. Faria, Jr., "Cuban psychiatry—The perversion of medicine," *Medical Sentinel* 2000;5(5):160-162, https://haciendapublishing.com/medicalsentinel/cuban-psychiatry-perversion-medicine.

44. Leo Alexander, "Medical science under dictatorship," *New England Journal of Medicine*, July 14, 1949. Reprinted by Bibliographic Press, Flushing, New York, 1996.

45. Wolfgang Weyers, *Death of Medicine in Nazi Germany* (Philadelphia, PA: LippincottRaven Publishers, 1998). Reviewed by Joseph M. Scherzer in *Medical Sentinel* March/April 1994, https://haciendapublishing.com/medicalsentinel/death-medicine-nazi-germany-wolfgang-weyers-md.

CHAPTER 25

1. Gary Kleck, "Crime control through the private use of armed force," *Social Problems*, February 1988;35:13 cited in "GOA Resources—1999 Firearms Fact Sheet," *Gun Owners of America*, December 24, 2008, https://www.gunowners.org/fs9901.htm. For the Macon-Bibb County crime problem and statistics, see Miguel A. Faria, Jr., "A citizen's solution to the problem of burglaries and home invasions," *Macon Telegraph*, March 4, 2012, https://haciendapublishing.com/randomnotes/faria-solution-problem-burglaries-and-home-invasions.

2. Gary Kleck, "Crime control through the private use of armed force," *Social Problems*, February 1988;35:15; See also the report of Chief Dwaine L. Wilson, City of Kennesaw Police Department, *Month to Month Statistics, 1991: Residential burglary rates from 1981-1991; Statistics for the months of March—October*, cited in "GOA Resources—1999 Firearms Fact Sheet," *Gun Owners of America*, December 24, 2008, https://www.gunowners.org/fs9901.htm.

3. Gary Kleck, *Point Blank: Guns and Violence in America* (New York: Aldine de Gruyter, 1991), p.140, cited in "GOA Resources—1999 Firearms Fact Sheet," *Gun Owners of America*, December 24, 2008, https://www.gunowners.org/fs9901.htm.

4. James Wright and Peter H. Rossi, *Armed and Considered Dangerous: A Survey of Felons and Their Firearms* (New York: Aldine de Gruyter, 1986). The updated edition is James Wright and Peter H. Rossi, *Armed and Considered Dangerous: A Survey of Felons and Their Firearms* (Piscataway, NJ: Aldine Transition, 2nd edition, 2008).

5. Kevin Johnson, "FBI will overhaul tracking report, add missing crimes," *USA Today*, April 2, 2015, http://www.usatoday.com/story/news/nation/2015/04/02/fbi-crime-report/70393428/; See also FBI, *Crime in the United States, 2013: Offenses Known to Law Enforcement, Expanded Homicide Data Table 6*, (Washington DC: Department of Justice, Federal Bureau of Investigation, 2013), http://www.fbi.gov/about-us/cjis/ucr/crime-in-the-u.s/2013/crime-in-the-u.s.-2013/offenses-known-to-law-enforcement/expanded-homicide/

expanded_homicide_data_table_6_murder_race_and_sex_of_vicitm_by_race_and_
sex_of_offender_2013.xls.

6. Gary Kleck, *Point Blank: Guns and Violence in America* (New York: Aldine de Gruyter,
1991), p.111-116, 148. For the armed citizen track record shooting more criminals
than the police, see: George F. Will, "Are we 'A Nation of Cowards'?," *Newsweek* 15
November 1993:93; and Edgar A. Suter, William C. Waters IV, George B. Murray, et
al., "Violence in America—effective solutions," *J Med Assoc Ga* 1995;84(6):254-256.
For the flawed *Los Angeles Times* and the VPC report see: Scott Martell, "Gun and
self-defense statistics that might surprise you—and the NRA," *Los Angeles Times*,
June 19, 2015, http://www.latimes.com/opinion/opinion-la/la-ol-guns-self-defense-
charleston-20150619-story.html. For the underreporting of justifiable homicides by
20 percent, and the rate of self-defense, see: Gary Kleck, "Crime control through the
private use of armed force, *Social Problems*, 1988;35:1-21, and Edgar A. Suter, "Guns in
the medical literature—a failure of peer review," *J Med Assoc Ga* 1994;83(3):137-148.
For the critique of NCVS underreporting gun uses, see: Edgar A. Suter, William C.
Waters IV, George B. Murray, et al., "Violence in America—effective solutions," *J Med
Assoc Ga* 1995;84(6):254-256, and Gary Kleck, "Guns and self-protection," *J Med Assoc
Ga* 1994;83(1):42.

7. Edgar A. Suter, "Guns in the medical literature—a failure of peer review," *J Med Assoc
Ga* 1994;83(3):137-148. For the study at the time of the Obama administration, see:
"Priorities for research to reduce the threat of firearm-related violence," Institute of
Medicine and the National Research Council of the National Academies, 2003, https://
www.nap.edu/read/18319/chapter/1; for foundational study, see: Gary Kleck and Marc
Gertz, "Armed resistance to crime: The prevalence and nature of self-defense with a
gun," *Journal of Criminal Law and Criminology* Fall 1995;86(1):182-183.

8. Erich Pratt, "Anti-gunners doubling down on gun control in wake of GOA victory,"
Action alert, *Gun Owners of America*, August 23, 2017, http://www.gunowners.org.

9. Timothy Wheeler, "A sweep of every house," *HaciendaPublishing.com*, July 12, 2016,
https://haciendapublishing.com/articles/sweep-every-house-dr-timothy-wheeler.

10. John Velleco, "Momentum growing for Hearing Protection Act," *The Gun Owners*,
newsletter for *Gun Owners of America* (GOA), Volume XXXVII, Number 1, March 31,
2017.

11. Timothy Wheeler, "Medicine's shameful silence on silencers," *Doctors for Responsible
Gun Ownership*, May 19, 2017, https://drgo.us/medicines-shameful-silence-on-
silencers/; For the latest news on this issue, see "Paul Ryan says NRA-backed bill
shelved indefinitely," *Associated Press*, October 3, 2017, http://www.gopusa.com/
paul-ryan-says-nra-backed-bill-shelved-indefinitely/.

12. "Paul's office tells GOA the senator is 'locked and loaded' for battle over anti-gun
Obamacare," *Gun Owners of America*, July 27, 2017, https://www.gunowners.org/
alert072717.htm.

13. AWR Hawkins, "Campus Carry: Nearly 15 years with zero crimes by concealed
carriers," *America's 1st Freedom*, September 22, 2017, https://www.americas1stfreedom.

org/articles/2017/9/22/campus-carry-nearly-15-years-with-zero-crimes-by-concealed-carriers/; Jason W. Swindle, law professor, quoted in AWR Hawkins, "Professor: Anti-campus carry arguments not 'based on logic, history, or verified facts.' " *Gun Owners of America*, July 9, 2017, https://www.gunowners.org/pro-gun-professor-campus-carry.htm.

14. Andy McClure, " 'Constitutional carry' or weapons license?" *The Telegraph (Macon)*, July 31, 2017, http://www.macon.com/opinion/opn-columns-blogs/article164507707.html.

15. "GOA-backed concealed carry bills gaining steam," *The Gun Owners*, newsletter for *Gun Owners of America* (GOA), Volume XXXVII, Number 1, March 31, 2017.

16. Stephen P. Halbrook, *That Every Man Be Armed: The Evolution of a Constitutional Right* (Albuquerque, NM: University of New Mexico Press, 1984).

17. Hollie McKay, "Concealed-handgun carry bill triggers pushback from coastal mayors, police chiefs," *Fox News*, August 2, 2017, http://www.foxnews.com/us/2017/08/02/concealed-handgun-carry-bill-triggers-pushback-from-coastal-mayors-police-chiefs.html.

18. Les Adams, *The Second Amendment Primer: A Citizen's Guidebook to the History, Sources, and Authorities for the Constitutional Guarantee of the Right to Keep and Bear Arms* (Birmingham, AL: Palladium Press, 1996), p. 52.

19. William Blackstone, *Commentaries on the Laws of England* (1755) (Birmingham, AL: The Legal Classic Library, Gryphon Editions, Ltd., 1983).

20. David T. Hardy, *Origins and Development of the Second Amendment*. (Chino Valley, AZ: Blacksmith Corporation, 1986).

21. Joseph Story, *A Familiar Exposition of the Constitution of the United States* (1840) (Birmingham, AL: The Library of American Freedoms, Palladium Press, 2001).

22. Andrew Branca, "GA 16-3-23.1, No duty to retreat prior to use of force in self-defense," *The Law of Self-Defense*, January 8, 2013, https://lawofselfdefense.com/statute/ga-16-3-23-1-no-duty-to-retreat-prior-to-use-of-force-in-self-defense/.

23. "States that have stand your ground laws," *Thomson Reuters*, 2017, http://criminal.findlaw.com/criminal-law-basics/states-that-have-stand-your-ground-laws.html; At the time of this writing, 33 states have some form of "Stand Your Ground" legislation in place.

24. Jason L. Riley, "Race relations and law enforcement," *Imprimis*, January 2015, Volume 44, No 1, https://haciendapublishing.com/articles/race-relations-and-law-enforcement-jason-l-riley; See also Miguel A. Faria, Jr., "Police shootings and black on black crime," *GOPUSA.com*, April 27, 2015, https://haciendapublishing.com/articles/police-shootings-and-black-black-crime.

25. Concealed Carry Permit Reciprocity Maps, *USA Carry*, at https://www.usacarry.com/concealed_carry_permit_reciprocity_maps.html; Georgia now reciprocates in recognizing firearms licenses with the following states: Alabama, Alaska, Arkansas, Arizona, Colorado, Florida, Idaho, Indiana, Iowa, Kansas, Kentucky, Louisiana, Maine, Michigan, Mississippi, Missouri, Montana, New Hampshire, North Carolina, North Dakota, Ohio, Oklahoma, Pennsylvania, South Carolina, South Dakota,

Tennessee, Texas, Utah, West Virginia, Wisconsin, and Wyoming; See also Jim Morekis, "Georgia, S.C. now have firearm permit reciprocity," *CS News and Opinion*, June 6, 2016, https://www.connectsavannah.com/NewsFeed/archives/2016/06/06/georgia-sc-now-have-firearm-permit-reciprocity.

26. "Republicans coming under fierce pressure to buckle on gun rights," *Gun Owners of America*, October 4, 2017, https://gunowners.org/alert100417.htm.

27. S.A. Miller, "Trump, NRA open to ban on 'bump stocks' for guns," *Washington Times*, October 5, 2017; See also "Nancy Pelosi: 'I certainly hope' a ban on bump stock will lead to further gun restrictions," *Gun Owners of America*, October 6, 2017.

28. Douglas Ernst, "Gingrich open to new gun laws: 'As technology changes, sometimes we have to change the rules,' " *Washington Times*, October 4, 2017.

29. Miguel A. Faria, Jr., "The Las Vegas massacre and the Mass Shooting Derangement (MSD) syndrome," *The Telegraph* (Macon) and *HaciendaPublishing.com*, October 5, 2017, https://haciendapublishing.com/articles/las-vegas-massacre-and-mass-shooting-derangement-msd-syndrome-miguel-faria-md; see also: Miguel A. Faria, Jr., "The mass shooting derangement (MSD) syndrome, PC, and the modern liberalism (socialism) ethos that created them," *The Telegraph* (Macon) and *HaciendaPublishing.com*, November 9, 2017, https://haciendapublishing.com/articles/mass-shooting-derangement-msd-syndrome-pc-and-modern-liberalism-socialism-ethos-created-the.

30. Joyce Frieden and Molly Walker. "Calls Grow for CDC to Resume Gun Violence Research," *MedPage Today*, October 03, 2017, https://www.medpagetoday.com/publichealthpolicy/healthpolicy/68300

31. Miguel A. Faria, Jr., "Gun control: The assault on Congress by the medical journals (Part 1)," *The Telegraph* (Macon) and *HaciendaPublishing.com*, November 21, 2017, https://haciendapublishing.com/articles/gun-control-assault-congress-medical-journals-miguel-faria-md. And Miguel A. Faria, Jr., "Gun control: The assault on Congress by the medical journals (Part 2, JAMA)," *HaciendaPublishing.com*, December 4, 2017, https://haciendapublishing.com/articles/gun-control-assault-congress-medical-journals-part-2-%E2%80%94-jama-miguel-faria-md.

32. Miguel A. Faria, Jr., "Censorship: How the medical journals deny academic freedom," *The Telegraph* (Macon) and *HaciendaPublishing.com*, December 16, 2017, https://haciendapublishing.com/articles/censorship-how-medical-journals-deny-academic-freedom-miguel-faria-md.

33. Miguel A. Faria, Jr., "Concealed carry reciprocity coming soon to the U.S. Senate!" *The Telegraph* (Macon) and *HaciendaPublishing.com*, January 10, 2018, https://haciendapublishing.com/articles/concealed-carry-reciprocity-coming-soon-us-senate-miguel-faria-md.

34. "Why would anyone trust Feinstein and Schumer to support their gun rights?" *Gun Owners of America* (*GOA*), December 14, 2017, https://gunowners.org/why-would-anyone-trust-feinstein-and-schumer-to-support-their-gun-rights.htm.

35. Brandon Morse, "NRA fires back at misleading claims about the 'Fix NICS' bill attached to national reciprocity," *RedState*, December 6, 2017, https://www.redstate.com/

brandon_morse/2017/12/06/nra-fires-back-misleading-claims-fix-nics-bill-attached-national-reciprocity/.

EPILOGUE

1. " 'Poor track record,' GOA Resources—1999 Firearms Fact Sheet," *Gun Owners of America*, December 24, 2008, https://www.gunowners.org/fs9901.htm.

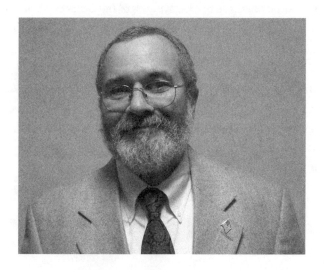

ABOUT THE AUTHOR

Miguel A. Faria, Jr., M.D. escaped with his father from communist Cuba at age 13 and came to the United States after a three-month odyssey through several Caribbean islands. They lived in "Little Havana" in Miami for two-and-one-half years before being reunited with the rest of their family. He grew up and was educated in Florida, South Carolina, and Georgia.

Presently, he is Associate Editor-in-Chief in Socioeconomics, Politics, Medicine and World Affairs of Surgical Neurology International (SNI), a peer-review, online, international journal for neurosurgeons and neuroscientists.

Dr. Faria is a former Clinical Professor of Surgery (Neurosurgery, ret.) and Adjunct Professor of Medical History (ret.), Mercer University School of Medicine.

Dr. Faria was appointed and served at the behest of President George W. Bush as a member of the Injury Research Grant Review Committee of the Centers for Disease Control and Prevention (CDC), 2002-2005.

He is the author of three books: *Vandals at the Gates of Medicine: Historic Perspectives on the Battle Over Health Care Reform* (1995); *Medical Warrior: Fighting Corporate Socialized Medicine* (1997); and *Cuba in Revolution: Escape From a Lost Paradise* (2002).

Dr. Faria has written over 200 medical, scientific and professional articles, letters or editorials published in the medical literature, including coauthoring several chapters in medical and neurosurgical textbooks. More than seventy of these articles are currently listed in PubMed under Faria MA Jr. as well as Faria MA or under his name at Google scholar listing. ResearchGate also cites some of his most recent peer-reviewed publications and citations in the medical literature.

BIBLIOGRAPHY

Beck, Glenn. *Control: Exposing the Truth About Guns.* (New York: Threshold Editions, 2013).

Bennett, James T. and DiLorenzo, Thomas J. *From Pathology to Politics: Public Health in America.* (New Brunswick, NJ: Transaction Publishers, 2000).

Bijlefeld, Marjolijn. *People For and Against Gun Control: A Biographical Reference.* (Westport, CT: Greenwood Press, 1999).

Blackstone, William. *Commentaries on the Laws of England (1755).* (Birmingham, AL: The Legal Classic Library, Gryphon Editions, Ltd., 1983).

Bovard, James. *The Destruction of American Liberty.* (New York: St. Martin's Press, 1995).

Clark, Juan M. *Castro's Revolution, Myth and Reality, Volume 1.* (CreateSpace Independent Publishing Platform, 1st edition, 2016).

Cook, Philip J. and Goss, Kristin A. *The Gun Debate: What Everyone Needs to Know.* (Oxford, UK: Oxford University Press, 2014).

Cornell, Saul. *A Well-Regulated Militia: The Founding Fathers and the Origins of Gun Control in America.* (Oxford, UK: Oxford University Press, 2008).

Courtois, Stéphane, Werth, Nicolas, Panne J. L., et al. *The Black Book of Communism: Crimes, Terror, Repression.* (Cambridge, MA: Harvard University Press, 1999).

Eakin, Lenden A. *Showdown: The Looming Crisis Over Gun Control.* (Herndon, VA: Mascot Books, 2014).

Egendorf, Laura K. *Guns and Violence: Current Controversies.* (Farmington Hills, MI: Greenhaven Press, 2005).

Encinosa, Enrique. *Cuba en Guerra.* (Miami, FL: Endowment for Cuban American Studies of the Cuban American National Foundation, 1st edition, 1994).

_____. *Unvanquished: Cuba's Resistance to Fidel Castro.* (Pureplay Press, 2004).

Faria, Miguel A. *Cuba in Revolution: Escape From a Lost Paradise.* (Macon, GA: Hacienda Publishing, Inc., 2002).

_____. *Medical Warrior: Fighting Corporate Socialized Medicine.* (Macon, GA: Hacienda Publishing, Inc., 1997).

_____. *Vandals at the Gates of Medicine: Historic Perspectives on the Battle Over Health Care Reform.* (Macon, GA: Hacienda Publishing, Inc., 1994).

Fumento, Michael. *The Myth of Heterosexual AIDS: How a Tragedy Has Been Distorted by the Media and Partisan Politics.* (New York: Basic Books, 1990).

Halbrook, Stephen P. *Target Switzerland: Swiss Armed Neutrality in World War II*. (Boston: Da Capo Press, 1998).

_____. *That Every Man Be Armed: The Evolution of a Constitutional Right*. (Albuquerque, NM: University of New Mexico Press, 1984).

Hardy, David T. *Origins and Development of the Second Amendment*. (Chino Valley, AZ: Blacksmith Corporation, 1986).

Horowitz, David. *Radical Son: A Generational Odyssey*. (New York: Free Press, 1997).

Kates, Don B. *Firearms and Violence: Issues of Public Policy*. (San Francisco: Pacific Research Institute, 1983).

Kleck, Gary and Kates, Don B. *Armed: New Perspectives on Gun Control*. (Amherst, NY: Prometheus Books, 2nd edition, 2001).

Kleck, Gary. *Point Blank: Guns and Violence in America*. (New York: Aldine de Gruyter, 1991).

_____. *Targeting Guns: Firearms and Their Control*. (New York: Aldine de Gruyter, 1997).

Kopel, David B. and Blackman, Paul H. *No More Wacos: What's Wrong With Federal Law Enforcement and How to Fix It*. (Amherst, NY: Prometheus Books, 1997).

Kopel, David B. *Guns: Who Should Have Them?* (Amherst, NY: Prometheus Books, 1995).

_____. *The Truth About Gun Control*. (New York: Encounter Books, 2013).

_____. *The Morality of Self-Defense and Military Action: The Judeo-Christian Tradition*. (Santa Barbara, CA: Praeger, 2017).

_____. *The Samurai, the Mountie, and the Cowboy: Should America Adopt the Gun Controls of Other Democracies?* (Amherst, NY: Prometheus Books; 1992).

LaPierre, Wayne. *Guns, Crime, and Freedom*. (Washington DC: Regnery Publishing, 1994).

_____. *Guns, Freedom and Terrorism*. (Washington DC: WND Books, 2003).

Lifton, Robert Jay. *The Nazi Doctors: Medical Killing and the Psychology of Genocide*. (New York: Basic Books, 1986).

Lott, John R., Jr. *More Guns, Less Crime: Understanding Crime and Gun Control Laws*. (Chicago: University of Chicago Press, 1998).

_____. *The Bias Against Guns*. (Washington DC: Regnery Publishing, 2003).

_____. *The War on Guns: Arming Yourself Against Gun Control Lies*. (Washington DC: Regnery Publishing, 2016).

Mack, Richard I. and Walter, Timothy R. *From My Cold Dead Fingers: Why America Needs Guns*. (Safford, AZ: Rawhide Western Publishing, 1994).

McGrath, Roger D. *Gunfighters, Highwaymen and Vigilantes: Violence on the Frontier*. (Berkeley: University of California Press, 1984).

Milloy, Steven J. *Junk Science Judo: Self-Defense Against Health Scares and Scams*. (Washington DC: Cato Institute, 2001).

Poe, Richard. *The Seven Myths of Gun Control: The Truth about Guns, Crime, and the Second Amendment*. (Roseville, CA: Prima Publishing, 2001).

Pratt, Larry. *Armed People Victorious*. (Springfield, VA: Gun Owners Foundation, 1990).

_____. *On the Firing Line: Essays in the Defense of Liberty*. (Franklin, TN: Legacy Communications, 2001).

_____. *Safeguarding Liberty: The Constitution & Citizen Militias.* (Franklin, TN: Legacy Communications, 1995).

Quigley, Paxton. *Armed & Female: Twelve Million American Women Own Guns. Should You?* (Boston: E.P. Dutton, 1989).

Rummel, R. J. *Death by Government: Genocide and Mass Murder Since 1900.* (Piscataway, NJ: Transaction Publishers; 1994).

Simkin, Jay, Zelman, Aaron S. and Rice, Alan M. *Lethal Laws: Gun Control Is the Key to Genocide.* (Milwaukee, WI: Jews for the Preservation of Firearms Ownership, 1994).

Smith, Guy. *Gun Facts. Version 6.2.* (CreateSpace Independent Publishing Platform, 1st edition, February 26, 2013). Available from: http://www.gunfacts.info/.

Solzhenitsyn, Aleksandr. *The Gulag Archipelago, 1918-1956: An Experiment in Literary Investigation, Parts I-II, The Prison Industry and Perpetual Motion.* (New York: Harper & Row Publisher, 1973).

_____. *The Gulag Archipelago, 1918-1956: An Experiment in Literary Investigation, Parts III-IV, The Destructive Labor Camps and The Soul and Barbed Wire.* (New York: Harper & Row Publisher, 1975).

Stolinsky, David C. and Wheeler, Timothy W. *Firearms: A Handbook for Health Professionals.* (Claremont, CA: The Claremont Institute, 1999).

Story, Joseph. *A Familiar Exposition of the Constitution of the United States, 1840.* (Birmingham, AL: The Library of American Freedoms, Palladium Press, 2001).

Utter, Glenn H. *Guns and Contemporary Society: The Past, Present, and Future of Firearms and Firearm Policy.* (Santa Barbara, CA: Praeger, 2015).

Walter, Timothy, R. and Mack, Richard I. *Government, God, and Freedom: A Fundamental Trinity.* (Safford, AZ: Rawhide Western Publishing, 1995).

Waters, Robert A. *The Best Defense: True Stories of Intended Victims Who Defended Themselves With a Firearm.* (Nashville, TN: Cumberland House, 1998).

Wheeler, Timothy W. and Wipfler, E. John, III. *Keeping Your Family Safe: The Responsibilities of Firearm Ownership.* (Bellevue, WA: Merrill Press, 2009).

Wolinsky, Howard and Brune, Tom. *The Serpent on the Staff: The Unhealthy Politics of the American Medical Association.* (New York: G.P. Putnam's Sons, 1994).

Wright, James D, Rossi, Peter, and Daly, Kathleen. *Under the Gun: Weapons, Crime, and Violence in America.* (New York: Aldine de Gruyter, 1983).

Wright, James D. and Rossi, Peter. *Armed and Considered Dangerous: A Survey of Felons and Their Firearms.* (New York: Aldine de Gruyter, 1986).

Zelman, Aaron and Stevens, Richard W. *Death by Gun Control: The Human Cost of Victim Disarmament.* (Hartford, WI: Jews for the Preservation of Firearms Ownership, Mazel Freedom Press, 2001).

INDEX

NOTE: *Insert page references are photographs.*

A

Abramski, Bruce, 226

abuse: domestic violence (*see* domestic violence); intimate partner, 187–91

Accidental Child Firearm Deaths, Insert page 9

accidental deaths, 202

accidents, guns, 117

activists, 11

Acute Care and Rehabilitation, 73

acute epidural hematoma (AEH), 218

acute subdural hematomas (ASH), 217, 218

Africa, 124, 215

African Americans, 114. *See* blacks

agriculture, Soviet Union, 30–32

AIDS, 35, 36

Alar, 98

Alcohol, Tobacco, Firearms, and Explosives (ATF), 224, 225, 226

Alexander, Leo, 172

Allen, Shaneen, 361

American Academy of Family Physicians (AAFP), 166

American Academy of Pediatrics (AAP), 165, 166, 354

American College of Physicians (ACP), 166, 354

American Journal of Epidemiology, 20

American Journal of Preventive Medicine, 123

American Medical Association (AMA), 6, 7, 15, 18, 61, 68, 101, 110, 117, 354; censorship of political incorrectness, 138–39; Council of Scientific Affairs, 24; ethics, 140–41, 159; gun control, 37–51, 165; membership, 137–45, 156; politics, 154, 162; privacy issues, 164–73; research (biases), 39–41; salaries, 142–45; sexual misconduct charges, 151–56; traditional medical ethics, 141–42

American Medical Women's Association (AMWA), 166

American Physician and Surgeons (AAPS), 55, 144

American Psychiatric Association (APA), 164, 166, 168

American Psychiatric Association Diagnostic and Statistical Manual of Mental Disorders, 236

American Public Health Association (APHA), 56, 92, 93, 94–96, 97, 98, 166

Americans for Gun Safety (AGS), 105

America's 1st Freedom (LaPierre), 253, 254, 301

Ammoland, Insert page 5, Insert page 6

analysis of statistics, 70

Anderson, E. Ratcliffe, 146, 149

Angell, Marcia, 141, 156

Ansell, Rodney William, 243

anti-communist insurgents (Cuba), Insert page 22

anti-gun: activists, 204; biases, 59; lobbying groups, 105; propaganda, 369–70

Antisocial Personality Disorder (APD; DSM-5), 309

a posteriori reasoning, 24

Appalachian School of Law, 284

a priori reasoning, 24, 34

Aquinas, Thomas, 212

AR-15s, 184, 185, 228, 325. *See also* assault weapons

Arias, Ileana, 85

Aristotle, 212

armed citizens, shooting rampages and, 282–87

Armed Citizens Legal Defense Network ejournal, 214

Armed People Victorious (Pratt), 343

armed self-protection ethics, 210–14

Arming America: The Origins of a Natural Gun Culture (Bellesiles), 303, 371–72

Arms Trade Treaty (ATT), 326

Asia, 215, 241

Asians, 115

Assam, Jeanne, 284, 288

assault weapons, 24, 54–55, 182; Bureau of Justice Statistics, 183; confused with assault rifles, 184-85, 324-25; constitutionality of, 192, 324; in Fast and Furious Operation, 265; in self-defense, 284; in self-defense during national emergencies, Insert page 7, Insert page 8, 181-85, 300-302; in the hands of citizens,

181–84; views of organized medicine and public health, 98

Assault Weapons Ban (Maryland [2013], and other states), 184-185, 324-325

Assault Weapons Ban of 2012, 54, 270, 272, 300

Association of American Physicians and Surgeons (AAPS), 139, 354

assumptions, 24

Attkinson, Sharyl, 299

Aurora Colorado shooting (2012), 64, 281, 284, 285, 332, 337

Ausman, James, I., 379

Australia, 339; ban on firearms, 249; Contact Crime Victimization Rates, Insert page 17; crime waves, 246–49, 329, 339; gun control, 244–51, 329, 339; homicide, 245, 246; homicide rates, Insert page 15; overview, 241-260; women and guns, 190

authoritarian states, 33, 34

availability: children and guns, 201; of firearms, 105–12; of guns, 25, 26, 177, 370–71 (see also guns)

B

background checks, 194–95; and mass shooting incidents, 198; National Instant Criminal Background Check System (NICS), 195–98

banning and confiscation of guns: efforts by public health establishment, 19; in Detroit, Washington, DC, California, Greece, Ireland, Jamaica, Bermuda, and throughout the world, 271; in police states, 273, 368-370; in the US, Washington, DC, Detroit, New York City, and California, 169

bans: AR-15s, 325; on gun research, 62, 63; guns, 245, 257, 300–302

Barr, Bob, 56, 57, 58

Batista, Fulgencio, 267, 318-19

Battle of New Orleans (1815), 316

Beck, Glenn, 437

Behavioral Risk Factor Surveillance System (CDC), 47

Belgium, 205, 233; suicides, 338; World War II, 343

Bellesiles, Michael A., 303-304, 371–72

Bennett, James T., 92, 93, 94, 95, 96, 97, 98, 99, 100

Berlin Wall, 32

The Best Defense (Waters), 291

The Bias Against Guns: Why Almost Everything You've Heard About Gun Control is Wrong (Lott), 50

biases, 34, 37, 83, 123; American Medical Association (AMA), 39–41; anti-gun, 59;

medical journalism, 146–63; minimization of, 70; surveys, 44 (*See also* surveys)

Bill of Rights, 192, 224, 226, 229, 243, 321–22

Birador, Roselle M., Insert page 12, 379

The Black Book of Communism (Courtois), 274, 342

Black Panthers, 268, 269

blacks, 114, 115, 151

Blackstone, William, 254, 359, 437

Blaylock, Russell, L., Insert page 12, Insert page 13, 379

Bloomberg, Michael, 18, 34, 67, 127, 357

blunt head trauma, 216–18, 220

Bowers v. DeVito (1982), 181, 360

Bowling Green State University, 290

Bowne, Carol, 195

Brady, Sarah, 59

Brady Law (1994–1998), 109, 193, 195

brain injuries, Insert page 12, Insert page 13

Brazil, 124, 215

Breivik, Anders Behring, 281, 334, 335

British Home Guard, 231

British National Health Service (NHS), 231, 256

Broun, Paul, 326

Brown, Michael S., 213-14, 299

Brune, Tom, 156

Bucknor, Cherrie, 115

Budapest, Hungary (1944), 317

Buffalo Bill Wild West Show, 304

Bukobsky, Vladimir, 33, 171

bump stocks, 363

Bureau of Alcohol, Tobacco, Firearms, and Explosives (ATF), 265, 326

Bureau of Crime Statistics and Research, 248

Bureau of Justice Statistics, assault weapons, 183

burglaries, 346–47

Burke, Edmund, 275

Bush, George H.W., 265

Bush, George W., 68

Buxton, George E., 232

C

California: gun registration, 271; loss of freedom in, 352

Campbell, Carroll, Jr., 182

Canada: burglaries, 347; comparing to United States, 19; gun control, 241; homicide rates, 19, 20, 109, 110

Canadian Outreach, 272

Carson, Ben, 64

Carter, Jimmy, 321

Case Control Studies, 78, 84

Castle Doctrine, 178, 345, 358–61

Castro, Fidel, 2, 267, 318

Castro, Raúl, 319
Cattledge, Haile, 85
celebrating shooters, 280–81
censorship, 54, 138–39
Center for Economic and Policy Research, 115, 116
Center for Gun Policy Research, 86
Center for Injury Control at Emory University, 179
Centers for Disease Control and Prevention (CDC), 3, 5, 12, 13, 15, 17, 19, 27, 35, 39, 47; ban on gun research, 62, 63; Behavioral Risk Factor Surveillance System, 47; epidemiology, 84; Grant Review Committee, 68; gun control, 206; *Injury Prevention Newsletter,* Insert page 2; investigations, 53–57; National Center for Injury Prevention and Control (NCIPC), 52, 53, 58, 59, 60, 61, 67, 71, 79; National Violent Death Reporting System, 98; restriction of funds for political lobbying, 86; tax dollars spent by, 72–73
Centerwall, Brandon, 19, 20, 109, 110, 299
Chamberlain, Neville, 327
charity, 23
Charleston, South Carolina incident (2015), 250, 287
Charlton, Bruce G., 69, 71, 81, 120, 121
Chavez, Hugo, 344
Chicago Tribune, 143
children, 200–209; death from firearms, 107, 338, 339; and guns, 201–2; homicide rates, 114; moral societal decline, 206–9; perpetrators of violence (per PHE), 200–201. *See also* juvenile delinquency
China, 234, 342
Christianity, 232, 233, 235, 269
Christoffel, Katherine, 58
chronic subdural hematomas (CSH), 217, 218
Churchill, Winston, 231
Cicero, 212
Cicilline, David, 270
civilian disarmament, 13, 49, 165, 183, 256, 264; in tyranny and freedom, 341-344; in Weimar Republic and Nazi Germany, Poland, Hungary, Soviet Union, China, Cuba, 273-74; UN attempts, 327
Clackamas Town Center incident (2012), 228
Clinton, Hillary, 11, 96, 193, 364
Clinton, William J. (Bill), 38, 67, 95, 106, 149, 152, 224, 225, 351
clusters, diseases, 99
CNN, 337
Cohort Studies, 78, 84
Coke, Edward, 253, 254, 359
Cold War, 125, 229-231, 372
Coleman, Loren, 299

collectivism, 33
college campus concealed carry, 355–56
Colt AR-15, 184
Columbine School shooting (1999), 11, 49, 288, 300
Columbus, Christopher, 319
Committees for the Defense of the Revolution (CDR), 261
communism, 171
Communist Manifesto (Marx), 95
Concealed Carry and Violent Crime, Insert page 23
concealed carry reciprocity (CCR), 11, 361–65
concealed carry weapons (CCW), 180, 260, 290, 294, 295, 302, 333; on college campuses, 355–56; constitutional, 357–58; legislation, 49, 345; licenses, 220; shall issue, 357–58
confidence intervals (CIs), 73, 76, 77, 80, 82
confiscation: gun registration and, 271; during natural disasters, 300–302
Congressional Research Service, 226
congressional subcommittee hearings, 57–60
Conklin, Larry, Insert page 8
Conklin, Marjorie, Insert page 8
Constitutional Carry (CC): laws, 302; rights, 260
constitutional concealed carry, 357–58
Constitutional Concealed Carry Reciprocity Act of 2017, 362
Contact Crime Victimization Rates, Insert page 17
control groups, 81
Conyers, John, 270
Cook, Philip J., 48
Cook's Index, 119, 120
Corlin, Richard F., 137, 138
Cornyn, John, 362, 363
Council of Scientific Affairs (AMA), 24
Courtois, Stéphane, 274, 342, 437
Crapo, Mike, 353
crime: firearm ownership and violent, 123–27; guns as deterrent to, 43; prevention, 50–51; statistics (FBI), 49
Crime Prevention Research Center, 109
crimes of passion, 25–26, 189, 333. *See also* domestic violence
Crime Survey (UK), 257
crime waves (Australia), 246–49
criminology, 26
Cuba, 95, 171, 265, 269, 318–19, 344; civilian disarmament, 342; anti-communist insurgents, Insert page 22; in revolution, 272, 318-19; media support, 261, 265, 267
Cuba in Revolution: Escape From a Lost Paradise (Faria), 2, 267, 318-319
Cuomo, Andrew, 293
Curfman, Gregory, 161

Czech Republic,, mass shootings, 205; in the EU and World War II, 327

D

Darwin, Charles, 30
Davis, Devra Lee, 151
day care, 96
Death by Government (Rummel), 274, 342
death from firearms: Accidental Child Firearm Deaths, Insert page 9; children, 107; U.S. Accidental Firearms Deaths, Insert page 9
de Blasio, Bill, 293
Deep State, 266, 321
defensive lethal force, 218–20, 349. *See also* self-defense
defensive uses of firearms, 45
de-institutionalization of the mentally ill, 294–98
democracy, 242, 330
Democratic Party, 216, 263, 337
Denmark (Danes): suicides, 25, 338; World War II, 233
Department of Health and Human Services (HHS), 72, 83, 85
Dependent Personality Disorder, 236
der staat über alles (State), 60
Diagnostic and Statistical Manual of Mental Disorders (DSM-5), 308
Dick, Cressida, 258
Dickey, Jay, 61, 64
Dickey, Nancy, 149
Dickey Amendment, 57, 64
DiLorenzo, Thomas, 92, 93, 94, 95, 96, 97, 98, 99, 100, 437
Dinkins, David, 271
disarmament: civil, 273–74; civilian, 341–42
Disaster Recovery Personal Protection Act (2006), 301
diseases: clusters, 99; Soviet Union, 34–36
District of Columbia v. Heller (2008), 322, 323
Doctors Against Handgun Injury, 164, 165
Doctors for Integrity in Policy Research (DIPR), 7, 16, 27, 44–45, 53, 57
Doctors for Responsible Gun Ownership (DRGO), 3, 45, 54-57, 126, 129, 133-34, 151, 166, 168, 170, 209, 213, 214, 236, 296, 299, 353, 379
domestic abuse and women, 54–55
domestic violence, 18, 187–91; crimes of passion, 25–26; self-defense by women, 42
Drega, Carl, 225
Drug Enforcement Administration (DEA), 265
Duncan, Jeff, 353
du Plessis, Armand Jean (Cardinal Richelieu), 226
Durbin, Dick, 177

E

Earp, Wyatt, 304
Eastern Europe, 215
ecologic fallacy, 120
ecologic studies, 84, 123–27
The Economist, 119, 124, 147
Eddie Eagle *GunSafe* program (NRA), 202
Edeen, John, 356
Edinboro, Pennsylvania, 336
Edmonton Journal, 272
education statistics, 113–22, 116
Einstein, Albert, 24
Eisenhower, Dwight D., 320–21
Elmasri, Bonnie, 194
Encinosa, Enrique, Insert page 22, 437
end-of-life care, 154
English Bill of Rights of 1689, 243
Environmental Protection Agency (EPA), 99, 100
epidemiology, 69, 72, 75, 80, 84–86, 87, 120, 123
epidural hematomas, 217
ergo propter hoc reasoning, 25
errors, 5
Escambray rebellion, 319
ethics: American Medical Association (AMA), 140–41, 158; armed self-protection, 210–14; flexible (medical), 140, 141–42; Hippocrates, 87; medical, 153; organized medicine, 167–69; traditional medical, 141–42
European Firearms Directive, 327
European social democracies: American gun culture and, 229–33; anti-gun culture, 234–35; gun control, 223–39; *Hogs Gone Wild*, 235–37; laws, 226–29; loss of liberty, 224–26; trapping feral hogs, 237–39
European Union (EU), 205, 315, 327; Brexit, 262; gun control, 315; legal challenge by EU members, 327; mass shootings, 205
Evaluation & Management (E&M) guidelines, 154
Ezell, Edward, 184

F

Fackler, Martin, 24
family protection, 348–52
Faria, Miguel A., Jr., 1, 2, 3, 30, 52, 57, 67, 267, 318, Insert page 1
far left politics, 94–96, 101. *See also* politics
FBI Uniform Crime Reports, 45, 208, 282, 349
Federal Bureau of Investigation (FBI), 256; crime statistics, 49; National Instant Background Check System (NICS), 363, 364; statistics, 368
Federal Bureau of Justice Statistics, 46, 350
Federalist Paper #62, 227
Federalist Papers, 357

Feinstein, Dianne, 177, 270, 272, 300, 364
feral hogs, 237–39, Insert page 24
Ferguson, MO riots (2014), 181, Insert page 5
Fifth Amendment (U.S. Constitution), 226
Findley, Patricia, 84
Fine, Russ, 56
Finland, 205
firearms, 15; accidents, 117; availability and
    violence statistics, 105–12; death from
    (children), 107; defensive uses of, 45, 97;
    ignoring benefits of, 179–81; mass shooting
    incidents, 107–9; neglected benefits of, 44–50;
    number of in homes, 118; ownership, 38,
    118; ownership and violent crime, 123–27;
    protective benefits of, 42–43; research, 2; and
    the U.S. Constitution, 319–21. See also guns
Firearm Act of 1934, 184, 307
Firearm Act of 1968, 184
Firearm Act of 1986, 184
Firearm Safety Act of 2013 (Maryland), 185, 325
Firearms Law and the Second Amendment (Kopel,
    Johnson, Moscary, O'Shea), 296
First Baptist Church incident (2017), 285
Fishbein, Morris, 148, 149
flexible (medical) ethics, 140, 141–42
Florida's Firearm Owners' Privacy Act (FOPA),
    169–71
forced entries, 346–47
Fort Hood, Texas incident (2014), 228
Founders, 58, 81, 131, 213, 224, 226, 265, 322, 357
Fourteenth Amendment (U.S. Constitution), 192,
    323
Fourth Amendment (U.S. Constitution), 226
Fowler, Katherine, 206
Fox, James, 203, 205
France, 204-5, 327; mass shootings, 228; suicides,
    241; World War II, 232-33"
Franklin, Benjamin, 225
freedom, 251, 343; international perspective,
    331–44; personal, 241; protection of, 126. See
    also liberty
French and Indian War (1756–1763), 303
From Pathology to Politics: Public Health in America
    (Bennett/DiLorenzo), 92, 93
FrontPage Magazine, 342
Fumento, Michael, 150, 151
Fund, John, 289

G

General Accounting Office (GAO), 197
genetics (Soviet Union), 30–32
genocide, 273–74, 341–42

Germany, 342; mass shootings, 289; Nazi doctors,
    171-73, 344; suicides, 25, 338; World War II
    and totalitarianism, 232-33, 270-73, 316-17,
    342-43"
Gertz, Marc, 180, 351
Giffords, Gabrielle, 280
Gift, Thomas, E., 133
Gillibrand, Kirsten, 364
Gingrich, Newt, 11, 363
Glorious Revolution of 1688, 243
Goethe, Johann Wolfgang von, 5, 6, 299
Good Samaritans, 216
Gorbachev, Mikhail, 33
Gorsuch, Neil M., 320, 323, 324
Graeco-Roman legacy, 212
Grant Review Committee (CDC), 68
grants, 71, 100
Great Britain, 327, 335, 340; ban on guns, 257;
    burglaries, 347; Contact Crime Victimization
    Rates, Insert page 17; gun control, 240–44,
    252–58; homicide rates, Insert page 16; self-
    defense, 347
Greenlee, Joseph, 170
Guatemala, 343
Guevara, Che, 310
The Gulag Archipelago (Solzhenitsyn), 258–62
gun activists, research and, 106–7
gun buyback programs, 340
gun control: American Medical Association
    (AMA), 37–51, 137, 165; Australia, 244–51;
    Canada, 241; CDC investigations, 53–57;
    Centers for Disease Control and Prevention
    (CDC), 206; civil disarmament, 273–74;
    congressional measures, 11; congressional
    subcommittee hearings, 57–60; creating and
    sustaining tyranny, 264–66; crime prevention,
    50–51; European social democracies, 223–39;
    Great Britain, 240–44, 252–58; The Gulag
    Archipelago (Solzhenitsyn), 258–62; gun
    registration, 271–72, 274–75; Japan, 241;
    laws, 226–29; legislation and, 272–73; loss of
    liberty, 224–26; mainstream liberal media,
    268–69; medical journalism, 158–61; and
    medical politics, 15–21; methodologies,
    41–43; misuse of public funds, 61–62;
    neglected benefits of firearms, 44–50;
    overview of, 52–64; politics of, 22–28;
    propaganda, 67, 68; and public health, 19–21,
    63, 97–98; public health establishment
    (PHE), 37, 367–68; research, 264; scientific
    survey problems, 43–44; socialism and
    critical thinking, 269–71; state-controlled
    media, 266–67; tyranny and, 263–75; viable
    solutions, 198–99

Gun Control, 187
Gun Control Act of 1968, 201, 334, Insert page 10
gun culture, 229–33, 303–6, 331, 371–72
Gunfighters, Highwaymen, and Vigilantes: Violence on the Frontier (McGrath), 305
gun free zones (GFZs), 294, 337, 356
gun ownership: benefits of, 328–30; privacy, 164–73; as risk factor for homicides, 42
Gun Owners of America (GOA), 194, 195, 210, 243, 245, 246, 326, 327, 343, 346, 352, 353, 361
gun-related suicides, 337. *See also* suicides
gun research, 62, 63
gun rights: advocating, 345–65; Castle Doctrine, 358–61; college campus concealed carry, 355–56; concealed carry reciprocity (CCR) legislation, 361–65; constitutional concealed carry, 357–58; hearing protection legislation, 353–55; home invasions, 346–47; Martin, Trayvon, 361; promoting family and home protection, 348–52; shall issue concealed carry, 357–58; stand-your-ground legislation, 358–61; Zimmerman, George, 361
guns: accidental deaths, 202; accidents, 117; availability of, 25, 26, 177, 201, 370–71; bans, 245; children and, 201–2; demonization of, 236, 237; as deterrent to crime, 43; international perspective, 331–44; linking homicide to, 125; need for self-protection, 177–99; portrayal of (in medical literature), 17; rights, 243; roles of in society, 6; safe-handling of, 169; self-protection, Insert page 14; suicide and, 25–26
gunshot wounds, 216
Guns: Who Should Have Them (Kopel), 330
Gunter, Lorne, 272
gun violence, 6, 8, 16, 38; and civil liberties, 339–41; medical journalism, 147; as public health issue, 11–13
gun-violence restraining order (GVRO), 296, 298

H

Halbrook, Stephen P., 192, 438
Halloween truck attack (2017), 292, 293, 363
Hamilton, Alexander, 357
Handgun Control, Inc. (HCI), 59
Handgun Epidemic Lowering Plan (HELP), 58, 59
handguns, 15, 184. *See also* firearms; guns
Hardy, David T., 438
Harris, Eric, 288
Harvard School of Public Health, 16, 106, 113, 124, 283
Havana, Cuba (1959), 318–19
Haynes v. United States (1968), 274

head trauma, Insert page 12, Insert page 13
health care, 156–58
Health Care Financing Administration (HCFA), 144
"Health for All" strategy (WHO), 80
Healthy People 2000, 73
Healthy People 2010, 73, 80–82, 88
Hearing Protection Act or the Silencers Helping US Save Hearing Act (SHUSH), 353
hearing protection legislation, 353–55, 363
Hegel, Georg, 263, 271
Heller decision (2008). *See District of Columbia v. Heller* (2008)
hematomas, 217, 218
Hemenway, David, 124
Henry, Patrick, 254
Hideyoshi, Toyotomi, 242
high school mass shootings, 289. *See also* mass shooting incidents
Hippocrates, 87, 141, 148, 153, 162, 167–68
Hispanics, 115, 124
history of public health, 90–101
Hitler, Adolf, 273, 317. *See also* Nazis
HIV/AIDS, 35, 158–61
Hobbes, Thomas, 212
Hodgkinson, James, 294
hogs, trapping, 237–39
Hogs Gone Wild, 235–37
Holland (Dutch): World War II, 233, 343
Holliday, Doc, 304
Holmes, James, Insert page 19
home invasions, 346–47
home protection, 348–52
Homestead Air Force Base (Florida), 182
homicides: Australia, 245, 246, Insert page 15; Canada, 19, 20; children, 114; domestic violence and, 42, 189; by family members, 179; Graeco-Roman legacy, 212; Great Britain, Insert page 16; gun ownership as risk factor for, 42; Judeo-Christian tradition, 211; justifiable, 46, 349; linking to guns, 125; prevention, 166; rates of, 41, 109, 110, 305, 333; U.S. Homicide Rate, Insert page 10. *See also* violence
Horowitz, David, 270, 438
House Appropriations Subcommittee on Labor, Health, Education, and Human Services (1996), 67
households, violence in, 179
Hudson, Richard, 362
humanitarianism, 23
Hungary: civilian disarmament, 273, 342; in the EU, 327; suicides, 25, 338; World War II (1944), 317

hunting and trapping feral hogs, 137, Insert page 24, 235-39
Hurricane Andrew (1992), 182, 300, Insert page 7, Insert page 8
Hurricane Hugo (1989), 182, 300
Hurricane Irma (2017), 183, 301
Hurricane Katrina (2005), 300, 301
hypotheses, 24, 81

I

ideology in public health, 16–18, 27–28
Ieyasu, Tokugawa, 242
income levels, 116, 117
individualism, 241
Initial Review Group (IRG), 82, 83
Injury Prevention Network Newsletter, 54
Injury Prevention Newsletter (CDC), Insert page 2
Injury Rate by Self Protection Mode, Insert page 14
Injury Research Centers (IRGs), 68
Injury Research Grant Review Committee (IRGRC), 68, 82
Institute of Genetics of the Soviet Academy of Sciences, 30
Institute of Medicine and National Research Council, 350
Internal Revenue Service (IRS), 224
International Firearm Ownership and Homicides, Insert page 11
international perspective (guns, freedom), 331–44; armed citizens, 342–43; civilian disarmament, 341–42; gun violence and civil liberties, 339–41; media sensationalism, 336–37; shooting rampages, 334–35; suicides, 337–39; violence, 332–34
International Suicide Rates and Firearms Ownership, Insert page 11
intimate partner abuse, 187–91
investigations (CDC), 53–57
Islamic State (IS), 234
Islamic terrorism, 130, 234, 252, 291-92, 308. *See also* terrorism
Israel, 118, 205, 334
Istook, Jim, Jr., 57, 58
Italy: fascism, 270

J

Jackson, Andrew, 316
Japan, 118, 241-43, 332, 337, 343; democracy in, 242; gun control, 241; suicides, 25, 338
Jefferson, Thomas, 275
Jenner, Edward, 23, 90
jihad, 291–94, 308

Johns Hopkins Bloomberg School of Public Health, 67, 86, 282, 283
Johns Hopkins Center for Gun Policy and Research, 64, 86
The Journal of Criminal Law and Criminology, 180
Journal of the American Medical Association (JAMA), 8, 12, 16, 27, 39, 44, 59, 118, 138, 147, 148–51; national health care reform, 156–58; objectives, 152, 153
Journal of the Medical Association of Georgia (JMAG), 2, 3, 6, 7, 37, 38, 39, 43, 55, 67, 138, 146, 147, 192
Journal of Trauma, 106, 110, 113, 120, 121
Joyce Foundation, 18, 127
Judeo-Christian tradition, 211
Junk Science Judo (Milloy), 76
justifiable homicides, 349
juvenile delinquency, 109–12, 114, 115, 200–209, 203–6

K

Kassirer, Jerome, 54, Insert page 3
Kastigar v. United States, 406 U.S. 441 (1972), 274
Kates, Don B., 19, 41, 44, 57, 139, 185, 186, 274, 290, Insert page 1
Kavanaugh, Brett, 323
Kellermann, Arthur, 7, 25, 39, 40, 41, 42, 44, 48, 59, 61, 62, 112, 179, 180, 187, 329
Kelley, Devin Patrick, 285
Kennesaw, Georgia, 347
Kerner Report of 1968, 92
KGB (Soviet Union), 265
Khan, Sadiq, 258
Khrushchev, Nikita, 33
Kimoon, Ban, 326
King, Rodney, 181, 182, 300, Insert page 5
Klarevas, 283
Klebold, Dylan, 288
Kleck, Gary, 7, 41, 44, 45, 46, 47, 118, 126, 179, 180, 185, 186, 202, 290, 347, 348, 349, 350, 351, 370, 371–72
Koch, Robert, 23, 26, 38, 74, 81, 83, 91, 178, Insert page 3
Koop, C. Everett, 159, 160
Kopel, David, 2, 7, 44, 187, 190, 192, 233, 255, 257, 296, 330, 331, 339, 371–72, 438
Koresh, David, 225
Kouri, Jim, 290
Kübler-Ross, Elisabeth, 306
Kukla, Robert J., 187
Ku Klux Klan (KKK), 268

L

Lago, Armando M., 319

Lamarck, Jean Baptiste, 30

Lamarckian theory, 30, 31

Lancet, 12, 161

Langendorff, John, 363

Langendorff, Johnnie, 285

Lanza, Adam, 280, 281, Insert page 19

LaPierre, Wayne, 253, 438

Las Vegas shooting (2017), 11, 306–11, 355, 363

Latin America, 124, 214; violence, 241

laws: concealed carry weapons (CCW), 49;
 Constitutional Carry, 302; U.S. Constitution,
 226–29

Lee, Robert W., 187

legislation: concealed carry reciprocity (CCR),
 361–65; concealed carry weapons (CCW),
 345; gun control, 272–73; hearing protection,
 353–55, 363; stand-your-ground, 358–61

Lenin, Vladimir Ilyich, 30, 268

Lenin Academy of Agricultural Science, 30

lethal force, 218–20. *See also* self-defense

Lethal Laws, 273, 341

Lewinsky, Monica, 149

Lewis, John, 11, 364

liberalism, 34

liberty: benefits of gun ownership, 328–30; Bill of
 Rights, 321–22; Budapest, Hungary (1944),
 317; firearms and the U.S. Constitution,
 319–21; gun violence and civil liberties,
 339–41; Havana, Cuba (1959), 318–19; loss
 of, 224–26, 265; recapitulation of, 315–30;
 Second Amendment decisions (Supreme
 Court), 322–25; Small Arms Treaty (2013
 [UN]), 279, 325–27; Warsaw, Poland (1943),
 316–17

limitations on ownership, 180

Lincoln, Abraham, 316

Lincoln County, New Mexico, 305

Lister, Joseph, 90

literacy, 114

Lithuania: suicides, 338

Littleton, Colorado, 288

Locke, John, 213, 275, 358

Loft, John, 125

London, England, 258

London Daily Telegraph, 257

London Sunday Times, 252, 256

Lopey, John, 197

Lopez, Ivan, 228

Los Angeles, CA riots (1992), 181, 182, 300, Insert
 page 5

Los Angeles Times, 45, 46, 348, 349, 350

Lott, John R., Jr., 44, 46, 48, 49, 109, 126, 201, 284,
 329, 330, 347, 349, 371–72

Loughner, Jared, 280, Insert page 19

Ludwig, Jens, 48

Lundberg, George D., 146, 147, 151, 152, 153, 159;
 *Journal of the American Medical Association
 (JAMA)*, 148–51; national health care reform,
 156–58

Luxembourg, 343

Lysenko, Trofim Denisovich, 30, 31, 32, 89

M

Maalot Massacre, 334

MacCallum, Martha, 306

Macon, Georgia, 335; crime, 346; local newspaper,
 223-224, 364; looting, 183; self-defense, 335;
 wild hogs, 237

Macon-Bibb County, Georgia, 346

Madison, James, 193, 321, 357

Maduro, Nicolas, 344

mainstream liberal media (mass media), 38, 63,
 140-141, 147-48, 160-61, 177-79, 183-84, 198,
 233-37, 264-65, 268-69, 280-81, 290-91, 311,
 338, 351, 355, 367, 371

Malec, James F., 84

malpractice statistics, 70

management (AMA), 137

Margulies, Robert A., 214

marijuana use, 197

Marshall, John, 321

Martin, Tony, 229, 252, 253, 254, 260, 335

Martin, Tracy, 186

Martin, Trayvon, 361

Marx, Karl, 95, 263

Marxism, 30, 269

Mass Shooting Derangement (MSD) syndrome,
 306–11

mass shooting incidents, 107–9, 334–35, Insert page
 18, Insert page 19; background checks and,
 198; banning weapons, 300–302; celebrating
 shooters, 280–81; de-institutionalization of
 the mentally ill, 294–98; European Union
 (EU), 205; instructive cases, 287–91; juvenile
 delinquency and, 203–6; Mass Shooting
 Derangement (MSD) syndrome, 306–11;
 mental health, 279–311; revising American
 history, 303–6; sensationalizing violence,
 298–300; statistics, 203; terrorism, 291–94.
 See also specific incidents

Mateen, Omar, 292

McCabe, Andrew, 266

McCain, John, 355

McDonald v. Chicago (2010), 322, 323

McGrath, Roger D., 305, 438
media: mainstream liberal, 268–69; mass shooting
    incidents, 279–311 (*see also* mass shooting
    incidents); propaganda, 236; sensationalism,
    336–37; sensationalizing violence, 298–300;
    state-controlled, 266–67; violence, 109–12
medical costs: cost of gun violence, 47, 48; saved
    by guns, 45
medical discoveries, 90, 91
medical ethics, 153
medical journalism, 161–63; biases, 146–63; gun
    control, 158–61; gun violence, 147; HIV/
    AIDS, 158–61; Lundberg, George D., 148–51;
    national health care reform, 156–58; sexual
    misconduct charges, 151–56
medical politics, 141; gun control and, 15–21;
    ideology in public health, 27–28; suicide and
    guns, 25–26
medical science: recognition of true science, 23–25;
    subversion of, 22–28
Medical Sentinel, 23, 44, 55, 138, 139, 167
Medical Society of New Jersey, 148
*Medical Warrior: Fighting Corporate Socialized
    Medicine* (Faria), 2, 67, 139
Medicare, 155
Medicare For All, 155
Meiji Restoration of the Mikado (1867), 242
membership, American Medical Association
    (AMA), 137–45, 156
memory holes, 110
Mendel, Gregor, 30
Mengele, Joseph, 32
mental health: de-institutionalization of the
    mentally ill, 294–98; mass shooting incidents,
    279–311 (*see also* mass shooting incidents)
Mercer University School of Medicine, 56
methodologies, 23, 79; epidemiology, 84–86; gun
    control, 41–43
Mexico: violence, 124
militias, 192, Insert page 6
Miller, Matthew, 111, 114, 118, 119, 121
Miller v. U.S. (1938), 185
Milloy, Steven, 76, 79, 438
minorities, statistics, 114–17
Mitchell, Elena Faria, Insert page 4
morality, 23
moral relativism, 140-42, 207, 341, 372
*The Morality of Self-Defense and Military Action:
    The Judeo- Christian Tradition* (Kopel), 233
moral societal decline, 206–9
*More Guns, Less Crime—Understanding Crime and
    Gun Control Laws* (Lott), 48
Mother Jones, 198, 282, 286, 328, 329
Mouzos, Jenny, 251

murders. *See also* homicide
Murphy, Chris, 204, 270
Myrick, Joel, 286, 289, 336

N

Nagin, Ray, 301
Nash, Ryan, 293
National Center for Education, 115
National Center for Injury Prevention and Control
    (NCIPC), 17, 27, 34, 52, 53, 58, 59, 60, 61, 67,
    68, 71, 79
National Committee on Violence (NCV), 190
National Crime Victimization Survey (NCVS), 46,
    350
National Education Association (NEA), 162
National Empowerment Television (NET), 53
National Firearms Agreement (NFA), 245
national health care reform, 156–58
National Instant Criminal Background Check
    System (NICS), 195–98, 363, 364
National Institute of Justice, 105
National Institute of Mental Health, 110
National Institutes of Health (NIH), 60
National Review Online (NRO), 289
National Rifle Association (NRA), 12, 62, 105, 126,
    186, 198, 231, 243, 246, 247, 253, 290, 339,
    346, 361, 365; *America's 1st Freedom,* 301;
    Eddie Eagle *GunSafe* program, 202
National Safety Council, 339
National Socialists (Germany), 270
National Victims Data, 186, 219
National Violent Death Reporting System (CDC),
    98
Nation's Health, 56
natural disasters, 300–302, Insert page 6, Insert
    page 8
Nazis, 124, 171-73, 230-33, 270, 272, 273, 316-17,
    342-43, 372
Neel, Travis Dean, 284
Neo-Nazis, 268
Netherlands: burglaries, 347
New Deal, 91
The New England Journal of Medicine (NEJM), 7–8,
    19, 25, 39, 40, 54, 148, 329
The New Jersey Medicine, 147, Insert page 2
New Socialist Man, 32
Newsweek, 147
New York Observer, 165
New York Times, 282
New Zealand, 118
Nicaragua, 95, 344
Ninth Amendment (U.S. Constitution), 192
Nobunaga, Oda, 242

No Child Left Behind, 115
Norman, Dale, 324
Northern District of Texas, U.S. v. Emerson (1999), 193
North Atlantic Treaty Organization (NATO), 229-230
North Korea, 268
Norway, 205, 281, 343; suicides, 338
Norway shooting incident (2011), 281, 289, 332, 334-35
NRA-ILA report (2017), 251

O

Oath of Hippocrates, 141, 148, 167–68
Obama, Barack, 12, 63, 142, 144, 224, 225, 250, 263, 264, 265, 267, 270, 272, 295, 320
ObamaCare, 140, 155, 295, 345, 355
O'Carroll, Patrick, 16
Occupational Safety and Health Administration (OSHA), 60
October Revolution (1917), 30
Old West, 304
O'Leary, Daniel, 84
Omnibus Appropriations Bill (1996), 61
open carry, 324
organized medicine, 165, 167–69
Orient, Jane, 23, 24
Orlando, Florida, 346, 347
Orlando nightclub shooting incident (2016), 292
Ortega, Daniel, 344
ownership: firearms, 38, 118; limitations on, 180; privacy, 164–73; protection of property and freedom, 126; and violent crime, 123–27

P

Paddock, Stephen, 307, Insert page 19
Palestine Liberation Organization (PLO): terrorism, 205
Palmer v. District of Columbia (2014), 324
Parkland, Florida incident (2018), 204, 290
partisan politics, 92–93. *See also* politics
Pasteur, Louis, 23, 90, 91
pathology of blunt head trauma, 216–18
patients: advocacy, 153; privacy, 164–73
Patriot's Day (April 19, 1775), 303, 343
Paul, Rand, 355
Pax Americana, 231
Pediatrics, 206
Pelosi, Nancy, 11, 364
personal freedom, 241
Peters, C. J., 17
philanthropy, 23

Philippines, Insert page 12, 343, 379
physicians: aligning with the State, 171–73; privacy, 164–73
Poe, Richard, 342, 438
Point Blank: Guns and Violence in America (Kleck), 45, 179
Poland: civilian disarmament, 273, 342; in the EU, 327; public executions, Insert page 20; resistant fighters, Insert page 21; suicides, 338; World War II (1943), 316-17
political hatred, 291–94
political incorrectness, censorship of, 138–39
political lobbying, restriction of funds for, 86
politics, 11, 12, 13; American Medical Association (AMA), 18, 154, 162; far left, 94–96, 101; of gun control, 22–28; gun control and medical, 15–21; history of public health, 90–101; ideology in public health, 27–28; medical, 141; recognition of true science, 23–25; science, 34, 35; Soviet Union (research and diseases), 34–36; suicide and guns, 25–26
popular culture, 125, 227, 235, 264, 280, 291, 298, 306, 309-11
Port Arthur, Tasmania incident (1996), 243, 245, 329, 339
post hoc ergo propter hoc reasoning, 43
post hoc reasoning, 25
poverty levels, 116, 117
Pratt, Erich, 196-197, 379
Pratt, Larry, 210-11, 265, 343-44, 438
prevention: crime, 50–51; homicide, 166
Price, Tom, 140, 141
privacy: American Medical Association (AMA), 164–73; Florida's Firearm Owners' Privacy Act (FOPA), 169–71
private sector, 91, 92
progressives, 34
propaganda, 7, 13, 336–37; anti-gun, 369–70; gun control, 67, 68; media, 236; public health establishment (PHE), 117–20
property, protection of, 126
protective benefits of firearms, 42–43
Prothrow-Stith, Deborah, 16
Przebinda, Arthur, Z., 133
psychiatry, 25; in Cuba and other totalitarian countries, 28, 171; in gambling, 308; in mass shootings, 280-81, 296-97, 306, 309; in Soviet Union, 32-34; in suicide, 337; in US, 168-69, 236
public executions (Poland), Insert page 20
public funds, misuse of, 61–62
public health: congressional authorization, 72–73; consensus, 82–84; and far left politics, 94–96; golden age of, 90–92; gun control and, 63,

97–98; gun violence as issue, 11–13; history of, 90–101; ideology in, 27–28; and partisan politics, 92–93; premature disclosure of scientific findings, 75; relative risks (RRs), 75–78; researchers and gun activists, 106–7; and science, 99–101; science and, 67–78; science or ideology in, 16–18; searching for social problems, 74–75; social science and, 79–89; as tool for gun control, 19–21

public health establishment (PHE), 6, 11, 13, 17, 18, 52, 56, 72, 74, 92, 93, 95; defensive uses of firearms, 97; domestic violence and, 187, 188; gun control, 37, 367–68; limiting gun availability, 178; propaganda, 117–20; structure of, 101

Putin, Vladimir, 239

p-values, 73, 75, 77, 79, 80, 81

Q

Quinn, John Gerald, 225

R

RAND Corporation, 62

randomization, 81

reading proficiency, 111

Reagan, Ronald, 321

Reason (Kopel), 206, 339

Reay, Donald T., 329

recapitulation of liberty, 315–30; benefits of gun ownership, 328–30; Bill of Rights, 321–22; Budapest, Hungary (1944), 317; firearms and the U.S. Constitution, 319–21; Havana, Cuba (1959), 318–19; Second Amendment decisions (Supreme Court), 322–25; Small Arms Treaty (2013 [UN]), 279, 325–27; Warsaw, Poland (1943), 316–17

reform, national health care, 156–58

registration, gun, 271–72, 274–75

Registration of firearms: analogy to automobiles, 159-160; constitutionality, 274; in Australia, 244-45; in Canada, 272-73; in Cuba, 318; in Great Britain, 254; in Greece, Ireland, Jamaica, Bermuda, 271; in tyranny, 341-42; prelude for banning and confiscation, 197-98, 264-65

regulations, 93

rehabilitation (Soviet Union), 32–34

Rehnquist, William, 193

Reid v. Covert (1957), 326

relative risks (RRs), 73, 75–78, 80, 81, 99, 100

religion, 212

Republican congressional baseball practice incident (2017), 294, 295

Republican Party, 268

research: American Medical Association (AMA), 39–41; firearms, 2; gun, 62, 63; and gun activists, 106–7; gun control, 264; social, 84; Soviet Union, 34–36; violence, 13

research and development (R&D), 92

resistant fighters (Poland), Insert page 21

Reuter, Peter, 251

Revere, Paul, 304

Revised Organic Act of the Virgin Islands (1954), 302

revising American history, 303–6

Revolutionary Directorate (RD), 318, 319

Reynolds, Gleen Harlan, 192

Richardson, H.L., 245

rights: Bill of Rights, 192; Constitutional Carry (CC), 260; guns, 243 (*see also* gun rights); reaching consensus of, 191–93; Second Amendment (U.S. Constitution), 196

Rigsby, Brian, 283

RINO (Republican in name only), 265

robbery (Great Britain), 257, 258

Robinson, Victor, 88–89

Roof, Dylan, 287, 288

Roosevelt, Franklin D., 91, 320

Rosenberg, Mark, 17, 61, 368

Rosenberg, Mark L., 59

Rosenstein, Rod, 266

Ross, Rayna, 194

Rossi, Peter, 46, 347, 349

Rummel, R.J., 274, 342

Russia, 230, 261. *See also* Soviet Union

Russian AK-47, 184

Rwanda massacre (1994), 341

Ryan, Paul, 11

S

Safeguarding Liberty: The Constitution and Citizens Militias (Pratt), 210

salaries (AMA), 142–45

Sammons, James H., 144

The Samurai, the Mountie, and the Cowboy: Should America Adopt the Gun Controls of Other Democracies? (Kopel), 190, 331

San Bernardino terrorist attack (2015), 291, 292

Sanders, Bernie, 269

Sandy Hook tragedy (2012), 11, 12, 62, 63, 280, 284, 290

San Francisco Examiner, 59

Santana School shooting (2001), 108

Satcher, David, 12

Scalia, Antonin, 320

Scalise, Steve, 294, 306, 308, Insert page 18

Scandinavia: gun control, 281, 335; suicides, 25, 338; World War II (1944), 229, 233

Schlafly, Andrew L., 144

Schlafly, Roger, 119

Scholastic Assessment Test (SAT), 116

school shootings, 108, 205. *See also* mass shooting incidents

Schuman, Stanley, 96

Schumer, Charles, 177, 270, 300

Schwam, Wallace, 236

science: congressional authorization, 72–73; history of public health, 90–101; missing statistical tools, 73–74; politics, 34, 35; premature disclosure of scientific findings, 75; and public health, 67–78; public health and, 99–101; recognition of true science, 23–25; relative risks (RRs), 75–78; searching for social problems, 74–75; social science and public health, 79–89; Soviet Union, 29–36 (*see also* Soviet Union); *versus* statistics, 69–72; subversion of medical, 22–28

science in public health, 16–18

Scipione, Andrew, 249

Second Amendment (U.S. Constitution), 2, 20, 64, 142, 170, 279, 315, 321, 322–25, 323, 324, 358; militias, 192; need for self-protection, 177–99; rights, 196

Segal, Steven P., 296

self-defense, 179, 186, 210–20, 345, 350; defensive lethal force, 218–20; domestic violence, 187–91; ethics of armed self-protection, 210–14; Graeco-Roman legacy, 212; Great Britain, 347; international perspective (guns, freedom), 332–34; Judeo-Christian tradition, 211; killings, 348; pathology of blunt head trauma, 216–18; problem of physical violence, 214–16; by women, 219

self-protection, 177–99, Insert page 14

semi-automatic civilian firearms, 184. *See also* assault weapons; guns

sensationalizing violence, 298–300

September 11, 2001, 105, 234, 292. *See also* terrorism

The Serpent on the Staff (Brune/Wolinsky), 156

sexual misconduct charges: American Medical Association (AMA), 151–56

shall issue concealed carry, 357–58

shooters, celebrating, 280–81

shooting rampages, 279–311, 282–87, 334–35. *See also* mass shooting incidents

shotguns, 184. *See also* firearms; guns

silencers, 353

Simone, Ginny, 248

Simpson-Istook Amendment, 58

single payer health care systems, 95, 155

Sloan, John H., 19, 25

Small Arms Treaty (2013 [UN]), 279, 325–27

The Smear (Attkinson), 299

Smith, Guy, Insert page 9, 379, 439

Smoak, Randolph, Jr., 143

social democrats, 34

social engineering, 36, 82

socialism, 269–71, 344

Socialist Workers Party (SWP), 268

social justice, 80

social problems, searching for, 74–75

social research, 84

social responsibility, 153

social science: availability of taxpayer money, 87–88; epidemiology, 84–86; Healthy People 2010, 80–82; and public health, 79–89; public health consensus, 82–84; *The Story of Medicine* (Robinson), 88–89

socioeconomic factors, statistics, 113–22

sociology, 26

Solzhenitsyn, Aleksandr, 33, 258–62, 439

Soros, George, 18, 34, 127

Soul on Fire (Cleaver), 269

Soul on Ice (Cleaver), 269

South Africa: homicide rates, 109

Soviet Red Army, 125, 317

Soviet Union, 171, 224, 233, 258, 259, 265, 270, 342; genetics, 30–32; in Cold War, 229-231; politics (research and diseases), 34–36; psychiatry and rehabilitation, 32–34; science, 29–36

Specter, Arlen, 53, 61

Sports Shooting Association, 339

Sri Lanka: suicides, 25, 338

Stalin, Joseph V., 30, 341

stand-your-ground legislation, 345, 358–61

State (*der staat über alles*), 60

State, physicians aligning with, 171–73

state-controlled media, 266–67

statistics, 79; assault weapons, 183; education, 116; education and socioeconomic factors, 113–22; Federal Bureau of Investigation (FBI), 368; firearm availability and violence, 105–12; gun activists, 106–7; malpractice, 70; mass shooting incidents, 107–9, 203; media violence, 109–12; minorities, 114–17; missing statistical tools, 73–74; National Crime Victimization Survey (NCVS), 350; public health establishment propaganda, 117–20; science *versus*, 69–72

Stevens, Richard Gable, 287, 336

Stolinsky, David C., 48, 160
Stoneman Douglas High School, 290. *See also* Parkland, Florida incident (2018)
Story, Joseph, 321, 322, 439
The Story of Medicine (Robinson), 88–89
Strand, James, 286
street crime, 332–34
Styer, Tom, 283
subdural hematomas, 217, 218, Insert page 12, Insert page 13
suicides, 97, 106, 133-34, 159, 161, 204, 206, 299 333, 337–39, 371, Insert page 10; children, 114; and guns, 25–26
Sullum, Jacob, 339
Sunbeam Corporation, 154
The Sunday Times, 340
Supremacy Clause, Article VI (U.S. Constitution), 325
Supreme Court (United States), 192, 320, 321, 322–25
surveys, 351; *Journal of the American Medical Association (JAMA)*, 44; National Crime Victimization Survey (NCVS), 350; problems, 43–44
Suter, Edgar, 2, 7, 8, 27, 39, 40, 41, 47, 48, 159 189, 350, 369
Sutherland Springs, Texas, 285
Sweden, 228; suicides, 338
Swindle, James W., Jr., 356
Switzerland, 118, 242, 332, 334, 343
The Sydney Morning Herald, 247

T

tax dollars spent by the CDC, 72–73
taxpayer money, availability of, 87–88
Taylor County, Georgia, 238
The Telegraph, 223, 224
television: distraction for kids, 110-11; violence on, 20, 109-112, 311, 371
Temple University (Philadelphia, PA), 88
Tennessee Law Review, 19
Tenth Amendment (U.S. Constitution), 193
terrorism, 291–94, 308. *See also* specific attacks
Texas Department of Public Safety, 285
Their Finest Hour (Churchill), 231
theories, 24, 30, 31
Third Way, 105
Thomas, Clarence, 324
Thomas, Ernest, 238
Thompson, Tommy, 68
The Time Machine (Wells), 229, 234
Tingle, John, 248
Tokugawa Shogunate (1600—1867), 242

Tombstone, Arizona, 304
tools, statistics, 79. *See also* statistics
totalitarianism, 172
traditional medical ethics, 141–42
trapping feral hogs, 237–39
Traumatic Brain Injury, 73
Truman, Harry, 320
Trump, Donald, 11, 73, 142, 204, 234, 267, 270, 290, 293, 310, 321, 323, 336, 362, 365
tyranny and gun control, 263–75, 341–42; civil disarmament, 273–74; creating and sustaining, 264–66; gun registration, 271–72, 274–75; legislation and, 272–73; mainstream liberal media, 268–69; socialism and critical thinking, 269–71; state-controlled media, 266–67

U

United Kingdom (UK), 257; burglaries & self-defense, 347; gun control, 240-44, 252-262; mass shooting, 289, 340; War of 1812, 316; World War II, 327. *See also* Great Britain
United Nations (UN), 279, 315, 325–27
United States, 334; burglaries, 347; comparing to Canada, 19; homicide rates, 109, 255; Supreme Court, 192; Virgin Islands, Insert page 6; women and guns, 190
United States Code, 226
United States Department of Justice, 340, 368
University of Alabama at Birmingham, 56
University of California at Berkeley, 296
University of Iowa Injury Prevention Research Center, 59
University of Texas Tower shooting incident (1966), 307
University of Washington, 109
University of Washington School of Public Health, 299
University of West Georgia, 356
University of Wisconsin, 290
U.S. Accidental Firearms Deaths, Insert page 9
U.S. Bureau of Justice Statistics.(10,11,12), 282
U.S. Constitution: amendments (*See* specific amendments); Bill of Rights, 321–22 (*see also* Bill of Rights); *Federalist Paper #62*, 227; firearms and the, 319–21; laws, 226–29; Supremacy Clause, Article VI, 325
U.S. Department of Education, 298
U.S. Department of Justice, 45, 208, 251
U.S. Homicide Rate, Insert page 10
U.S News and World Report, 147
U.S. Public Health Service, 15
U.S. Secret Service, 298

U.S. Supreme Court. *See* Supreme Court (United States)
U.S. v. Lopez (1995), 193
U.S. v. Miller (1938), 192, 193
U.S. v. Verdugo-Urquidez (1990), 191

V

Vandals at the Gates of Medicine (Faria), 30, 52
Vaughan, Tom, 128-29, 132, 201
Venezuela, 344
Verret, Adam "Tad," Insert page 7
video games, violence, 110
violence, 6; domestic, 187-91 (*see also* domestic violence); firearm ownership and violent crime, 123-27; firearms and, 105-12; in households, 179; international perspective (guns, freedom), 332-34; media, 109-12; pathology of blunt head trauma, 216-18; perpetrators of (per PHE), 200-201; problem of physical, 214-16; rates of, 41; research, 13; school shootings, 205; sensationalizing, 298-300; serialization of, 279-311; video games, 110. *See also* gun violence
Violence Policy Center (VPC), 45, 46, 105, 106, 107, 109, 113, 114, 348

W

Wainwright, Robert, 246, 247
waiting periods, 194, 195
Wakefield, Massachusetts, incident (2000), 108
The Wall Street Journal, 150, 289
War of 1812, 316
The War on Guns: Arming Yourself Against Gun Control Lies (Lott), 50
Warren, Elizabeth, 270
Warsaw, Poland (1943), 316-17
Warsaw Ghetto, 316
Washington, George, 303
Washington, Stacy, 301, 302
Washington Post, 204, 284
The Washington Post, 186, 351
The Washington Times, 255
Waters, Robert A., 291
Waters, William C., IV, 7, 16, 53, 57, 139, Insert page 1
Weatherburn, Don, 247
Weather Underground, 268
Weaver, Vicky, 225
Webster, Daniel, 64, 282, 283
Weingarten, Dean, Insert page 5
welfare reform (1996), 95
Wells, H.G., 229, 234

Wheeler, Timothy W., 7, 27, 48, 54, 57, 68, 139, 151, 152, 167, 352, 353, 354, Insert page 1, Insert page 3, 379, 439
whites, 115
Whitman, Charles, 307
Willeford, Stephen, 285, 363
Wintemute, Garen J., 161
Wipfler, John, E., 3, 209, 439
Wisconsin Medical Journal, 147
Wolinsky, Howard, 156
women: domestic abuse and, 54-55; domestic violence, 187-91; Second Amendment (U.S. Constitution), 177-99; self-defense by, 42, 219
Woodham, Luke, 286
Workers World Party (WWP), 268, 269
World Health Organization (WHO), 80, 337
World Net Daily, 252
World Resources Institute, 151
World War I, 232, 233
World War II, 124, 230, 242, 341
Wright, James D., 46, 347, 349, 439
Wurst, Andrew, 286, 336

X

Xerox workplace incident (1999), 107

Y

York, Alvin (sergeant), 232-33
Young, Robert B., 170-71, 296-97, 329

Z

Zelman, Aaron S., 439
Zhukov, Georgi, 317
Zimkin, Jay, 439
Zimmerman, George, 361
Zrinzo, Ludvic, 230, 231